ANNUAL REVIEW OF WOMEN'S HEALTH

Volume III

ANNUAL REVIEW OF WOMEN'S HEALTH

Volume III

Edited by

Beverly J. McElmurry

and

Randy Spreen Parker

National League for Nursing Press • New York
Pub. No. 14-672X

ISBN 0-88737-672-X
ISSN 1073-1695

The views expressed in this publication represent the views of the authors and do not necessarily reflect the official views of the National League for Nursing.

Cover illustration: *Dreamcatcher*, by Maxine Noel-Ioyan Mani.

This book was set in Aster and Trump by Publications Development Company. The editor was Maryan Malone and the designer was Nancy Jeffries. The cover was designed by Lauren Stevens.

Printed in the United States of America

To Wynne Spreen,
a woman for all the seasons of life.

Contributors

Lynne T. Braun, PhD, RN
Associate Professor
College of Nursing
Rush University
Chicago, Illinois

Jacquelyn Campbell, PhD, RN, FAAN
Anna D. Wolf Endowed Professor
Johns Hopkins University
School of Nursing
Baltimore, Maryland

Roberta Cassidy, MSN, RN
Graduate Student
Department of Public Health, Mental Health,
    and Administrative Nursing
University of Illinois at Chicago
Chicago, Illinois

Carol D. Christiansen, PhD, RN
Post Doctoral Fellow
University of Illinois at Chicago
Chicago, Illinois

Carol J. Collins, PhD, RNC
Assistant Head Nurse
Psychiatric Nursing
University of Illinois Hospital
Chicago, Illinois

Claudia Cotes, BA
Medical Student
University of Illinois at Chicago
Chicago, Illinois

M. Ryan Gantes, PhD, RN
Associate Director, Ambulatory Services
University of Illinois at Chicago Medical
    Center Hospitals
Chicago, Illinois

Janet Grossman, DNS, RN
Assistant Professor of Nursing and Psychiatry
University of Illinois at Chicago
Chicago, Illinois

Donna S. Huddleston, PhD, RN
President/Executive Director
BHM Health Associates, Inc.
Home Health Care and Premier Hospice, Inc.
Crown Point, Indiana

Tonda L. Hughes, PhD, RN
Assistant Professor
Department of Public Health, Mental Health,
    and Administrative Nursing
University of Illinois at Chicago
Chicago, Illinois

Ayhan Aytekin Lash, PhD, RN
Associate Professor of Nursing
School of Nursing
Northern Illinois University
Dekalb, Illinois

Agatha Lowe, PhD, RN
Director of Women and Children's Health
    Programs
Chicago Department of Public Health
Chicago, Illinois

Joan N. Martellotto, MS, RN, CS
Doctoral Candidate in Nursing Science
College of Nursing
University of Illinois at Chicago
Chicago, Illinois

Beverly J. McElmurry, EdD, FAAN
Professor and Associate Dean
College of Nursing
University of Illinois at Chicago
Chicago, Illinois

Christine Miaskowski, PhD, RN, FAAN
Associate Professor and Chair
Department of Physiological Nursing
University of California
San Francisco, California

Kathleen Fordham Norr, PhD
Associate Professor
College of Nursing
University of Illinois at Chicago
Chicago, Illinois

Barbara Parker, PhD, RN, FAAN
School of Nursing
University of Virginia
Charlottesville, Virginia

Randy Spreen Parker, PhD, RN
Research Specialist
College of Nursing
University of Illinois at Chicago
Chicago, Illinois

Kathleen Potempa, DNS, RN, FAAN
Professor and Dean
Oregon Health Sciences University
School of Nursing
Portland, Oregon

Judith A. Roos, MSN, RN
Associate Professor
College of Nursing
University of Illinois at Chicago
Chicago, Illinois

Beth A. Staffileno, MS, RN
Doctoral Candidate
College of Nursing
Rush University
Chicago, Illinois

Phyllis Noerager Stern, DNS, RN, NAP,
    FAAN
Council General
International Council on Womens Health
    Issues (ICOWHI)
Professor and Chair
School of Nursing
Indiana University

Nancy Fugate Woods, PhD, RN
Professor, Family and Child Nursing Director
Center for Women's Health Research
University of Washington
Seattle, Washington

Contents

Preface

After reading the draft of the *Annual Review of Women's Health, Volume III*, I tuned in to National Public Radio on my drive home from the office the other day. The narrator told of her fears when her teenage daughter took a job delivering pizza. "Don't worry," said the girl, "If it looks dangerous, they send one of the guys." The mother then mused at how casually women accept from men the gift of safety, and perhaps the gift of life as they protect us. Which gives us both a different slant on a difficult problem, and explains in part why women around the world are subject to social and cultural controls that, at first, and even second glance, seem unreasonable. It is also why books such as this one before you are so important.

Women are highly prized in all countries for their fecundity. In turn, women are socialized to expect that men will protect them from murder, rape, and mayhem, so the species will survive. And it is true that men are stronger physically than women. At least in the short run.

However, there are dangers in engendered cultural expectations and practices. This may also explain to us, why this protection sometimes takes on such bizarre forms. Female circumcision is but one such form. In countries where genital mutilation of young girls is the cultural norm, the cultural reasoning behind the practice is to curb women's inborn reckless sexual activity, and thus to keep them safe from promiscuity with its attendant diseases and the danger of bearing a child by other than their lawful mate. The practice is so culturally ingrained that most women insist that the ritual be performed on their daughters, so that they will be marriageable.

Too often, women's only other course for financial security in these countries is prostitution.

The social and cultural value placed on fecundity may also explain why older women tend to have lower social value than their younger sisters, after all we are the only mammal on the planet that lives beyond its ability to reproduce. Crooks (1994) illustrates the relative social value of older women in her study of breast cancer treatment. Women younger than 80 were given the choice of lumpectomy or mastectomy. Women over 80 were simply told, "It has to come off." This may also explain the widespread use of hormone replacement therapy. If our bodies think we are still fecund, perhaps we will be more socially acceptable. On the other hand, perhaps mother nature expected us to die at 45, and hadn't made plans to protect our hearts and bones beyond that time. She certainly prepared us poorly for the autoimmune disease of degenerative arthritis, from which 80% of older women suffer. Ironically, relief comes from chemical substances that scientists, often men, have invented to ease calcified joints and allow us to perform the activities of daily living.

The value society places on women's fecundity may explain why lesbians (and gay men for that matter) are placed far down on the social scale by the general populace. It also explains why many men and women in the Western World believe that a woman's right to abortion should be amended from "pro-choice" to "no choice."

The cultural belief that men need to protect women could account for the fact that one of my students tells me she too often hears from men that, "Ninety-five percent of women are nuts," because women have said, "Enough already—I want to be free." Is the abusive man's need to control "his woman's" every action a distorted perception that he is being protective?

It *is* noted that gender driven cultures may pose particular dangers, and if protected, women tend to live long, productive lives. We also know that social rules and cultural beliefs are resistant to change. Will casting aside unexamined norms, such as men will protect us, leave us vulnerable to rape, carnage and death? Or, will systematic examination of women and their health help us live to be wiser, older women, the "Crones" (Walker, 1985) who have been around long enough to advise us on life? The authors in this Annual Review, while not all qualifying as "Crones," have a handle on how our social and cultural position came to be and that knowledge is essential in transforming culture. In our efforts to make social change, we risk loss and must weigh freedom against danger. From my point of view, urging men and women to read this Review is a means for building respect between the sexes that allows us our freedom, and our chance at "cronehood." But I am rarely opinion free, and I am the first to admit that using knowledge to challenge engendered health beliefs and practices is a conundrum.

REFERENCES

Crooks, D. (1994, June). *The process of survival in older women with breast cancer.* Paper presented at the Second International Qualitative Health Research Conference, Hershey, PA.

Walker, B. G. (1985). *The Crone: Women of age, wisdom, and power.* San Francisco: Harper & Row.

Phyllis Noerager Stern, DNS, RN, FAAN, NAP

Introduction

Beverly J. McElmurry
and Randy Spreen Parker

The cover of this *Annual Review of Women's Health* depicts a woman weaving a dreamcatcher. The art by Maxine Noel-Ioyan Mani symbolizes the work of the editors and contributing authors as they weave a web for the future of women's health.

The legend of the dreamcatcher is found throughout Indian history and culture, particularly among the Sioux, Ojibway, and Oneida Indians. It was their belief that good and bad dreams fill the night air. Dreamcatchers were hung over babies' cradles and lodges to capture the dreams. The good dreams, knowing their way, slipped through the web and floated to the dreamer below. The bad dreams (nightmares), not knowing their way, became entangled in the web and subsequently perished at the light of day.

The wisdom of the legend is relevant for future directions in healthcare delivery. Participating authors of each *Annual Review of Women's Health* are part of a community of professional scholars who are committed to healthcare that addresses the uniqueness of women. The web of the dreamcatcher has yet to be completed. Many of the values we hold about healthcare are challenged in a time of rapid change in healthcare systems. It is encouraging that women are more frequently included in various research endeavors and programs. On the other hand, healthcare for women is increasingly focused on the treatment of diseases through managed care systems that do not profit from an emphasis on increasing health promotion and disease prevention services. As editors, our web is constructed on a primary health care (PHC) frame. Incorporating new knowledge about women's health within a PHC perspective is not an elusive goal if we work together with others in positions of influence on healthcare policy in efforts to achieve legislative actions that support PHC. If we act as a unified, empowered community, we will be able to weave a web that is strong enough to filter such healthcare nightmares as racism, inequality, and poverty.

The analogy of PHC as the frame for weaving a web of women's health knowledge emphasizes several concepts, including:

1. Accessibile health services to all of the population;
2. Maximum individual and community involvement in the planning and operation of healthcare services;
3. Emphasis on services that are preventive and promotive;
4. The use of appropriate technology with local resources and government support;
5. The integration of health development with total overall social and economic development;
6. Provision of culturally acceptable health activities; and
7. A focus on the health concerns of highest priority for the community residents and health system.

As with earlier volumes of the *Annual Review of Women's Health,* the use of our preferred classification system for organizing women's health knowledge represents the web to be woven. (See Table 1.) These categories and access words for women's health provide a guide for reading this and other sources of information on women's health. The following brief overview of each chapter categorizes the content under this classification system.

DEVELOPMENT ACROSS THE LIFE CYCLE

The women's health research community has worked for some time to have women included in clinical trials. Therefore, it is a distinct pleasure to offer readers the chapter by Nancy Woods, a leader in both the methodology of clinical trials and the study of hormonal therapy with older women. The historical perspective in Woods' chapter provides a useful anchor for this rapidly changing research area for women. For older women, understanding the decision for inclusion/exclusion in clinical trials requires recognition of the triple jeopardy they face when racism, ageism, and sexism interact. Attention is drawn in this chapter to ethical and legal concerns for investigators and trial participants as well as clinicians. A relatively unexplored issue is how to accurately and effectively report results of these large clinical trials to lay women.

Table 1
Categories and Access Words for Women's Health

Characteristics of Women	**Physical Diseases and Health Problems**
Development Across the Life Cycle	substance abuse/addiction
menstrual cycle	osteoporosis
sexuality	STD
physiology	gynecological issues
child-rearing/	cancer
parenting	
relationships	**Mental Health/Illness**
family	violence/abuse
	body image
Health Promotion and Maintenance	eating disorders
nutrition	
lifestyles	**Drugs, Devices, Therapeutic Interventions**
risk factors	
screening	**Economics, Ethics, Policy, Legislation**
status/assessment	
environmental health	**Research/Theoretical Issues**
	methods
Women as Providers of Health Care	theories
professional providers	scales/instruments
non-professional	lived experience
providers	feminism
work of the nurse	
	Additional/Alternative Access Words:
Delivery of Health Care to Women	
	_____
Health and Work	
	_____
Reproductive Health	
maternal-fetal	_____
health/illness	
intrapartum	_____
postpartum	

HEALTH PROMOTION AND MAINTENANCE

We have come to rely on Donna Huddleston for her ability to raise important questions in women's health. She does just that in her chapter about the relationship of hormone replacement therapy for the promotion of health and prevention of disease. Pointing out the profits for drug companies in marketing hormone replacement therapy (HRT), Huddleston notes that popular magazines now include coupons for prescription discounts. She also reminds us that working with women to help them decide on HRT requires that women are able to make informed decisions. Even the

Healthy People 2000 documents infer that counseling perimenopausal women about the benefits and risks of HRT improves the quality of life (QOL) of women. It is interesting that the database Huddleston uses for the review of HRT decisions comes from professional and lay sources, as well as computer-accessed online publications and discussion groups. The varied positions and distortions of data relative to HRT are serious threats to women's ability to choose an appropriate course of action relative to the management of menopause symptoms and prevention of diseases specific to aging. Huddleston emphasizes the importance of advancing a national research agenda for menopause by citing the proposed 1993 NIH agenda. Overall, the relationship of each woman's response to menopause and efforts to achieve a desired QOL are complex factors to weigh in decisions about HRT.

WOMEN AS PROVIDERS OF HEALTHCARE

We thought it appropriate that sexual harassment be classified as an experience of most women. It is an experience particularly rampant in settings where the power differences between men and women are unequal. Therefore, Judith Roos' comprehensive discussion of this topic is long overdue. Although there have been differences in the legal and empirical definitions of harassment, Roos notes that more recent work favors distinguishing gender harassment, unwanted sexual attention, and sexual coercion as categories for examining the experiences and the scholarship on this topic. Key to understanding this topic is our willingness, whether men or women, to examine the effect of sex role socialization and gender stereotyping in society, particularly work and learning environments. A focus of Roos' review includes what we know about women at risk and those who perpetuate harassment. It is particularly helpful to understand that sexual harassment is both an event and a process. The materials abstracted by Roos are drawn from many disciplines and include both historical overviews of the topic as well as practical guides for parents wishing to ensure that their children's rights are protected. In delineating the implications that can be drawn from the literature, Roos stresses that in addition to strengthening means for addressing this issue, we can all work to strengthen policies and procedures in the work settings that are sensitive to women's models for resolving conflict. Educational programs, including those for counselors, are important in helping women who have suffered the effects of harassment and in finding ways to create change. Women should not have to resort to resigning their positions or becoming whistleblowers in order to escape such intolerable situations.

Carol Collins also deals with issues relevant to women's healthcare providers as she covers the topic of violence against women health workers. While this topic has been a concern for decades, Collins draws upon the literature to illustrate how reticent we have been in examining the effect of violence on health providers. Over the years, more attention has been placed on managing and preventing violent behaviors of patients. The conflicting positions on this topic are illustrated by the tendency of health professionals to identify the risk for violence in healthcare settings, yet criticize clinicians who use chemical and physical restraints on violence-prone individuals. How we define and cope with victimization is important in making sense of violent experiences. It is important to recognize the gendered nature of violence and the tendency to blame the victims of violence. We have been slow to accept the idea of violence as a workplace hazard. Collins cites several authors who identify possible institutional structures and mechanisms that would help address potential and actual hazards. One question she raises is whether cost containment efforts in healthcare create environments that are more prone to violence. This is an important issue for all of us to consider, whether we are providing or seeking healthcare.

DELIVERY OF HEALTHCARE TO WOMEN

The comprehensive chapter by Roberta Cassidy and Tonda Hughes is extremely useful. While the authors primarily address the barriers in accessing healthcare for lesbian women, the cumulative goal of their chapter is to help everyone understand how to enhance the care of lesbians. The chapter is a resource for clinicians, researchers, and educators. This topic is especially important in understanding how oppressive social systems are reflected in health services when there is potential for interaction between all of the "isms" in societal stereotyping of groups according to race, sex, class, and sexual orientation. This review of literature is divided into healthcare experiences, lesbian health overviews, adolescent health, aging, alternative, i.e., insemination/childbearing/parenting issues, cancer, mental health, substance use and abuse, violence/abuse, HIV, and healthcare providers. These authors also list additional references that are not reviewed but may be of interest to readers. Other resources identified for readers are community clinics and service groups for lesbians as well as research networks and newsletters. Some practical implications are identified by the authors after completing their review of the status of lesbian healthcare. For example, they suggest including questions about sexual orientation in major surveys of women's health. While some of the suggestions seem simple, acting on them may require major social breakthroughs in order to realize health-care that is respectful of the diversity in people.

HEALTH AND WORK

Latex allergy is a rapidly emerging threat to the health of women and others. Joan Martellotto is courageously pursuing this topic in her writing and research. It is not always the case that the pursuit of truth is desired, especially if knowledge threatens company profits, increases the likelihood of lawsuits, or requires massive changes in how we conduct our service agencies. The recent emphasis on the use of latex gloves and other latex products to protect self and others from blood-borne diseases has intensified the allergy issues for many patients, health workers, and others who serve the public. Martellotto describes the development of sensitization risk for exposure and identification, and management of sensitivity once the allergic response becomes apparent. Readers will be surprised at the many ways women and healthcare providers can be exposed to latex products. Important advice is offered in this chapter on correct diagnostic tests, sources of accurate information about the allergy, management of the environment to reduce risk, and centers of excellence working on this general issue. The implications for policy, education, and research about latex allergy are compelling. We must become knowledgeable about latex allergies and speak up about the mechanism that will reduce this environmental, occupational, and recreational threat to health.

REPRODUCTIVE HEALTH

Kathleen Norr, M. Ryan Gantes, and Agatha Lowe tackle a very difficult topic—prenatal AIDS testing for pregnant women. Their review of this topic is extraordinary and thoughtful. The common wisdom is that prenatal testing for AIDS is performed in order to determine whether there is a need to treat an infected woman with drugs in order to avoid the transfer of this deadly disease to the infant. However, the reality is much more complicated than merely ordering a test. The authors of this chapter frame their discussion in terms of the ethical, policy, and cost issues that accompany the procedure of prenatal testing for AIDS. As the knowledge of this topic is rapidly unfolding, the chapter's format differs from others in the *Annual Review*. The authors provide an extensive integrative review of the available research on prenatal testing and then provide a brief segment on ways to locate the latest information on this topic. After reading this chapter, most readers will understand the importance of working to ensure the prevention of perinatal AIDS infection.

PHYSICAL DISEASE AND
HEALTH PROBLEMS

The diseases specific or more prevalent in women are not always the diseases that receive high levels of funding from a national research agenda or even those most often covered in the lay health media. We truly hope that Ayhan Lash's chapter brings greater awareness to our lay and professional readers about the serious threats to women's health from the group of diseases known as autoimmune diseases, particularly systemic lupus erythematosus (SLE). These conditions occur when the immune system turns on the body and begins to destroy its own tissues. Lash focuses on SLE as a prototype example of this serious phenomenon for women. However, she includes a list of diseases by prevalence in women that highlights the devastation of this group of chronic conditions which are grave and difficult to manage. Interestingly, SLE is even more prevalent in African American and Hispanic American women than in Caucasians. Lash points out that self-care is important in achieving a quality of life consistent with symptoms and disease progression. To this end, she presents recent literature about areas such as accurate and early identification of SLE, the relationship of disease progression to pregnancy, hormonal therapy and fatigue, as well as comprehensive books written specifically for lay and professional audiences.

For another problem important to women, we asked Braun, Staffileno, and Potempa to examine hypertension in women because of the known prevalence of this disease. In particular, we were concerned that women have sufficient knowledge to pursue the management of this condition, by self and/or health professionals. We are pleased that the authors emphasize hypertension as both a disease and a risk factor for other cardiovascular conditions such as coronary heart disease and stroke. Comparisons of the differences between genders is important in understanding the cause, treatment, and effects of hypertension. In addition, the authors of this chapter note differences between races in terms of prevalence, treatment, and control. The inclusion of information on prevention, risk appraisal, reduction of risk, lifestyle modifications, and drug therapy are very useful to professional and lay readers, as well as the tables that explain blood pressure classifications and categories of drugs used to treat hypertension. Braun, Staffileno and Potempa review the recent clinical trials using hormonal replacement therapy (HRT) for postmenopausal women, an important topic when women weigh the cardiovascular effects of hormonal therapy. The importance of including hypertension screening in areas where women naturally congregate is stressed as well as ways for lay and professional groups to work together to achieve communities conducive to cardiovascular health. Women are underrepresented in the clinical research on cardiovascular disease, including hypertension. Many interesting questions are raised by these authors for future areas of research.

MENTAL HEALTH AND ILLNESS

The highest rate for attempted suicide is found in Latina high school students. While these adolescent females do not have the highest rate for completed suicides (that rate is found in Caucasian males), there are many factors to consider before launching programs for prevention and early identification of risk conditions. Janet Grossman and Claudia Cotes draw on extensive experience and expertise in framing a perspective for examining this topic. In developing a public health approach to suicide prevention, the authors explore the context of Latino-American culture, the mortality and morbidity on suicide in Latina youth, and risk factors for suicide in this group. Their chapter offers information on suicide prevention intervention combining mental health and public health perspectives. Nontraditional settings are identified as settings that can effectively house prevention programs for Latinas, a minority group that is known to underutilize traditional health services. Thus, emergency rooms and school-based health programs are important areas for integrating prevention services. Attention is paid to programs for youth as well as families. This is an extremely important population where parents are immigrants and have adolescents experiencing acculturation stress. For any suicide prevention program to work, communities as well as families must stress injury prevention and restrictions of those means by which children and youth often commit suicide, such as ensuring the removal of firearms from the home.

DRUGS, DEVICES, AND THERAPEUTIC INTERVENTIONS

Strange as it may seem, we have little research specific to gender differences in pain management. Christine Miaskowski helps us begin to address the lack of databased information to guide pain management in women. She draws our attention to important dimensions to consider in the experience of pain; the physiological, sensory, affective, emotional, behavioral cognitive, and sociocultural factors that influence pain. While some studies of pain have been conducted, they often take place in laboratory settings rather than clinical settings. There are many fascinating questions raised as Miaskowski reviews studies, but it is startling that to date, definitive conclusions cannot be drawn about women's sensitivity, response, and perceptions of pain due to menstrual and hormonal fluctuations. Pain syndromes with a specific gender distribution are noted in this review and interesting questions are raised about the expectations for and acceptance of these differences. In a practical way, how women's pain is treated and managed may be more reflective of unexamined gender stereotypes held by care providers than the scientific competence of the professionals.

ECONOMICS, ETHICS, POLICY, LEGISLATION

Campbell and Parker have recently published several literature reviews of research about battered women and their children. Therefore, the format for their chapter details the rationale for an extensive list of policies recommended for the care of women who have been subjected to abuse. These policies cover universal screening for all women entering the health system, the screening tools to use, and service points at which the potential for uncovering violence are particularly important (family planning, treatment of sexually transmitted diseases, and depression). How health professionals handle the treatment of women who have been abused is emphasized with attention to disclosure, lethal risks, and avoidance of victim blaming. There is a flexibility in the authors' approach to this topic in the recognition that some abusive relationships can be changed and that the process of leaving abusive and violent relationships sometimes occurs over time. The importance of health professional leadership in dealing with this problem is noted and ideas are provided about the content to include in the basic education programs. It is important to note the link of professional responses to domestic violence as a global problem that requires human rights initiatives.

RESEARCH AND THEORETICAL ISSUES

Female genital mutilation is a topic of urgent international concern for the health of young girls. Carol Christiansen offers an overview of this topic and covers what is known historically about female circumcision, the classifications for this ritual act, its geographic prevalence, and health risks/outcomes for young girls and women. This practice is deeply rooted in certain cultures. Whenever we have discussed the practice in diverse groups, the dialogue has become quite intense. However, we urge readers to talk about the topic and to understand it at the same time that you work to end the practice. When you encounter a circumcised woman seeking healthcare, find a way to provide sensitive care and an opportunity for her to tell her story. Most certainly, refer to this chapter when you are considering how to help others understand the practice.

CONCLUSION

Overall, as we look toward the coming year, we urge all of you to raise questions about the health of women. Do you find the information you need on a given subject area? Further, do the systems of care you participate in or read about provide women an option for informed choice and control over their bodies?

We do hope that after reading the following chapters you will agree that the material provided in this volume of the *Annual Review of Women's Health* is extremely important to the healthcare of women. As before, we continue to be grateful for the support of the National League for Nursing Press in making this material available. In particular, the sensitivity of Allan Graubard and the editing skill of Nancy Jeffries continue to grace our existence. They add extraordinary skills in moving the creative process forward.

Part I

Development Across the Life Cycle

Chapter 1

Clinical Trials with Older Women

Nancy Fugate Woods

Women account for a substantial majority of the population living into old age. Indeed, the life expectancy for women born in the decade after World War II (the Baby Boomers) is nearly 80 years (National Center for Health Statistics, 1993). Increasing concern about costs necessary for healthcare for the elderly has stimulated interest in the optimal ways to promote health and prevent disease for this population. Because of exclusion of women from clinical trials in the past, women now face uncertainty about the optimal ways to promote their health and prevent disease as they age. Past exclusionary practices have produced a significant deficit in knowledge about the optimum ways to treat diseases of midlife and older women.

The purposes of this review are to:

1. Examine issues related to inclusion and exclusion of women from clinical trials;

2. Explore the historical events that preceded U.S. National Institute of Health (NIH) and Food and Drug Administration (FDA) policy changes regarding inclusion of women and the social context for those policies;

3. Review exemplars of recently completed and ongoing clinical trials that focus on the health of older women (midlife and older women);

4. Discuss implications of women's representation in clinical trials for clinical practice with older women, education of clinicians about older women's health, and health policy related to older women and research.

Material included in this review were identified initially through a Medline Search for the period 1990 to the present and references cited in these materials were also reviewed. In addition, the Office of Women's Health of the NIH graciously provided the prepublication copies of their forthcoming papers assessing NIH's experience in responding to legislative mandates about inclusion of women and minorities in clinical trials (Hayunga, Costello, & Pinn, in press; Hayunga & Pinn, in press; Rothenberg, Hayunga, Rudick, & Pinn, 1996).

CLINICAL TRIALS: INCLUSION, EXCLUSION, AND CONSEQUENCES FOR OLDER WOMEN

Clinical trials constitute an important subset of clinical studies. In general, clinical trials are experiments whose purpose is to test the safety and efficacy of one treatment in comparison to another in (at least) two comparable groups of people who have been assigned at random to receive the experimental treatment, or to receive the standard care, or a placebo. The experimental treatment is given according to a specific protocol and a comparison or control protocol is also carefully specified, often the standard approach to care. Usually both the people receiving the experimental or comparison treatment (participants) are unaware of the treatment status of the individuals; that is, the treatment status is masked from both participants and trial personnel. Some trials are termed crossover trials. Participants in these trials receive two or more treatments (or an experimental treatment and control or standard treatment) in a designated order. Also common are parallel trials in which only one treatment is administered to each participant.

Clinical trials are designed to optimize internal validity. This means that the study design emphasizes controlling for factors that could interfere with the interpretation of treatment effects (the effect of the treatment on the health outcome). When studies are designed to maximize internal validity, they often compromise on external validity, or the ability to apply the results of the study to a larger reference population. One way investigators have enhanced the internal validity of their studies is by restricting the sample studied in a variety of ways, for example by limiting the study to one gender, age group, or ethnic group. In an effort to restrict variability in the health outcome being influenced by the treatment being studied, investigators often excluded people with certain characteristics, such as women and people from ethnic groups underrepresented in the U.S. population. Although this strategy may have enhanced the homogeneity of the sample and may have contributed to internal validity of the study design, the consequences for women are problematic. Compromising on the ability to generalize to a larger population, investigators have omitted people of one gender (often women) in favor of studying a more homogeneous group of people (often men) and thus have emphasized internal validity at the expense of external validity.

Omissions of women from studies becomes increasingly problematic when it occurs during a series of trials such as those necessary for drug development and approval that are carried out over a lengthy period (approximately twelve years). The series of studies required for FDA approval begins with a three- to four-year period of preclinical testing involving laboratory and animal studies to assess the safety and biological activity of a drug. Clinical trials begin with Phase I trials in which a drug is tested with 20 to 80 healthy humans to determine safety and dosage levels. In Phase II trials, the drug is studied with 100 to 300 patients to determine its efficacy and side effects. Phase III trials involve 100 to 300 patients to determine effectiveness and adverse reactions with long-term use. Finally, Phase IV trials may be required after FDA approval during a postmarketing testing period. When women have been omitted from Phases I and II of drug studies, they may eventually be studied in Phase III trials of a drug never before studied in women or after Phase III trials are completed, they may have been treated with a drug never tested on women. Consequences may have included inappropriate dose due to the differences in weight and metabolism between men and women, unanticipated pharmacokinetic effects in women, unanticipated side effects, toxic effects, or ineffectiveness (American College of Clinical Pharmacy, 1993; Mastroianni, Faden, & Federman, 1994).

SHIFTING POLICIES:
AN HISTORICAL PERSPECTIVE

The history of omission of women from clinical trials is a long and complicated one. Dating to the early 1980s (Kinney, Trautmann, Gold, Vesell, & Zelis, 1981), policies influencing women's participation in clinical trials reflect several changing perspectives. Overall, there has been a shift from viewing women's participation in research as a burden to their participation as a benefit. As appreciation grew of the inadequate knowledge base for caring for women, exclusionary policies have been viewed increasingly as depriving women of the potential health benefits accruing from the advancement of knowledge about women's health and optimum healthcare. As the NIH guidelines shifted from encouraging investigators to include women in clinical research to requiring it as a condition of research funding, FDA regulations have changed from excluding certain groups of women from research for the purposes of protecting the fetus, to encouraging inclusion of women in drug testing (Rothenberg, 1996).

NIH Policy

A series of events led to the NIH Guidelines on the Inclusion of Women and Minorities in Clinical Research (Federal Register, 1994). As chronicled in the 1985 Report of the U.S. Public Health Service (USPHS) Task Force on Women's Health Issues (USPHS, 1985) the task force recommended that "biomedical and behavioral research should be expanded to insure emphasis on those conditions and diseases unique to, or more prevalent in, women in all age groups." In addition, the Task Force emphasized those conditions where circumstances for women were unique, the interventions were different for women than for men, or the health risks were greater for a woman than for a man (USPHS, 1985, p. 6). In 1986, the NIH Advisory Committee on Women's Health recommended the policy that investigators include women in studies, especially in clinical trials; explain exclusion of women from their proposals when that was seen as appropriate; and evaluate gender differences in their findings. In 1989, a U.S. Government Accounting Office (GAO) study of the NIH implementation of this policy was requested. In 1990, the GAO report, "Problems in Implementing Policy on Women in Study Populations" revealed that the policy was not being implemented. In 1990, the Congressional Caucus on Women's Issues drafted the Women's Health Equity Act and the House and Senate conducted hearings on women's health research being funded by the NIH. In 1990, the Office of Research on Women's Health (ORWH) was created within the Office of the Director, NIH, to strengthen and enhance prevention, diagnosis, and treatment of illness in women and to enhance research related to diseases and conditions that affect women. During the same year, NIH established an Office of Research on Minority Health. Among the objectives of the ORWH is ensuring appropriate participation of women in clinical research, especially clinical trials (NIH, 1992). The Office of Research on Minority Health has a similar charge. In 1990, Dr. Ruth Kirschstein, who had co-authored the USPHS Task Force on Women's Health Report, became acting director of the ORWH. In August 1990, the NIH Guide to Grants and Contracts published the NIH policy on inclusion of women in studies, strengthening guidelines on inclusion of women and minorities in study populations. Beginning in February 1991, no PHS grant applications were accepted unless women were adequately represented in clinical research, except in cases where their exclusion was justified. In 1991, the Institute of Medicine (IOM) convened a meeting to assess the adequacy of existing knowledge for formulating gender-specific hypotheses and to consider the advisability of conducting a study to explore further women's participation in clinical studies. In 1992, in response to a request from NIH, the IOM convened the Committee on the Ethical and Legal Issues Relating to the Inclusion of Women in Clinical Studies. In March 1991, Dr. Bernadine Healy assumed the directorship of NIH, the first woman to be appointed to the post. In Fall 1991, Dr. Vivian Pinn assumed the directorship of the Office for Women's Health Research (NIH, 1992).

In 1991, the ORWH named an NIH Task Force on Opportunities for Research on Women's Health and charged it with assessing the current status of women's health research, identifying research opportunities and gaps in knowledge, and a cross NIH plan for future directions for women's health research. The Task Force, in conjunction with ORWH staff, invited public and scientific deliberations in developing the research agenda published in 1992 (NIH, 1992). The Workshop on Opportunities for Research on Women's Health held in Hunt Valley, MD, September 1991, included experts in basic and clinical sciences, women's health clinicians, and representatives of women's organizations. The goal was to develop recommendations for research activities on behalf of all U.S. women. The framework for development of a research agenda involved working groups to address major divisions of the lifespan and scientific areas that cut across women's health throughout life (NIH, 1992).

In 1993, Congress mandated specific NIH action regarding women and minorities as participants in NIH supported clinical research in the NIH Revitalization Act of 1993 (Public Law 103-43). The NIH responded by revising its policy which is published in the Federal Register as the NIH Guidelines on the Inclusion of Women and Minorities as Subjects in Clinical Research (NIH Guidelines, 1994). Statutory requirements are that women and minorities and their subpopulations shall be included as subjects in clinical research and that in the case of clinical trials, they should be included in such ways that valid analyses can be conducted to test differences among participating groups. Moreover, NIH must engage in outreach efforts to recruit these groups into clinical research studies. Four new requirements of NIH are reflected in the guidelines. NIH must ensure that women and minority group members and their subpopulations are: included in human subject research and included in Phase III clinical trials such that valid analyses testing differences in intervention effects can be accomplished. In addition, NIH must prohibit cost considerations as an acceptable reason for excluding certain groups, and initiate and support efforts for recruitment and retention of participants (La Rosa, Seto, Caban, & Hayunga, 1995).

The 1993 legislation and current NIH policy raised several considerations for Phase III clinical trials. The legislation explicitly requires that trials are designed and conducted in a way to provide for valid analysis of whether variables being studied have a different effect on women or members of minority groups. NIH defines clinical trials as investigations for the purpose of evaluating an experimental intervention in comparison with a standard or control intervention or comparing two or more existing treatments. Their definition includes pharmacological, nonpharmacological, and behavioral interventions given for disease prevention, prophylaxis, diagnosis, or therapy and includes community trials and other population-based intervention trials (La Rosa et al., 1995). Two additional components of this definition specify the NIH interpretation of valid analysis and significant differences. NIH defines valid analysis as that assessment that will produce the correct estimate of the difference in outcomes between two groups of participants and significant differences as those of clinical or public health importance. The latter are not always synonymous with statistical significance (La Rosa et al., 1995).

FDA Policy

A chronology of FDA policy changes has also been reported by several authors (Mastroianni et al., 1994; Merkatz & Junod, 1994; Rothenberg, 1996; Rothenberg et al., in press). The Food and Drug Administration regulates privately funded research with humans that is intended to introduce new drugs or medical devices. The policies on inclusion of women are set forth in guidelines that are not mandatory interpretations but advisory opinions on meeting regulatory requirements. In the FDA guidelines for 1977, women of childbearing potential were advised to be excluded from earliest dose ranging studies. Although this guideline largely excluded women from clinical trials, three exceptional circumstances were considered for inclusion of women of childbearing potential. Those circumstances included situations where the purpose of the drug was to save or prolong life, the drug belonged to a class for which teratogenic potential had been established in animals, or institutionalization of the woman allowed investigators to determine she was not pregnant. The FDA allows drug manufacturers to market drugs without reproductive testing, as long as notice is included on the product label. Moreover, when stipulating guidelines for males, a risk/benefit approach is used, even when male reproductive abnormalities may result from the drug (Rothenberg, Hayunga, Rudick, & Pinn, 1996).

In 1992, the Congressional Caucus for Women's Issues urged the GAO to audit the FDA with respect to inclusion of women in drug development studies. The GAO study found that women were underrepresented in drug trials, especially in the early phases of testing of new drugs (U.S. General Accounting Office, 1990). In 1993, the FDA issued a new guideline for the inclusion of women in drug research, "Guideline for the Study and Evaluation of Gender Differences in the Clinical Evaluation of Drugs" (Food and Drug Administration, 1993). This guideline lifted the blanket ban on the inclusion of women of childbearing potential in new drug research. Instead, sponsors of drug research are expected to include a broad range of patients in their studies, conduct appropriate analyses to evaluate potential subset differences in patients they have studied, study possible pharmacokinetic differences in patient subsets, and carry out targeted studies for subset pharmacodynamic differences that are especially likely or that would be especially important if present. The distinction in this new guideline is FDA's recognition that women are competent to give informed consent for their participation in research and that informed consent provides the necessary insulation to protect researchers and manufacturers from suits by the mother or possible child for all except negligent enrollment practices (Rothenberg, 1996; see Merkatz, Temple, Subel, Feiden, & Kessler, 1993, for further discussion of the FDA policy changes). Although the FDA guidelines represent an important advance for inclusion of women in clinical trials, they do not mandate inclusion of women.

SOCIAL CONTEXT FOR REGULATION OF WOMEN'S PARTICIPATION IN CLINICAL TRIALS

Regulation can only be understood by considering the social context in which it evolves. Early attempts to regulate women's participation in clinical trials reflected themes of protectionism. Women were perceived to need protection from burdens of participating in research and not judged able to give informed consent for their participation or that of their fetus. This orientation to women's participation was grounded in assumptions about women as reproductive instruments rather than as individuals with inherent worth and a conflation of women's health with reproductive and fetal health (Johnson & Fee, 1994). Despite the fact that heart disease is the leading cause of death for women, the Multiple Risk Factor Intervention Trial included only men. More recently, the study of aspirin prophylaxis for heart disease included only men. Because men are assumed to be the normal income generating unit in the society, exclusion of women, particularly elderly women with heart disease from such studies may reflect not only sexism but also ageism and classism. Elderly women are not judged economically productive. Even more recently, exclusion of younger women from drug trials using AZT for HIV/AIDS has resulted in a lack of information about appropriate dosing for women and may be responsible for some experiences of drug toxicity. The exclusion of women from early HIV research may reflect the assumption that HIV, like heart disease, is a health problem for men alone.

No doubt some concerns of regulators reflected past injustices and oppression of research participants; for example, pregnant women included in studies of DES without their informed consent or women included in contraceptive trials in a control group without their knowledge and without access to pregnancy termination. (See Rothenberg, 1996, for a discussion of the history of regulating human subjects research.)

Gender composition of the nation's scientists and the subset of scientists who shape science policy also may have influenced exclusion of women from trials. Bias in allocating research funds to topics thought to be important by those making funding decisions may have discouraged investigators from studying topics of greater importance to women than men. Moreover, viewing women as instruments of reproduction versus individuals with inherent value and worth has limited the kinds of questions studied in populations of childbearing women.

Scientific infeasibility is a reason frequently given for the exclusion of women from studies. Consideration of a woman's menstrual cycle is one such factor believed to complicate research designs. Alternatively, a woman's menstrual cycle phase should be considered as a factor that furthers understanding of the phenomenon (e.g., drug) being studied. Difficulty in recruitment is another basis for concern about including women in clinical trials. Gender specific strategies for enhancing recruitment need to be developed to enhance inclusion (see Mastroianni et al., 1994, for ideas). The need to increase sample sizes to include women in trials is raised as a basis for excluding women. Although cost of including additional groups (gender or ethnic groups) in research has been given to justify their exclusion, exclusionary practices carry the cost of ignorance. Despite women's greater longevity than men's, the Baltimore Longitudinal Study on Aging did not include women during the first twenty years of data collection. Consequences include a lack of information about health and normal aging among women, the substantial majority of elderly citizens!

PERSPECTIVES FOR CONSIDERING WOMEN'S REPRESENTATION IN CLINICAL TRIALS

Both ethical and legal perspectives contribute to understanding the issue of representation of women in clinical trials. Sherwin (1994) has explored two specific ethical concerns. First, some or all women have been excluded unjustly from clinical trials and suffer as a result. She suggests that women should be represented in future trials proportionate to their health risks or have privileged places in such trials. Second, women may be unjustly enrolled in studies exposing them to risks without appropriate benefits accruing to them. For example, poor women may be studied to test treatments only available to women who can pay for the treatment when it becomes available for purchase. Thus Sherwin cautions us against wholesale endorsement of using women in studies.

Principles of respect for persons, beneficence, and justice have been proposed to analyze the ethical problems regarding exclusion of women from clinical trials. Respect for persons is a concern for the inherent value of the individual and has been used in consideration of human subjects' issues related to informed consent. Beneficence in research requires not only concerns regarding harm to participants, but the loss of the substantial benefits that may accrue to women from the research. In some cases, the benefit may have been direct, as in access to treatment for a fatal disease, while in others it may accrue to future generations of women. Justice concerns would dictate that women and men should have equal opportunities to participate in trials and that those who participate in the trials are those who stand to benefit from the results. Under-representation yields unequal distribution of benefits of biomedical research (Mastroianni, Faden, & Federman, 1994, p. ix).

Rothenberg (1996) has explored an array of legal perspectives that help address the issue of exclusion of women from clinical trials. Denying women access to participation in clinical research raises questions of gender discrimination. She reviews Supreme Court decisions affirming women's right to decision making about their reproductive behavior as it affects reproductive status, including the Johnson Controls Court decision that supported women being trusted in the decision they make about exposing themselves and their fetuses to risk. Constitutional issues related to privacy and liberty interests and equal protection, and federal and state antidiscrimination statutes are also relevant to the problem of exclusion. Tort liability, including liability for exclusion as well as inclusion, is another framework for the legal analysis of exclusion of women from clinical trials.

FUTURE CONSIDERATIONS REGARDING WOMEN'S PARTICIPATION IN CLINICAL TRIALS: CONCERNS ABOUT AGING WOMEN

In addition to reviewing the literature about past exclusionary practices and the policies that sustained exclusion of women, it is important to anticipate changing practices. As investigators develop studies of midlife and older women, it will be important to consider strategies that support their representation through recruitment and retention efforts. Specific strategies have been suggested for a number of ethnic groups of women in the publications cited in the following review.

Consequences of past exclusion may include knowledge gaps in diagnosis and treatment, inadequate protections from hazards including those to the fetus, and lack of access to future benefits from participation in trials. Many older women will live with the consequences of past omissions. Clinicians need to be alert to the problems that this situation may create, such as unanticipated drug side and toxic effects. Educators of future clinicians need to alert their students to the risk inherent in the lack of information about older women, including normal aging processes, health problems and treatments that have been studied only with samples of men, and other unknowns. Moreover, educators need to prepare the next generation of researchers, and retrain the current ones, regarding how to design studies that optimize women's opportunities to participate while respecting their right not to do so.

REFERENCES

American College of Clinical Pharmacy. (1993). Women as research subjects. *Pharmacotherapy, 13*(5), 534–542.

Federal Register (1994). The NIH guidelines on the inclusion of women and minorities as subjects in clinical research. *Federal Register, 28,* 14508–14513.

Food and Drug Administration. (1993). Guideline for the study and evaluation of gender differences in the clinical evaluation of drugs. *Federal Register, 39,* 406.

Hayunga, E., Costello, M., & Pinn, V. (in press). Inclusion of women and men in clinical research: Demographics of study populations. *Applied Clinical Trials.*

Hayunga, E., & Pinn, V. (in press). Including women and minorities in clinical research: Implementation of the 1994 NIH guidelines. *Applied Clinical Trials.*

Johnson, T., & Fee, E. (1994). Women's participation in clinical research: From protectionism to access. In A. Mastroianni, R. Faden, & D. Federman (Eds.), *Women and health research: Ethical and legal issues of including women in clinical studies* (Vol. 2, pp. 1–10). Washington, DC: National Academy Press.

Kinney, E., Trautmann, J., Gold, J., Vesell, E., & Zelis, R. (1981). Underrepresentation of women in new drug trials. *Annals of Internal Medicine, 95*(4), 495–499.

La Rosa, J., Seto, B., Caban, C., & Hayunga, E. (1995). Including women and minorities in clinical research. *Applied Clinical Trials, 4,* 5, 31–38.

Mastroianni, A., Faden, R., & Federman, D. (Eds.). (1994). *Women and health research: Ethical and legal issues of including women in clinical studies* (Vol. 1). Washington, DC: National Academy Press.

Merkatz, R., & Junod, S. (1994). Historical background of changes in FDA policy on the study and evaluation of drugs in women. *Academic Medicine, 69,* 703–705.

Merkatz, R., Temple, R., Subel, S., Feiden, K., & Kessler, D. A. (1993). Women in clinical trials of new drugs: A change in Food and Drug Administration policy. *New England Journal of Medicine, 329,* 292–295.

National Center for Health Statistics. (1993). *Current estimates from the National Health Interview Survey, 1992* (Series 10). Hyattsville, MD: U.S. Department of Health and Human Services.

National Institutes of Health. (1992). *Opportunities for research on women's health.* Bethesda, MD: Author.

Rothenberg, K. (1996). Gender matters: Implications for clinical research and women's health care. *Houston Law Review, 32*(5), 1201–1272.

Rothenberg, K., Hayunga, E., Rudick, J., & Pinn, V. (1996). The NIH inclusion guidelines: Challenges for the future. *IRB, 18*(3), 1–4.

Sherwin S. (1994). Women in clinical studies: A feminist view. In A. Mastroianni, R. Faden, & D. Federman (Eds.), *Women and health research: Ethical and legal issues of including women in clinical studies* (Vol. 2, pp. 11–17). Washington, DC: National Academy Press.

U.S. General Accounting Office. (1990). *National Institutes of Health: Problems in implementing policy on women in study populations.* Washington, DC: Author.

U.S. General Accounting Office. (1992). *Women's health: FDA needs to ensure more study of gender differences in prescription drug testing.* Washington, DC: Author.

U.S. Public Health Service Task Force on Women's Health Issues. (1985). *Women's health: Report of the Public Health Service* (Vol. 2, DHHS Publication No. PHS-85-50206). U.S. Department of Health and Human Services, Washington, DC: Public Health Service.

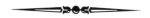

Abstracts of articles included in this review are in two sections. The first set of works addresses the issues and approaches to inclusion of women in clinical trials. The second contains reports of two studies exemplifying the currently funded NIH trials with women. Other examples include studies of urinary incontinence management in community dwelling women, therapies for osteoporosis, and breast cancer treatment trials. The first exemplar is the completed Postmenopausal Estrogen and Progestin Intervention (PEPI) trial. Several publications about the trial and its results are cited. The second exemplar is the Women's Health Initiative (WHI) trial, the largest, multisite clinical trial in history begun in 1992. Papers related to the design of the trial are reviewed here. Results of the trial will be published in future years, with some not available until 2005. Both the PEPI and WIU trials are excellent examples of research designed to address the complexity of midlife and older women's health.

Clinical Trials with Women: Issues and Approaches

American College of Clinical Pharmacy. (1993). Women as research subjects. *Pharmacotherapy, 13*(5), 534–542.

This article includes a position statement from the American College of Clinical Pharmacy advocating inclusion of women in every stage of drug development and provides useful background information about the effects of gender on pharmacokinetics and pharmacodynamics. In addition to recommendations for regulatory agencies, the article includes recommendations for policy makers, those involved in drug development, and investigators.

Controlled Clinical Trials: Design, Methods and Analysis, 16(5). (1995). The entire issue of this journal focuses on the inclusion of women and minorities in clinical trials and the consequences of the NIH Revitalization Act of 1993. It provides perspective of NIH Clinical Trialists, and includes commentary and discussion from investigators regarding specific aspects of the guidelines, such as the valid analysis requirement.

Hayunga, E., Costello, M., & Pinn, V. (in press). Inclusion of Women and Men in Clinical Research: Demographics of Study Populations. *Applied Clinical Trials.*

It is now possible to track demographic data for the NIH study populations and preliminary analyses showed substantial numbers of women and minorities included in Phase III trials and other clinical research studies. The tracking system implemented in October 1994 will support analyses of progress in implementation of the NIH Revitalization Act (1993-PL103-43) in future years.

Hayunga, E., & Pinn, V. (in press). Including Women and Minorities in Clinical Research: Implementation of the 1994 NIH Guidelines. *Applied Clinical Trials.*

This investigation reveals evidence that compliance with new guidelines for inclusion of women in clinical research is high. Initial review groups view the inclusion of women and minorities as a criterion for evaluating scientific merit. Projects not meeting this standard are identified in the initial review and administrative procedures are used to promote resolution of problems. Institutional Review Boards (IRBs) have traditionally focused on protecting the right of humans not to participate in research and are now having to think about the right of humans to participate in research. Respect for persons, beneficence, and justice are guiding principles in this matter. NIH staff reviewed 52 Phase III clinical trials pending award prior to the date specified in the Revitalization Act, and found 24 appropriate as submitted, 25 in compliance when investigators furnished additional information about the study populations, and only 3 found to have inadequate representation of women or minorities. Two of the latter were brought into compliance through instituting changes in study population and one with inadequate representation was justified on the basis of portfolio balance. Concerns voiced by the scientific community included barriers to recruiting participants, potential costs associated with expanding clinical trials, and requirements for including minority subpopulations. For two Council meetings (1/95 and 5/95) 92 percent of applications met inclusion requirements as submitted, 4 percent did not meet gender inclusion requirements, and 7 percent did not meet minority inclusion requirements.

Mastroianni, A., Faden, R., & Federman, D. (Eds.). (1994). *Women and health research:*

Ethical and legal issues of including women in clinical studies (Vol. 1). Washington, DC: National Academy Press.

The first volume of this two-volume report of the Institute of Medicine Committee on the Ethical and Legal Issues Relating to the Inclusion of Women in Clinical Studies contains the executive summary and an overview of issues related to women's participation in clinical trials. Individual chapters address the historical and contemporary status of women's participation in clinical studies, justice in clinical studies and guiding principles, scientific considerations related to gender differences and methodological implications, social, ethical, and legal considerations, and implementation issues. Appendices address reports on women's participation in clinical studies from 1977 to 1993, the NIH Revitalization Act of 1993 regarding the issue, a DES case study, and a review of compensation systems for research injuries.

Mastroianni, A., Faden, R., & Federman, D. (Eds.). (1994). *Women and health research: Ethical and legal issues of including women in clinical studies* (Vol. 2). Washington, DC: National Academy Press.

The second volume of the report contains papers presented at an invited workshop at George Washington University Conference Center March 24-25, 1993. Contributions to this workshop included papers addressing women's participation in clinical research from a variety of perspectives: policy analysts, feminist theorists, ethicists, legal analysts, public health researchers, and research methodologists. These papers included:

- Johnson, T., & Fee, E. *Women's participation in clinical research: From protectionism to access* (pp. 1–10). Chronicles the historical events leading to the current policies of inclusion.
- Sherwin, S. *Women in clinical studies: A feminist view* (pp. 11–17). An analysis of

exclusion from a feminist perspective, advocates a justice model recognizing oppression of women.

- Robertson, J. *Ethical issues related to the inclusion of pregnant women in clinical trials* (Vol. 1, pp. 18–22).
- Steinbock, B. *Ethical issues related to the inclusion of pregnant women in clinical trials* (Vol. 2, pp. 23–28).
- Moreno, J. *Ethical issues related to the inclusion of women of childbearing age in clinical trials* (Vol. 3, pp. 29–34). These 3 papers together provide contrasting opinions about inclusion with respect to paternal interests in the health of the fetus.
- Weisman, C., & Cassard, S. *Health consequences of exclusion or underrepresentation of women in clinical studies* (Vol. 1, pp. 35–40). Reviews information deficits and consequences with respect to morbidity and mortality, diagnosis and treatment patterns, treatment outcome, and provider perceptions.
- Benet, L. *Health consequences of exclusion or underrepresentation of women in clinical studies* (Vol. 2, pp. 41–44). Discusses possible types of gender differences in drug metabolism.
- Stoy, D. *Recruitment and retention of women in clinical studies: Theoretical perspectives and methodological considerations* (pp. 45–51). Recommends: 1) providing young women with children and older women with very specific information regarding requirements of study, 2) offering flexible scheduling and child care, 3) offering assistance with transportation, 4) allowing extra time to carefully review study's risks and benefits, 5) designing recruitment materials to be sensitive to women, and, 6) recognizing women's contributions to research.
- Mitchell, J. *Recruitment and retention of women of color in clinical studies* (pp. 52–56). Recommends we answer

these questions first: 1) Do women of color feel participation in clinical studies is important? 2) Do they feel their participation is important? 3) For women who were offered an opportunity to participate but declined, why? 4) For women who were not offered an opportunity to participate, why did they feel they were not offered the opportunity? 5) For the provider, why were these women not offered the opportunity?

- Levine, R. *Recruitment and retention of women in clinical studies: Ethical considerations* (pp. 57–64). Addresses problems associated with incentives, dropout, costs, and special issues regarding women in developing countries.

- Merton, F. *Impact of current federal regulations on the inclusion of female subjects in clinical studies* (pp. 65–83). Examines regulations that limit versus encourage inclusion and recommends changes in the law.

- Charo, R. *Brief overview of constitutional issues raised by the exclusion of women from research trials* (pp. 84–90). Review of applicable constitutional law.

- Flannery, E., & Greenberg, S. *Liability exposure for exclusion and inclusion of women as subjects in clinical studies* (pp. 91–102). Discussion of tort liability.

- Clayton, E. *Liability exposure when offspring are injured because of their parents' participation in clinical trials* (pp. 103–112).

- Mariner, W. *Compensation for research injuries* (pp. 113–126). Reason for compensation and types of compensation plans.

Commissioned papers included were:

- De Bruin, D. *Justice and the inclusion of women in clinical studies: A conceptual framework* (pp. 127–150). Discusses injustices of our practices and remedies.

- Bird, C. *Women's representation as subjects in clinical studies: A pilot study of research published in JAMA in 1990 and 1992* (pp. 151–173). Finds that women were underrepresented in medical studies and in studies that included women, analysis by gender was not done or not reported.

- Gamble, V., & Blustein, B. *Racial differentials in medical care: Implications for research on women* (pp. 174–191). Discusses the social construction of race and the dangers inherent in looking for difference in medical research, ending with a cautionary note on what it means to study racial differences.

- Lex, B., & Norris, J. *Health status of American Indian and Alaska Native women* (pp. 192–215).

- Yu, E. *Ethical and legal issues relating to the inclusion of Asian/Pacific Islanders in clinical studies* (pp. 216–231).

- Zambrana, R. *The inclusion of Latino women in clinical and research studies: Scientific suggestions for assuring legal and ethical integrity* (pp. 232–240). These three chapters contain reviews of specific issues for each ethnic population of women.

Merkatz, R., & Junod, S. (1994). Historical background of changes in FDA policy on the study and evaluation of drugs in women. *Academic Medicine, 69,* 703–705.

Merkatz, R., Temple, R., Subel, S., Feiden, K., & Kessler, D. A. (1993). Women in clinical trials of new drugs: A change in Food and Drug Administration policy. *New England Journal of Medicine, 329,* 292–295. These two articles track the changes in FDA policy regarding inclusion of women.

Rothenberg, K. (1996). The Institute of Medicine's report on women and health research: Implications for IRBs and the research community. *IRB, 18*(2), 1–3.

This article includes a discussion of the implications of the recently published IOM report for IRBs, particularly their responsibility for ensuring the just selection of persons to be participants in studies and their accountability to ensure adequate representation of gender, racial, and ethnic groups for studies. Rothenberg points out that IRBs and the research community need to think and believe that pregnant women should be given the opportunity to benefit from clinical research and that they can be trusted to make good decisions for themselves and their offspring.

National Institutes of Health. (1994). *Outreach notebook for the NIH guidelines on the inclusion of women and minorities as subjects in clinical research.* Washington, DC: U.S. Department of Health and Human Services, National Institutes of Health, Office of Women's Health Research.

This notebook contains a wealth of information designed to support investigators in their efforts to include women (and underrepresented ethnic groups) in clinical research. A decision tree to guide investigators in considering inclusion of women and minority populations, particularly in assessing to what extent subgroup analyses are necessary and sample size needs to be estimated accordingly. Elements of outreach, ethical issues, sources of help, an interpretation of the review criteria for inclusion of women and minorities is included.

Rothenberg, K., Hayunga, E., Rudick, J., & Pinn, V. (in press). The NIH inclusion guidelines: Challenges for the future. *Applied Clinical Trials.*

This article focuses on challenges presented by the new 1994 NIH Guidelines for Inclusion of Women and Minorities as Subjects in Clinical Research. It includes a report of the 1996 Office of Research on Women's Health workshop in which NIH staff reviewed their experiences with implementation of the new guidelines. Evidence also is presented that suggests IRBs have incorporated the inclusion requirements into their review processes. They are defining to what extent they should require

information from investigators to determine whether the proposed study is equitable, and how actively they should monitor and collect enrollment data to evaluate whether recruitment and retention goals are being met.

Society for the Advancement of Women's Health Research. (1995). *Toward a women's health research agenda: Risk and liability: What are the implications for women's health research?* Washington, DC: Author.

This volume contains proceedings of the corporate advisory council of the society. It includes perspectives of several different stakeholders in the policy regarding inclusion of women in clinical trials, including the impact of liability on women, legal perspectives on federal regulations and product liability, specific drugs and biomaterials issues, and an ethicist's perspective on risk, liability, and business ethics. The FDA perspective is included in a paper by Merkatz.

Exemplars from Contemporary Clinical Trials

Postmenopausal Estrogen and Progestin Intervention (PEPI) Trial

The recently completed PEPI study assessed estrogen and estrogen and progestin therapy with respect to their capacity to reduce cardiovascular disease risk factors. In this study, the effects of estrogen and various combined hormone therapy combinations on LDL and HDL cholesterol levels and other risk factors were examined. The trial included 875 healthy postmenopausal women aged 45 to 64 years who had no known contraindication to hormone therapy who were randomized to placebo, conjugated equine estrogen (CEE), .625mg, CEE 0.625mg plus cyclic medroxyprogesterone acetate (MPA) 10 mg/day for 12 days per month, CEE .625mg plus consecutive NTA 2.5 mg per day; or CEE .625 mg plus cyclic micronized progesterone (NT) 200 mg/day for 12 days per month (The PEPI Trial, 1995). Because the PEPI trial followed women for only three years, it was not possible to estimate how the treatments affected the incidence of disease (such as heart disease), but it was possible to estimate effects of hormone therapy on risk factors. A much longer follow-up period and larger sample size (as in the Women's Health Initiative) would be necessary to assess the actual risk of development of heart disease.

Bush, T., Espeland, M., & Mebane-Sims, I. (1995). The Postmenopausal Estrogen/Progestin Interventions (PEPI) trial. Introduction. *Controlled Clinical Trials, 16*(Suppl. 4), 1s–2s.

An overview of the goals and conduct of the study. Note: This issue contains a series of papers describing the PEPI trial.

Espeland, M., Bush, T., Mebane-Sims, I., Stefanick, M., Johnson, S., Sherwin, R., & Waclawiw, M. (1995). Rationale, design, and conduct of the PEPI trial. *Controlled Clinical Trials, 16*(Suppl. 4), 3s–19s.

Description of the PEPI objectives, primary endpoints (HDL cholesterol, systolic blood pressure, insulin, fibrinogen), secondary endpoints, and detailed description of the study design.

Greendale, G., Bodin-Dunn, L., Ingles, S., Haile, R., & Barrett-Connor, E. (1996). Leisure, home, and occupational physical activity and cardiovascular risk factors in postmenopausal women. *Archives of Internal Medicine, 156*(4), 418–424.

Cross-sectional analysis of baseline data from PEPI trial participants. In white women, leisure physical activity was positively associated with HDL cholesterol, and inversely associated with levels of insulin and fibrinogen. Home physical activity was positively related to HDL cholesterol level. Systolic blood pressure did not vary by leisure, occupational, or home physical activity. Unique relationships between types of physical activity and cardiac risk factors make it important to consider multiple domains of activity in women.

Greendale, G., Wells, B., Barrett-Connor, E., Marcus, R., & Bush, T. (1995). Lifestyle factors and bone mineral density: The Postmenopausal Estrogen/Progestins Intervention study. *Journal of Women's Health, 4,* 231–245.

Report of a cross-sectional analysis of baseline data. In a multivariate model that included age, body mass index (BMI), years of former estrogen use, and all lifestyle factors under study, leisure time physical activity, dietary calcium, and alcohol intake were statistically significantly associated with higher bone mineral density (BMD) at one or more bone sites. Leisure time physical activity had the greatest effect on BMD. Among healthy postmenopausal women, higher levels of leisure time physical activity, dietary calcium, and alcohol intake (within a moderate range) were associated with higher BMD.

Johnson, S., Mebane-Sims, I., Hogan, P., & Stoy, D. (1995). Recruitment of postmenopausal women in the PEPI trial. *Controlled Clinical Trials, 16*(Suppl. 4), 20s–35s.

Discusses recruitment goals, planning, monitoring, recruitment strategies, screening process, and findings regarding recruitment across multiple sites.

Marcus, R., Greendale, G., Blunt, B., Bush, T., Sherman, S., Sherwin, R., Wahner, H., & Wells, B. (1994). Correlates of bone mineral density in the Postmenopausal Estrogen/Progestin Interventions trial. *Journal of Bone and Mineral Research, 9*(9), 1467–1476.

Report of results from baseline measures. Increased body mass was correlated with bone mineral density and heavier postmenopausal women may be protected by a higher BMI. Exposure for 5 years to exogenous estrogen was associated with significantly increased age- and BMI-adjusted bone mineral density.

Miller, V., Byington, R., Espeland, M., Langer, R., Marcus, R., Shumaker, S., & Stern, M. (1995). Baseline characteristics of the PEPI participants. *Controlled Clinical Trials, 16*(Suppl. 4), 54s–64s.

Provides a detailed description of the trial participants at the beginning of the trial including a demographic profile, primary and secondary outcome measures at baseline, gynecologic and obstetric characteristics, current medication use, and lifestyle characteristics.

Stefanick, M., Legault, C., Tracy, R., Howard, G., Kessler, C., Lucas, D., & Bush, T. (1995). Distribution and correlates of plasma fibrinogen in middle-aged women. Initial findings of the Postmenopausal Estrogen/Progestin Interventions (PEPI) study. *Arteriosclerosis, Thrombosis, and Vascular Biology, 15*(12), 2085–2093.

In a model that included age, smoking, alcohol intake, prior HRT, leisure time physical activity, and body mass index, leisure time physical activity was not a statistically significant predictor of fibrinogen level. However, leisure time physical activity did correlate with fibrinogen level when it was considered in the absence of the other factors.

Wood, P., Kessler, G., Lippel, K., Stefanick, M., Wasliauskas, C., & Wells, H. (1995). Physical and laboratory measurements in the PEPI trial. *Controlled Clinical Trials, 16*(Suppl. 4), 36s–53s.

A detailed description of the methods used in the trial.

The Writing Group for the PEPI Trial. (1995). Effects of estrogen or estrogen/progestin regimens on heart disease risk factors in post-menopausal women. The Postmenopausal Estrogen/Progestin Interventions (PEPI) trial. *Journal of the American Medical Association, 273*(3), 199–208.

Report of the primary endpoints. Results indicated that estrogen alone or in combination with a progestin improved lipoproteins and lowered fibrinogen levels without adverse effects on postchallenge insulin or blood pressure. Unopposed estrogen was the optimal regimen for elevating HDL-C. A high rate of endometrial hyperplasia occurred in the groups that used unopposed estrogen, restricting recommendations for its use to women without a uterus. In women who have a uterus, CEE with cyclic micronized progesterone had the most favorable effect on HDL-C and with no excess increased risk of endometrial hyperplasia. NTA had no detrimental effects on lipids compared with the risk for those not taking hormones.

The Writing Group for the PEPI Trial. (1996). Effects of hormone replacement therapy on endometrial histology in postmenopausal women. The Postmenopausal Estrogen/Progestin Interventions (PEPI) trial. *Journal of the American Medical Association, 275*(5), 370–375.

Report of the consequences of using estrogen alone versus estrogen and a progestin for women with a uterus. Women assigned to the estrogen alone group had a higher rate of simple, complex, and atypical hyperplasia than those given placebo. Those who received estrogen along with a progestin or micronized progesterone had similar rates of hyperplasia as those who were given placebo. Of women who developed hyperplasia, 94 percent had the hyperplasia revert to normal after stopping study medications and treating with progestin therapy. CEE therapy at .625 mg enhanced the development of endometrial hyperplasia, but CEE plus a progestin in cyclic or continuous administration protected the endometrium from hyperplasia.

Women's Health Initiative (WHI)

Cardiovascular disease, cancer, and osteoporosis are the most common causes of death, disability, and impaired quality of life in postmenopausal women. The Women's Health Initiative study is the largest U.S. preventive study of its kind. It includes a randomized controlled clinical trial that will enroll nearly 63,000 postmenopausal women 50 to 79 years of age. Three interventions will be tested and women can enroll in one or more. Effects of a low-fat dietary pattern on prevention of breast and colon cancer and coronary heart disease will be evaluated in the first. The second will evaluate the effect of hormone replacement therapy on prevention of coronary heart disease and osteoporotic fractures. Effects of calcium and Vitamin D on prevention of osteoporotic fractures and colon cancer will be evaluated in the third component. Nine years of follow-up will be carried out to evaluate the associations between the treatments and disease endpoints. Another component of this study is an observational study following approximately 100,000 women over time. This study is in progress.

Institute of Medicine. (1993). *An assessment of the NIH Women's Health Initiative.* Washington, DC: National Academy Press.

This report analyzes the benefits and problems associated with the WHI trial, including some questions that may or may not be able to be answered in the course of this study.

McTiernan, A., Rossouw, J., Manson, J., Franzi, C., Taylor, V., Carleton, R., Johnson, S., & Nevitt, M. (1995). Informed consent in the Women's Health Initiative clinical trial and observational study. *Journal of Women's Health, 4*(5), 519–529.

Discusses the challenges associated with obtaining informed consent for this complex clinical trial and observational study.

Prentice, R., Rossouw, J., Johnson, S., Freedman, L., & McTiernan, A. (1995). The role of randomized controlled trials in assessing the benefits and risks of long-term hormone replacement therapy: Example of the Women's Health Initiative. *Menopause: The Journal of the North American Menopause Society, 3*(2), 71–76.

A critical role for randomized controlled clinical trials of adequate size, duration, and quality in HRT research is justified. The HRT component of the Women's Health Initiative Clinical Trial and methods to be used for benefit-versus-risk monitoring and analysis of the trial are described.

Rossouw, J., Finnegan, L., Harlan, W., Pinn, V., Clifford, C., & McGowan, J. (1995). The evolution of the Women's Health Initiative: Perspectives from the NIH. *Journal of the American Medical Women's Association, 50*(2), 50–55.

This article charts the history behind the Women's Health Initiative from the point of view of the NIH scientists who collaborated on its development.

Tinker, L., Burrows, E., Henry, H., Patterson, R., Rupp, J., & Van Hom, L. (1996). The Women's Health Initiative: Overview of the nutrition components. In D. Krummel and P. Krisetherton (Eds.), *Nutrition in women's health* (pp. 510–542). Gaithersburg, MD: Aspen.

An in-depth review of the nutritional interventions being tested in the trial.

Part II

Health Promotion and Maintenance

Chapter 2

Menopause: The Hormonal Replacement Therapy Decision

Donna S. Huddleston

Hormonal replacement therapy (HRT) is the predominant theme in the discussion of women's health during the perimenopause and postmenopause years. Few HRT studies include women in the perimenopause; the time that spans the first sign of menopause until 12 months after the last menses. For the postmenopausal years, clinical HRT drug trials abound and date back to 1935. Estrogen replacement therapy (ERT) rather than HRT was the predominant theme until the middle 1970's. Then studies showed an increase in uterine cancer in women on ERT. Taken together, ERT and progestin are known as HRT. Adding progestin to the therapy prevented unopposed estrogen complications of heavy bleeding, hyperplasia, and cancer of the uterus.

Historically, researchers have often focused on the quality of life or benefits perceived by women versus the risks of HRT. Research studies provide evidence that perimenopausal and postmenopausal women take HRT to improve the quality of their lives (Perlmutter & Iconis, 1995; Skolnick, 1992), but only 15 percent to 33 percent continue the therapy for any length of time due to fear of breast cancer and uncomfortable and annoying side effects. In reviewing the HRT literature, extreme differences of opinion about women taking HRT were found. Considering that quality of life and its relationship to HRT follow a continuum, on one end of the continuum,

Connell and Grody (1995) espoused commitment to HRT that extends to death. Connell and Grody saw the menopause as a hormonal deficiency disease, similar to diabetes. On the other end of the HRT continuum, MacPherson (1993) argued that false promises were given to women over the years about the safe and positive effects of ERT and HRT; these promises were built on the medical ideology of menopause as a disease requiring ERT and HRT intervention. To further complicate matters, women can enter and exit at various points along the continuum. (See Figure 2.1.) Researchers and healthcare providers including physicians also mark their point of reference; as a group researchers and healthcare providers have not reached a consensus that risks outweigh improvement in quality of life.

The major benefits of HRT are total relief from hot flashes and night sweats, commonly called *vasomotor symptoms*. Researchers have reached a consensus that hot flashes and night sweats are the prevalent signs of the menopause experienced by many women. Researchers concur that HRT completely controls hot flashes and night sweats in most women. The emphasis for HRT sales has now shifted to prevention of osteoporosis and protection from heart disease. Another benefit is that HRT improves the turgor and elasticity of estrogen dependent tissue.

**Figure 2.1   A CONTINUUM DEPICTING THE
RELATIONSHIP OF QUALITY OF LIFE TO HRT FOR
PERI- AND POSTMENOPAUSAL WOMEN**

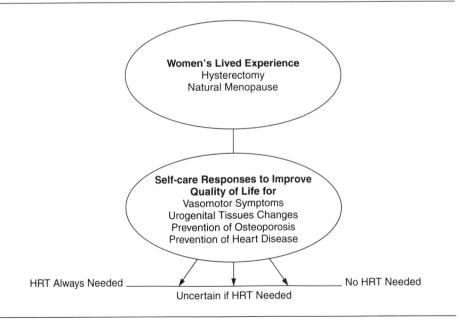

Studies also show that HRT prevents osteoporosis and the subsequent hip and spine fractures. HRT has been shown to slow down the rate of bone loss in the vertebrae (spine), proximal femur (hip), and wrists of women. However, HRT does not result in the replacement of bone loss.

Furthermore, studies have shown that ERT prevents heart disease. Recently, researchers have started to question the effects of HRT on prevention of heart disease (Skolnick, 1992), as progestin was shown to counteract the positive effects of HRT.

HORMONAL REPLACEMENT THERAPY IS BIG BUSINESS

American Home Products Corporation whose Premarin is the world's largest selling estrogen product had annual sales of almost $1 billion for that product alone (Tanouye, 1995). Wyeth Ayerest a major HRT drug company funds a chair for the University of Cleveland that oversees much menopausal research and houses the North American Menopause Society.

Drug companies market HRT directly to women; this year advertising in popular women's magazines offered $5.00 coupons toward prescriptions. This marketing is a change from the drug companies targeting physicians in medical journals. Over the years, the women pictured in these medical advertisements have changed—from a woman in a nightgown with a myriad of symptoms, to a harried housewife bathed in sweat beads trying to keep her husband happy, to a woman carrying a briefcase, to the perimenopausal woman—a much older model than in the 1980s—who is in top physical shape and depicted taking long thoughtful walks with her friends.

Informed Decision

In the United States in the year 2000, an estimated 20 million women will become menopausal. Multifaceted issues surround the decision to take HRT. The first issue is whose decision is it? The woman's or her healthcare provider's? A prescription is required, therefore, women must contact a physician to obtain either ERT or HRT. The woman must also enter a relationship which in the past has focused on the physician's dictates (Skolnick, 1992). A second issue is what reason does a woman have to take HRT—natural menopause symptoms, that is, hot flashes/night sweats or prevention of osteoporosis and/or heart disease. A third issue is whether to take HRT once it is prescribed. For women with hysterectomies who also have their ovaries removed, the hot flashes and night sweats can be severe. One gynecologist stated that if the woman does not want the HRT after a hysterectomy, he waited until the woman had the first hot flash and subsequent sweating. "They never forget their pills or patches again" (Huddleston, 1995, private correspondence). What happens to the women experiencing natural menopause who do not take hormonal therapy (Paier, 1996)? And if women do take HRT, do they need to live in fear of cancer or dread the side effects of the medications: nausea, edema, and continued menses? A fourth issue is other nonhormonal remedies for hot flashes, new medications to prevent osteoporosis, and lifestyle changes to prevent heart disease.

HEALTH PROMOTION AND MAINTENANCE FOR WOMEN: THE PERIMENOPAUSAL/ POSTMENOPAUSAL YEARS

Health promotion and maintenance for women during the perimenopausal and postmenopausal years, with the exception of osteoporosis and heart disease, have not been widely discussed. The lack of studies in health promotion and maintenance contrasts sharply with past research findings. Historically, myriad symptoms have been attributed to menopause. Researchers have found that women's experiences of menopause differ in meaning, culturally (Beyene, 1989; Flint & Garcia, 1979) and medically (McElmurry & Huddleston, 1991; Skolnick, 1992). In addition, HRT research is inexplicably bound to women who have had severe problems with menopause and women who have had hysterectomies.

The predominant theme of HRT prevails in *Healthy People 2000* (U.S. Public Health Service, 1991) objectives, although a significant goal of *Healthy People 2000* was an enhanced quality of life. The only objective for peri- and postmenopausal women was to increase to at least 90 percent the proportion of perimenopausal women who have been counseled about the benefits and risks of estrogen replacement therapy (combined with progestin, when appropriate) for prevention of osteoporosis. (Baseline data available in 1991, p. 118.)

Thus, restated, the question is, "Do perimenopausal women need HRT to improve the quality of their lives?" (See Table 2.1.) A related question is, "Should a perimenopausal woman continue taking HRT for the rest of her life to ensure health promotion and maintenance?"

For health promotion and maintenance during the perimenopause, Huddleston and McElmurry (1994) reported that women's self-care responses followed at least two paths. In one self-care response study, the authors found one group of perimenopausal women ($n = 102$) virtually ignored the passage. A second, smaller group of perimenopausal women

Table 2.1
Self-Care Decision Points for Peri- and
Postmenopausal Women Considering HRT

Women	Risks	Benefits*	Side Effects	Contra-indications
With hysterectomy	Increased risk: Breast cancer. Can take ERT without fear of uterine cancer.	Relief of hot flashes/night sweats. Improved tone and elasticity of the urogenital area. Prevention of osteoporosis. Reduce risk of heart disease—(ERT only).	Nausea & vomiting. Retention of excess fluid. Spotty darkening of the skin, particularly on the face. Breast tenderness or enlargement.	Breast cancer—self/family. Abnormal blood clotting. History of heart or circulation problems.
With natural menopause	Increased risk: Breast cancer. Need to take progestin with ERT to prevent uterine cancer.	Relief of hot flashes/Night sweats. Improved tone and elasticity of the urogenital area. Prevention of osteoporosis. Reduce risk of heart disease—(ERT only).	Nausea & vomiting. Retention of excess fluid. Spotty darkening of the skin, particularly on the face. Breast tenderness or enlargement. Enlargement of benign tumors of the uterus. Continued monthly menses, spotting, or breakthrough bleeding.	Pregnancy Breast cancer—self/family. Abnormal blood clotting. History of heart or circulation problems.

* *Physician's Desk Reference*, (1995). Nervous symptoms, depression—no evidence exists that estrogens are effective for such symptoms nor will ERT keep skin soft and supple for long periods (years) after the menopause or keep women feeling young.

($n = 41$) in the same study increased the number and frequency of their self-care responses in many areas of their lives as menopausal changes occurred.

REFERENCES

Beyene, Y. (1989). *From menarche to menopause: Reproductive lives of peasant women in two cultures.* Albany, NY: State University of New York Press.

Connell, E. B., & Grody, M. H. (1995). Estrogen: Major factor in pelvic reconstructive and urogynecologic surgery. In G. Gavert & S. Finn (Ed.), *Benign postreproductive gynecologic surgery* (pp. 1–32). New York: McGraw-Hill.

Flint, M. P., & Garcia, M. (1979). Culture and the climacteric. *Journal of Biosocial Science, 6*(Suppl.), 197–215.

Huddleston, D. S. (1995). Women & HIV/AIDS. In B. J. McElmurry & R. S. Parker (Eds.), *Annual review of women's health* (Vol. 2, pp. 221–239). New York: NLN Press.

Huddleston, D. S., & McElmurry, B. J. (1994a). Determinants of self-care responses of perimenopausal women. In D. Gilbert (Ed.), *Mind-body rhythmicity: A menstrual cycle perspective.* Seattle, WA: Hamilton & Cross.

Huddleston, D. S., & McElmurry, B. J. (1994b). Measuring vaginal tissue changes of the perimenopause. In D. Gilbert (Ed.), *Mind-body rhythmicity: A menstrual cycle perspective.* Seattle, WA: Hamilton & Cross.

MacPherson, K. I. (1993). The false promises of hormone replacement therapy and current dilemmas. In J. C. Callahan (Ed.), *Menopause: A midlife passage* (pp. 145–159). Bloomington: Indiana University Press.

McElmurry, B. J. (1993). Introduction. In B. J. McElmurry & R. S. Parker (Eds.), *Annual review of women's health.* New York: NLN Press.

McElmurry, B. J., & Huddleston, D. H. (1991). Self-care and menopause: Critical review of research. *Health Care International, 12*(1), 15–26.

Outreach. (1993, Fall). Bethesda, MD: National Institute of Health, Office of Information of the National Institute of Nursing, Research.

Paier, G. S. (1996). Specter of the crone: The experience of vertebral fracture. *Advances in Nursing Sciences, 18*(3), 27–36.

Perlmutter, C., & Iconis, R. (1995). Women's health. Do women doctors take estrogen? *Prevention, 47*(4), 65–75.

Skolnick, A. A. (1992). At third meeting, menopause expo makes the most of insufficient data. *Journal of the American Medical Association, 268*(18), 2483–2486.

Tanouye, E. (1995, June 15). Delicate balance. Estrogen study shifts ground for women—and for drug firms. *The Wall Street Journal,* pp. 1–2.

U.S. Public Health Service. (1991). *Healthy People 2000 National Promotion of Disease Prevention Objectives. Full report, with commentary.* Washington, DC: U.S. Department of Health and Human Services, Public Health Service.

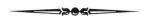

REVIEW OF THE LITERATURE

The literature was reviewed from a woman's health framework (Huddleston, 1995; McElmurry, 1993; McElmurry & Huddleston, 1994) and women's lived experiences of menopause rather than biological models of menopause when possible. In reviewing articles and studies, the major decision points were as follows: framework/theory, questions asked, methods, informed consent, tools used to collect data and measure, analysis appropriate to data, generalizable findings, and whether the information was useful to the healthcare provider in making a decision and/or to a woman making a self-care decision to take HRT.

The menopausal and HRT literature were reviewed from January 1994 to March 1996. Older literature was abstracted for background information. Several databases were used including CINAHL and Medline. In addition, general periodicals were reviewed from January 1995 to March 1996. Also, on-line publications were perused through Internet connections. Examples of on-going conversations about the menopause were found on America On Line in "Power Surge" and in *Woman's Day* magazine.

Connell, E. B., & Grody, M. H. (1995). Estrogen: Major factor in pelvic reconstructive and urogynecologic surgery. In G. Gavert & S. Finn (Eds.) *Benign postreproductive gynecologic surgery* (pp. 1–32). New York: McGraw-Hill.

The introduction to this gynecologic surgery text described the effects of estrogen on tissue. The authors from Temple University Hospital (TUH) saw menopause as an estrogen deficiency disease. In fact, the author required women to make a life time commitment postoperatively. This introductory chapter is one of the strongest statements for use of estrogen, from estrogen priming postoperatively to life time estrogen commitment. The authors also gave a strong argument for giving estrogen to women with cancer of the breast, thrombosis, and even uterine cancer. It should be noted that this introductory chapter was selected for review both for its 253 references and to demonstrate the complete medicalization of menopause and the total acceptance of the estrogen deficiency theory.

Knight, D. C., & Eden, J. A. (1995). Phytoestrogens—a short review. *Maturitas, 22,* 167–175.

This article provided a synopsis of the literature of phytoestrogens related to aging. Phytoestrogens are plant estrogens, found in cereals, vegetables, and medicinal plants. Soy flour and other soy products are high in biologically active isoflavines, a class of phytoestrogens. The author contends that phytoestrogens are at least part of the reason why vegetarians and Asian populations have a low incidence of menopausal symptoms and a low rate of cancer and heart disease.

LeBouef, F. J., & Carter, S. G. (1996). Discomforts of the perimenopause. *Journal of Obstetrics, Gynecology & Neonatal Nursing, 25*(2), 173–180.

For this article, the author used a self-help framework for promotion of comfort and a healthy lifestyle for women with perimenopausal discomforts. These include Speroff's (1994) four categories of symptoms, (1) disturbances in menstrual patterns, (2) vasomotor instability, (3) atrophic conditions, and (4) psychologic symptoms. A bleak picture is painted that virtually all women, within 4 to 5 years of cessation of menses, will experience urogenital atrophy. (Huddleston & McElmurry, 1994b, using a Vaginal Tissue Changes Index did not find this on inspection of several hundred women ages 45 to 85. Only in the women over 80 who were not sexually active was atrophy present.) A Self-Help Measures table is reprinted from Adams (1986), *Health Education for women: A guide for nurses and other health professionals*, pp. 336–337, Norwalk, CT: Appleton-Centruy-Crofts. There is also a useful table on cyclic and continuous HRT regimens.

Loprinzi, C. L., Michalak, J. C., Quella, S. K., O'Fallon, J. R., Hatfield, A. K., Nelimark, R. A., Dose, A. M., Fischer, T., Johnson, C., Klatt, N. E., Bate, W. W., Rospond, R. M., & Osterling, J. E. (1994). Megestrol acetate for the prevention of hot flashes. *New England Journal of Medicine, 331*(6), 347–352.

This study was a clinical trial for megestrol acetate, a progestational agent. The researchers wanted to know if megestrol acetate decreased the number and severity of hot flashes in both men and women. Although treatment with estrogens in women and androgens in men eliminates hot flashes altogether,

estrogen is contraindicated in women with breast cancer. Medical researchers have suggested that estrogen treatment combined with tamoxifen is a rational approach for women, although this treatment regimen is not widely accepted. Clonidine, methyldopa, and belladonna alkaloid studies have not proven to be effective in treating menopausal hot flashes. For this study, 97 women with a history of breast cancer and 66 men with prostate cancer with bothersome hot flashes participated in a double-blind study. Bothersome hot flashes were defined as at least one month duration, occurred at least seven times per week and were sufficiently severe that the patient desired therapeutic intervention. Informed consent was obtained. The participants were randomly assigned to group 1 or 2. Menopausal status and history of hysterectomy were not addressed. The antiestrogen agent, tamoxifen, 20 mg. per day was permitted. Nonparametric tests (Wilcoxon rank-sum, chi-square, and fisher's exact tests) were used. All P values were two-tailed. After 4 weeks, hot flashes were reduced by 85 percent in the group receiving megestrol acetate ($p < 0.001$). A side effect for women in this study was withdrawal menstrual bleeding, generally occurring one to two weeks after megestrol acetate had been discontinued.

Moore, A. A. (1996). A nurse's guide to hormone replacement therapy. *Journal of Obstetrics, Gynecology & Neonatal Nursing, 25*(1), 24–31.

Although the accompanying abstract stated that menopause is a natural event, the article is written from within a medical framework. A serious drawback to this article is the symptoms reported for groups of women by age. This list of symptoms by age is not supported by interviews or research studies. The article does have some useful tables about different preparations of HRT. The authors felt that evidence was compiling that indicated the benefits of HRT may outweigh concerns. A variety of symptoms throughout the perimenopausal transition were seen as treatable, i.e., vasomotor, urogenital, and emotional changes as well as sleep disturbances. The authors also pointed out that during peri-menopause a woman has contraceptive needs until both serum FSH and LH are elevated. When should a woman switch from low-dose birth control pills to HRT? The lowest dosage contraceptive is four times greater than needed for HRT. Based on a review of the literature, the authors recommend a FSH level of 30 mIU/ml (30.0 IU/L) or greater before initiating HRT. *Note:* Luteinizing Hormone (LH) stimulates the development of the corpus luteum in the ovary and together with FSH regulates the secretion of progesterone. Follicle-stimulating hormone (FSH) stimulates the growth of the Graafian follicles in the ovary. Both LH and FSH are in an estrogen feedback loop in pre-menopausal women.

Paier, G. S. (1996). Specter of the crone: The experience of vertebral fracture. *Advances in Nursing Sciences, 18*(3), 27–36.

The purpose of this study was to describe the meaning of the experience of five women living with spinal fractures secondary to post-menopausal osteoporosis. One woman was re-cruited from a southwestern city, and the other four were from a retirement community in the northeastern United States, informed consent was obtained. The women participants ages 58 to 86 were interviewed and audiotaped during a 60- to 90-minute interview. Broad data generat-ing questions with multiple probes were used to explore the experience and circumstances of the fracture including thoughts and feelings re-membered. Data were analyzed following Co-laizzi's eight-step procedure for data analysis and interpretation; 484 significant statements were extracted. Five major theme categories were (1) grappling with the forces of pain, (2) self-taught resilience, (3) specter of the crone, (4) vulnerability, and (5) contingent hope. Con-stant pain, loss of independent function, change in physical appearance, feelings of isola-tion, sense of vulnerability, and an uncertain future, suggest that nursing interventions for

postmenopausal osteoporosis need to have a broader definition.

Skolnick, A. A. (1992). At third meeting, menopause expo makes the most of insuffi-cient data. *Journal of the American Medical Association, 268*(18), 2483–2486.

The North American Menopause Society met and discussed the lack of conclusive data for HRT. No true consensus was found among the attendees about the protection from heart disease after reviewing the results of a nation-wide study of 140,000 women 50 years of age or older. W. Utian, chair of the Department of Reproductive Biology at Case Western Reserve University, pointed out that we do not have any prospective studies. The relative risk of breast cancer was higher with ERT at 30 per-cent to 40 percent increased risk. The author pointed out that the estrogen dosage was higher in previous years. The consensus was that breast cancer patients were at great risk for secondary breast cancer. From the confer-ence came a comment that U.S. Representative Pat Schroeder made to *Newsweek* (May 25, 1992, p. 71) that, "If you get six menopausal women together, you'll find that their doctors are doing six different things. Our joke is that you might as well go to a veterinarian." Al-though the researchers at the conference con-curred that variation in treatment may reflect differences in patients as well as differences in medical opinions; the researchers favored the premise that the women would be more differ-ent than the physicians. The suggestion for women was to have a reassessment on a regular basis, perhaps annually. Osteoporosis leads to debility and life threatening bone fractures. The two main problems identified were (1) pa-tients discontinue therapy and (2) physician's try to dictate to women and fail to identify individual needs and concerns and do not adequately discuss treatment options. Another drawback to this conference was that re-searchers extrapolated findings about estro-gen's effect on monkeys and rats to women.

U.S. Public Health Service. (1991). *Healthy People 2000 National Promotion of Disease Prevention Objectives. Full report, with commentary.* Washington, DC: U.S. Department of Health and Human Services, Public Health Service.

This article summarizes Healthy People 2000 objectives for perimenopausal women. Osteoporosis affects 50 percent of women over age 45 and 90 percent of women over age 75. Of these women, over half will have fractures related to osteoporosis. Currently there are 1.3 million bone fractures per year in the United States. Of these fractures, the proximal femur, or hip fracture, numbers around 250,000. These fractures are associated with a 12 percent to 20 percent greater risk of dying within the following year than otherwise expected. One out of three women will experience a hip fracture by age 90. The total cost in 1986, for osteoporosis and associated fractures was estimated at $7 to $10 billion. The costs are estimated to increase as the population ages. As ERT slows bone loss, Healthy People 2000 authors recommend ERT be initiated as soon after menopause as possible and maintained for 5 to 10 years as it is the most effective intervention for postmenopausal osteoporosis. In addition, ERT was also recommended for its other uses, i.e., hot flashes, vaginal discomfort, vaginal and urinary infections, and perhaps anxiety and depression. Also, ERT was recommended to reduce cardiovascular mortality in postmenopausal women—after balancing the risk, i.e., endometrial hyperplasia, carcinoma, and abnormal vaginal bleeding. Bone mass measurements were recommended to provide useful information but mass screening of women was seen as not warranted. Risk factors for osteoporosis include women who have had their ovaries removed prior to menopause, take corticosteroid medication chronically, require extreme immobility, history of anorexia nervosa or chronic amenorrhea, and are postmenopausal with a history of osteoporosis. Other factors include thinness, white ethnicity, alcohol consumption, and cigarette smoking. Exercise, dietary calcium, fluoride, and vitamin D were other modes of therapy for retarding or preventing bone loss.

Wardell, D. W., & Engebretson, J. C. (1995). Women's anticipations of hormonal replacement therapy. *Maturitas, 22,* 177–183.

This focused ethnographic study conducted at the University of Texas interviewed 12 women individually and 40 women in a group setting to expand the understanding of women's anticipation of perimenopausal use of HRT. The perimenopausal middle class Caucasian women ranged in age from 40 to 53. All had been taking HRT for no more than 6 months. The typologies of anticipation follow: (1) Trusting in nature, (2) Skeptical experimentation, (3) Fixing (damage done by menopause), (4) Restabilizing (return to "normal"), (5) Life enhancing (fear of crippling disease), and (6) trusting in science. Two of the six anticipations directly challenged assumptions of the medical model, and four were congruent with it.

Pertinent Lay Literature

Study shows acupuncture mitigates hot flashes. (1995). *Menopause News, 5*(3), 2–3. This article gave a synopsis of a Swedish study that showed acupuncture mitigates hot flashes. The study was small, $n = 21$, ages 47 to 62. Both classical acupuncture and superficial needle insertion decreased the frequency of hot flashes by 50 percent. But the group that had classical acupuncture showed a significant decrease that continued three months after treatment was stopped.

MacPherson, K. I. (1993). The false promises of hormone replacement therapy and current dilemmas. In J. C. Callahan (Ed.), *Menopause: A midlife passage* (pp. 145–159). Bloomington: Indiana University Press.

MacPherson described three false promises made to women by biomedical researchers, physicians, and mass media about the benefits of HRT. These promises were (1) eternal beauty and femininity (1966–1975), (2) safe, symptom-free menopause (1975–1981), and (3) escape from chronic diseases (1980–present). MacPherson's premise is that menopause is a natural event rather than the medical ideology of menopause as a disease requiring hormonal intervention. The current dominant medical trend is to link osteoporosis and heart disease to menopause. Careful scrutiny should be made of the promise of HRT for osteoporosis prevention and heart disease. An ethical issue is raised by asking is it appropriate to give a potentially dangerous drug to 75 percent of women who never will have osteoporosis. One dilemma was whether women with an intact uterus should risk endometrial cancer and take estrogen to reduce their risk of cardiovascular disease. Other dilemmas to taking HRT were discussed: uterine cancer, breast cancer, HRT versus ERT, and duration of treatment from the start of menopause until death.

Molvig, D. (1995). 41 ways to cope with menopause naturally. *Natural Health, 25*(3) 88–93.

This article provides an overview of the current thinking in HRT to help a woman decide if HRT is right for her. The author discusses HRT as a treatment with a past, personal choices, and homeopathy and herbs. A table of natural products and therapies is included.

Homeopathy. (1995). *Menopause News, 5*(5), 1–2.

Homeopathic remedies for menopause are based on the assumption that the disease symptoms are the body's attempts to cure itself. Much like traditional allopathic medicine, homeopathy views menopause as a disease to be cured and provides over-the-counter and homeopathic medicinal remedies for menopausal symptoms.

Estrogen replacement therapy: Is it right for you? (1995). *Mayo Clinic Health Letter, 2*, 4–5.

This two-page article covers benefits now and later, the health benefits with type of supplement, i.e., pill, patch, or cream, when ERT

is not the best choice, the alternatives—other medications and lifestyle changes. Women are advised to ask the following questions and talk with a physician:

1. Do menopause symptoms disrupt my life?
2. Am I at increased risk for osteoporosis or cardiovascular disease?
3. Is my risk for breast cancer relatively low?
4. Am I free of liver disease, gallstones, high blood pressure, or any other health problems that estrogen may aggravate?
5. Does estrogen offer more acceptable benefits than the alternatives?

If a woman answers "yes" to all five questions, ERT is recommended. The therapy begins at menopause and continues indefinitely.

Perlmutter, C., & Iconis, R. (1995). Women's health. Do women doctors take estrogen? *Prevention, 47*(4), 65–75.

How do women physicians decide for or against hormone replacement for themselves? The authors reported that they talked to dozens of women doctors and chose 8 of them to write about for this article. Most of the physicians that the authors interviewed who chose to take HRT had undergone hysterectomies. The most important factor in deciding for or against HRT was quality of life. Quality of life was defined as "Will HRT improve my life right now?" The personal interviews with the physicians run the gamut from never taking HRT to always taking it.

Savard, M. (1995). Your health. Should you take hormones? *Woman's Day, 9*, 34.

Dr. Savard is the Director of the Center for Women's Health at the Medical College of Pennsylvania. In this short article, Dr. Savard stated that the question she hears most often about HRT is, "Will it cause breast cancer?" As a woman she shares these fears. The Harvard Nurses' Health Study which followed 121,700 women found that long-term ERT use, 5 years or longer postmenopause, increases a woman's risk of breast cancer by 30 percent and HRT by 40 percent. To maintain heart disease and osteoporosis prevention benefits, the woman must keep taking the drug for life. Making a decision is based on steps. The first step is to become fully informed about your own individual risks, including family and personal history of breast cancer, heart disease, and osteoporosis. The second step is to determine if you have menopause symptoms. The third step is to seek the advice of a physician for long-term HRT use.

Tanouye, E. (1995, June 15). Delicate balance. Estrogen study shifts ground for women—and for drug firms. *The Wall Street Journal*, pp. 1–2.

This article detailed the battle of drug companies over the selling and developing of osteoporosis medicines with the new Harvard research linking long-term estrogen use to a higher risk of breast cancer. Merck has a new nonhormonal drug Fosomax that is effective against osteoporosis.

Tanouye, E. (1995, August 2). Health. New pill may offer safer alternative to estrogen-replacement therapies. *The Wall Street Journal*, pp. 1–2.

In this article, the new antiestrogen drugs are discussed. Initial tests suggested that these drugs, one is Tamoxifen, may prevent osteoporosis, heart disease, breast cancer, and in some cases uterine cancer. The drugs mimic estrogen in some organs, such as the liver and bones, while blocking cancer-promoting effects in other tissues.

IMPLICATIONS FOR EDUCATION, PRACTICE, RESEARCH, AND HEALTH POLICY

A standard of care cannot be adopted for education, practice, or health policy until a strong research agenda for menopause is initiated. Lack of research-backed information cannot be the basis for treating more than 20 million perimenopausal women with HRT. On the continuum for quality of life and its relationship to HRT, most women do not belong at either end of the continuum. Thus, for most women, they must weigh the quality of life versus their individual risks in making the self-care decision to take HRT. As it stands right now, there are clearly areas of uncertainty about HRT; what it is for, when to take it, and for how long.

In 1993, the National Institute of Health (NIH) proposed a research agenda for the menopause. This is an excellent agenda that was formed during a NIH Menopause Workshop chaired by Nancy Woods and Wulf Utian. In addition, Woods and Utian proposed long-term studies on large populations of women, such as the Women's Health Initiative. Such studies would include a strong menopause agenda in addition to HRT or osteoporosis topics. It would behoove drug companies and NIH to participate in the funding of this agenda. The NIH agenda is summarized below:

1. Distinguish menopause signs from other mid-life changes.
   a. Natural menopause.
   b. Surgical menopause (hysterectomy).
2. Design studies to collect data:
   a. About menopause in specific racial (including African-American women), ethnic, age, and socioeconomic groups where there is a (complete) lack of data.
   b. About culture and lifestyle that may affect menopause.
3. Change perception of menopause as a medical event to a normal life transition.
4. Adopt standards of care for how women can manage menopause.
   a. Symptom control.
   b. Enhance well-being.
   c. Reduce risk of osteoporosis.
5. Decrease women's dilemma in making decisions in conditions of uncertainty.

a. Benefits and risk of HRT.

b. Which hormones to take and in what dosages.

c. Why do women who are prescribed estrogen leave their prescriptions unfilled?

d. The decision-making process: How do women deal with the pros and cons of various approaches to the menopause?

6. Initiate educational programs for women where women can approach healthcare providers as active partners in making decisions.

7. Explore alternative therapies to HRT.

a. Exercise.

b. Behavioral techniques like stress management and participation in support groups.

c. Herbs and other potential sources of estrogen-like substances.

Part III

Women as Providers of Healthcare

Chapter 3

Violence Against Healthcare Workers

Carol J. Collins

As evidenced by recent reports in the media, violent incidents in healthcare settings are more prevalent than once thought and may be on the increase. Attacks both verbal and physical have occurred among staff and clients, staff and family members, and colleagues working in healthcare settings. Healthcare workers are at considerable risk of patient assault, for example, in mental health units and facilities (Poster & Ryan, 1989). To some extent, these incidents of violence can be attributed to increased violence in the general population, the widespread use of drugs, and the seemingly blurred boundaries between mental illness and criminal behavior. This chapter reviews current literature about factors that contribute to violence against healthcare workers and the physical, emotional, and psychological toll that such attacks take on workers.

While some research has been done to identify factors that trigger the violent-prone patient to assault another individual, many questions remain unanswered. Of particular interest is the effects of such assaults on patient caregivers. However, the personal and professional toll often is unacknowledged. One consequence is that healthcare workers abandon direct patient care for safer areas of clinical practice.

RESEARCH ON ATTACKS DIRECTED TOWARD HEALTHCARE PROVIDERS: SIGNIFICANT CONCEPTS

An incident of psychiatric patient assault was first documented in 1849 with the fatal attack on a psychiatrist by a mentally ill patient (Bernstein, 1981). The problem has been examined from a variety of perspectives that include exploring methods of predicting impending patient violence, examining effective aggression management strategies, noting structural changes that effect the physical safety of the healthcare setting, investigating the inter- and intrarelationships between patients and staff that potentially precipitate violence, assessing caregiver responses to violence-prone patients, and assessing the effectiveness of training and educational programs designed to promote safer management of aggressive patients.

Similar to other issues involving women's experiences the full extent and impact of assault by healthcare recipients on their caregivers has never been fully explored. Lanza (1983) reported that to examine the problem from the staff's perspective and from the recipients' perspectives is somehow detrimental to the patient. The pervasiveness of these attitudes may further complicate investigations of patient assault on healthcare workers. Professional nurses, in particular, practice under prevailing norms that the nurse is to provide care to the patient and that the nurse's needs are secondary to those of the patient, including the need for personal safety (Lanza, 1984).

The professional dilemma created by such attitudes is reflected in two recent publications. Illinois Nursing Association (INA) staff (INA meets with DMHDD director, 1993) and Cassetta (1993) posed conflicting points of view on the implications of managing violence with regard to staff safety in healthcare settings. The controversy centered around the use of physical and chemical restraints to subdue violence-prone behaviors in patients. INA staff supported the use of physical and chemical restraints to manage aggressive behavior. In contrast, the Cassetta (1993) article criticized the use of chemical and physical restraints to control aggressive behavior. Cassetta argued that nursing staff often used chemical and physical restraints in lieu of other more therapeutic verbal and behavioral interventions.

To more fully understand the impact of verbal and physical aggression on healthcare workers, it is helpful to review several concepts relating to victimization as a human experience such as vulnerability to human-induced events, responses to victimization, coping with victimization, and the victimization of women.

VICTIMIZATION

The theoretical underpinnings of victimization were examined extensively by sociologists and psychologists during the late 1960s through the mid-1980s. Janoff-Bulman and Frieze (1983) based their theoretical perspective on some of the earlier work of Lerner (1963) and others (Lerner & Lichtman, 1968; Lerner & Matthews, 1967; Lerner & Simmons, 1966; Wills, 1981) and noted that dimensions of the victimizing event varied and included both human-induced and naturally induced events. Victim responses to human-induced events often focused on the study of a particular type of victim, such as those who were criminally victimized (Wertz, 1983). Explorations of perceptions of vulnerability to victimization were conducted by Perloff (1983); victim responses to domestic violence were investigated by Campbell (1986a); survivors of childhood abuse victims were studied by Burgess, Hartman, and McCormack (1987), and women survivors of political torture were studied by Allodi and Stiasny (1985) and by Fornazzari and Freire (1990).

While each of these categories of individuals may have had a unique experience, there were common psychological sequelae shared across the population of victims. Blame placement and symptoms of post-traumatic stress were common responses experienced by victims whether the individual was a victim of spousal abuse (Walker, 1979), criminal assault (Wertz, 1983), or a patient attack (Caldwell, 1992).

Blaming the Victim

Lanza (1983), a predominant nurse investigator, conducted a series of studies in a Veterans' Administration Hospital designed to determine the nature of blame-placement along with the emotional, cognitive, social, and biophysiological reactions of nursing staff to physical assaults by patients. Attribution theory (Heider, 1958; Wortman, 1976) was the theoretical foundation for Lanza's (1984) work and suggests that individuals perceived events in unique ways based on needs, wishes, personalities, and environmental factors. She concluded that nurses were likely to assume that the nurse was to blame if a patient physically attacked him or her (Lanza, 1984). To test this notion, Lanza (1985, 1986, 1987, 1988, 1992) and Lanza, Milner, and Riley (1988) used three vignettes describing patient aggression (mild, severe, and control) to elicit nurses' reactions to victimization.

Lanza (1992) concluded that female victims received a higher degree of blame for the assault than did male victims. Victims who received less severe injuries were attributed higher levels of blame for the attack than those receiving more serious injuries. The mild assault situation was the only one in which gender did not play a role. An interesting finding surfaced in Lanza's 1984 study indicating that an individual assaulted by a patient in the past was less likely to blame another staff victim than a person who has never been assaulted.

Personal Assumptions of Vulnerability

Janoff-Bulman and Frieze examined victimization from the perspective of personal assumptions of vulnerability. These investigators noted that victims must not only deal with physical injury resulting from their experience but with tremendous psychological upheavals when basic assumptions are shattered. For example:

1. Belief in personal invulnerability ("it can't happen to me").
2. Perception of the world as meaningful and comprehensible.
3. View of self in a positive light.

Victimization does not make sense to victims who feel they are good and reasonably cautious people (Scheppele & Bart, 1983; Silver & Wortman, 1980). Victims may focus not on the question of why the event happened, but why the event happened to them (Janoff-Bulman & Frieze, 1983). If victims view themselves as decent individuals who do not take inordinate risks, they may be unable to explain what happened.

The trauma of victimization may also generate negative self-images (Horowitz, Wilner, Marmar, & Krupnick, 1980). Victims may perceive themselves as powerless and helpless against forces beyond their control (Peterson & Seligman, 1983). The fact that an individual has been "singled out" for misfortune, may lead to the belief on the victims part that they are different from others (Janoff-Bulman & Frieze, 1983).

Coping with Victimization

Coping with victimization entails rebuilding the assumptions that enabled the victim to function effectively. The state of disequilibrium following victimization is characterized by intense stress and anxiety and necessitates the re-establishment of a conceptual system that will allow the individual to function effectively again (Janoff-Bulman & Frieze, 1983). A valid way to redefine one's conceptual system is to incorporate the experience of victimization into a new model of reality (Horowitz et al., 1980). Researchers have explored methods victims use to redefine the victimizing event. One method is to minimize the event. This approach allows one's basic assumptions about the world to remain intact (Janoff-Bulman & Frieze, 1983). Taylor, Wood, and Lichtman (1983) discuss cognitive mechanisms designed to evaluate the event in terms of comparing it to those less fortunate or on the basis of a favorable attribute, creating hypothetically worse worlds, construing benefit from the experience, and developing normative standards of adjustment. All these strategies are designed to minimize the individual's perception of him- or herself as a victim.

An important aspect of coping with a victimizing experience is to attempt to make sense of the experience by searching for meaning in the experience (Bulman & Wortman, 1977; Silver & Wortman, 1980). In a study of incest victims by Silver, Boon, and Stones (1983), women who were able to make sense of their experience were less psychologically distressed than those unable to make sense of the experience. Following victimization, Janoff-Bulman and Frieze (1983) and Wortman (1976) found that self-blame can be functional, particularly if it is related to the individual's behavior rather than to the victim's personality. Behavioral self-blame enables the victim to believe that future events can be avoided if certain behaviors are changed (Janoff-Bulman & Frieze, 1983; Wortman, 1976). Conversely, self-blame attributed to a victim's personality trait can be associated with depression and a sense of helplessness (Janoff-Bulman & Frieze, 1983; Peterson & Seligman, 1983).

Victimization of Women

Since women make up approximately 80 percent of the workforce in healthcare and other health service industries (Worthington, 1994), no discussion of patient aggression directed toward healthcare workers would be complete without examining the literature concerning violence perpetrated toward women. Battered women's responses to abuse were examined from a women's health perspective in a series of descriptive studies by Campbell (1981, 1986a, 1986b, 1989) and by Campbell and Alford (1989). In Campbell's (1981) initial work, she examined the misogyny and homicide of women and concluded that everything that shapes the characteristics of women—biology, identification with the mother figure, promotion of empathy, emphasis on nurturance, ability to express positive emotions, and societal prescriptions of nonaggression—contribute to making women nonviolent except when "backed up against the wall" (p. 83). In follow-up citations, Campbell (1986b) described the benefits of survivor groups for battered women and designed the *Danger Assessment* tool to facilitate nurses' assessments of the potential for homicide by battered women directed toward their batterers and to assess male batterers as perpetrators of assault in intimate relationships (Campbell, 1986a).

The nature of nurse abuse from the context of a family violence model was addressed in an editorial by Chinn (1986) and in a descriptive study by Roberts (1991). Chinn (1986) noted that "just as family violence is 'privatized,' violence in the personal and work lives of nurses is silenced and denied" (p. ix). Roberts (1991) found that nurses tend to underreport incidents of abuse, feel blame for the incident, and receive little support from colleagues. Minimizing, denying, and forgetting the event were strategies nurses used to cope with the event. These behaviors paralleled women's ways of dealing with abuse in their personal lives (Roberts, 1991).

VIOLENCE IN THE WORKPLACE

A consideration of patient violence as a workplace hazard did not surface in the literature until 1987. In a survey of professional nurses conducted by *Nursing Times* (Vox Pop, 1987), it was concluded that at least one half of the subscribers believed that employing organizations had not taken measures to prevent violent acts toward nurses. Nurses recommended education designed to improve communication skills, to avoid potentially violent situations, and to teach self-defense skills (Vox Pop, 1987). Poster and Ryan (1989, 1994) were the first investigators to conduct a study of patient violence as a workplace hazard. Several gender issues emerged that are of particular interest. Male staff were more likely to believe that assaults were part of the job; that assaulted staff had characteristics that made them particularly vulnerable to attack; and that legal sanctions against assaultive patients might jeopardize their jobs more than female staff (Poster & Ryan, 1994). The study highlighted a nationwide concern for safety in the workplace among nursing staff (Poster & Ryan, 1994).

In a landmark study, Cox (1991a, 1991b) conducted a survey designed to investigate the effects of verbal abuse on nursing staff and to link the effects of verbal abuse on healthcare workers to those of oppressed group behavior. She defined verbal abuse as "any communication a nurse perceives to be a harsh condemnatory attack upon himself or herself, professionally or personally" (Cox, 1991a). Cox developed a questionnaire designed to identify the frequency, sources, nature of impact, and possible solutions for verbal abuse. Cox (1991a) suggested that nurse managers and administrators must re-evaluate management styles in terms of oppressed group behavior. Often what managers and administrators thought they were saying to nurses was not perceived in the same way by nurses. In her companion article dealing with verbal abuse between licensed and nonlicensed healthcare workers, Cox (1991b) found that respondents viewed verbal abuse as a coping mechanism often used by hospital staff following stressful situations. Not only do healthcare workers experience the threat of verbal and physical attack from their patients, patients' friends, and family members; but, from each other as well.

IMPLICATIONS AND RECOMMENDATIONS

While research has focused on predicting which patients are prone to act out aggressively, some studies suggest that aggressive attacks are unpredictable (Black et al., 1994). Placing blame on the victim can establish a false sense of security by creating a denial of the severity of problems experienced by healthcare workers and institutions (Lanza, 1992). Of far greater concern is the personal and professional costs of violence on providers of healthcare, particularly nurses. More indepth research is needed to examine the impact of patient violence on healthcare workers.

Greater attention is being drawn to the sequelae of patient violence and several recommendations have been proposed. Employee Assistance Programs (EAP) designed to meet the needs of employees in healthcare institutions have not been used by a sample of assaulted staff (Collins, 1996). Carmel and Hunter (1989) and Jones (1985) recommended more comprehensive documentation of patient-staff incidents. Such documentation should accurately define the scope of the problem and identify verbal and defensive techniques designed to defuse aggressive behavior. Roberts (1991) recommended debriefing sessions for all victimized staff and the development of peer support programs to assist staff dealing with the consequences of violence. Caldwell (1992) noted that debriefing sessions were rare and often focused on what the staff member had done wrong during the incident.

Caldwell (1992) recommended the development of programs designed to address symptoms of post-traumatic stress similar to the *Assaulted Staff Action Program* (ASAP) described in a study by Flannery, Fulton, Tausch, and DeLoffi (1991) and the *Staff Assistance for Employees* (SAFE), a program developed at the Mendota Mental Health Institute in Madison, Wisconsin (Caldwell, 1992). Murray and Snyder (1991) described the implementation of a *Nursing Consultation Service* (NCS) composed of qualified psychiatric staff nurses who had an interest in working on such a team and were recruited from each shift. A team member was designated to respond to any assault on their shift anywhere in the hospital. The victimized staff member is seen for counseling anywhere from one to four times. Consultation services were also made available to the unit housing the violent patient regarding resources and interventions (Murray & Snyder, 1991).

Finally, Morrison (1994) notes that personal attacks can occur even within programs designed to minimize aggressive behaviors. She suggests that "new interventions which take into account the social interactive nature of violence are needed to prevent aggression and violence and to limit the escalation process once aggression is initiated" (Morrison, 1994, p. 251). In a follow-up article, Harris and Morrison (1995) caution readers that norms against violence must be established in society as well as in healthcare facilities. The best strategy is to prevent violence from occurring in the first place.

REFERENCES

Allodi, F., & Stiasny, S. (1990). Women as torture victims. *Canadian Journal of Psychiatry, 35*(2), 144–148.

Bernstein, H. A. (1981). Survey of threats and assaults directed toward psychotherapists. *American Journal of Psychotherapy, 35*(4), 542–549.

Black, K. J., Compton, W. M., Wetzel, M., Minchin, S., Farber, N. B., & Rastogi-Cruz, D. (1994). Assaults by patients on psychiatric residents at three training sites. *Hospital and Community Psychiatry, 45*(7), 706–710.

Blair, D. T. (1991). Assaultive behavior: Does provocation begin in the front office? *Journal of Psychosocial Nursing, 29*(5), 21–26.

Braun, K., Christle, D., Walker, D., & Tiwanak, G. (1991). Verbal abuse of nurses and non-nurses. *Nursing Management, 22*(3), 72–76.

Briles, J. (1994). *The Briles report on women in healthcare: Changing conflict to collaboration in a toxic workplace.* San Francisco, CA: Jossey-Bass.

Bulman, R. J., & Wortman, C. B. (1977). Attributions of blame and coping in the "real world": Severe accident victims react to their lot. *Journal of Personality and Social Psychology, 35*(5), 351–363.

Burgess, A. W., Burgess, A. G., & Douglas, J. E. (1994). Examining violence in the workplace. *Journal of Psychosocial Nursing, 32*(7), 11–18, 53.

Burgess, A. W., Hartman, C. R., & McCormack, A. (1987). Abused to abuser: Antecedents of socially deviant behaviors. *American Journal of Psychiatry, 144*(11), 1431–1436.

Caldwell, M. F. (1992). Incidence of PTSD among staff victims. *Hospital and Community Psychiatry, 43*(8), 838–839.

Campbell, J. C. (1981). Misogyny and homicide of women. *Advances in Nursing Science, 3*(2), 67–85.

Campbell, J. C. (1986a). Nursing assessment for risk of homicide with battered women. *Advances in Nursing Science, 8*(4), 36–51.

Campbell, J. C. (1986b). A survivor group for battered women. *Advances in Nursing Sciences, 8*(2), 13–20.

Campbell, J. C. (1989). Women's responses to sexual abuse in intimate relationships. *Health Care For Women International, 10*, 335–346.

Campbell, J. C., & Alford, P. (1989). The dark consequences of marital rape. *American Journal of Nursing, 89*, 946–949.

Carmel, H., & Hunter, M. (1989). Staff injuries from inpatient violence. *Hospital and Community Psychiatry, 40*(1), 41–46.

Cassetta, R. A. (1993). Nurses grapple with restraints issue. *The American Nurse, 25*(1), 11.

Chinn, P. (1986). Violence and the health care family. *Advances in Nursing Science, 8*(4), ix.

Collins, C. J. (1996). Patient assault and its impact on psychiatric nursing practice. Unpublished manuscript.

Conn, L. M., & Lion, J. R. (1983). Assaults in a university hospital. In J. R. Lion & W. H. Reid (Eds.), *Assaults within psychiatric facilities* (pp. 61–69). New York: Grune & Stratton.

Cox, H. (1987). Verbal abuse in nursing: Report of a study. *Nursing Management, 18*(11), 47–50.

Cox, H. (1991a). Verbal abuse nationwide: Part 1. Oppressed group behavior. *Nursing Management, 22*(2), 32–35.

Cox, H. (1991b). Verbal abuse nationwide: Part 2. Impact and modifications. *Nursing Management, 22*(3), 66–69.

Flannery, R. B., Fulton, P., Tausch, J., & DeLoffi, A. Y. (1991). A program to help staff deal with psychological sequelae of assaults by patients. *Hospital and Community Psychiatry, 42*(9), 935–938.

Fornazzari, X., & Freire, M. (1990). Women as victims of torture. *Acta Psychiatrica Scandinavia, 82*, 257–260.

Gasparis, L., & Swirsky, J. (Eds.). (1990). *Nurse abuse: Impact and resolution.* New York: Power.

Harris, D., & Morrison E. F. (1995). Managing violence without coercion. *Archives of Psychiatric Nursing, 9*(4), 203–210.

Heider, F. (1958). *The psychology of interpersonal relations.* New York: John Wiley & Sons.

Horowitz, M. J., Wilner, N., Marmar, C., & Krupnick, J. (1980). Pathological grief and the activation of latent self images. *American Journal of Psychiatry, 137,* 1137–1162.

INA meets with DMHDD director McDonald: Demands improved safety and staffing in DMH facilities. (1993). *Chart, 89*(8), 12.

Janoff-Bulman, R. (1979). Characterological versus behavioral self-blame: Inquiries into depression and rape. *Journal of Personality and Social Psychology, 37*(10), 1798–1809.

Janoff-Bulman, R., & Frieze, I. H. (1983). A theoretical perspective for understanding reactions to victimization. *Journal of Social Issues, 39*(2), 1–17.

Jones, M. K. (1985). Patient violence: Reports of 200 incidents. *Journal of Psychosocial Nursing, 23*(6), 12–17.

Landau, J. (1993). The experiences of seven nurses who relate with violence-prone psychiatric inpatients. *Dissertation Abstracts International, 54*(2), 744B.

Lanza, M. L. (1983). The reactions of nursing staff to physical assault by a patient. *Hospital and Community Psychiatry, 34*(1), 44–54.

Lanza, M. L. (1984). Nursing staff as victims: Implications for a nursing diagnosis. In M. Kim, G. K. McFarland, & A. M. McLane (Eds.), *Proceedings from the fifth national conference on nursing diagnosis* (pp. 361–363). St. Louis: C.V. Mosby.

Lanza, M. L. (1985). How nurses react to patient assault. *Journal of Psychosocial Nursing, 23*(6), 6–11.

Lanza, M. L. (1986). Approaches to studying patient assault. *Western Journal of Nursing Research, 8*(3), 321–328.

Lanza, M. L. (1987). The relationship of the severity of assault to blame placement for assault. *Archives of Psychiatric Nursing, 1*(4), 269–279.

Lanza, M. L. (1988). Factors relevant to patient assault. *Issues in Mental Health Nursing, 9,* 239–257.

Lanza, M. L. (1992). Nurses as patient assault victims: An update, synthesis, and recommendations. *Archives of Psychiatric Nursing, 6*(3), 163–171.

Lanza, M. L., Milner, J., & Riley, E. (1988). Predictors of patient assault on acute inpatient psychiatric units: A pilot study. *Issues in Mental Health Nursing, 9,* 259–270.

Lerner, M. J. (1963). Evaluation of performance as a function of performer's reward and attractiveness. *Journal of Personality and Social Psychology, 1*(4), 355–360.

Lerner, M. J., & Lichtman, R. R. (1968). Effects of perceived norms on attitudes and altruistic behavior toward a dependent other. *Journal of Personality and Social Psychology, 9*(3), 226–232.

Lerner, M. J., & Matthews, G. (1967). Reactions to suffering of others under conditions of indirect responsibility. *Journal of Personality and Social Psychology, 5*(3), 319–325.

Lerner, M. J., & Simmons, C. H. (1966). Observer's reaction to the "innocent victim": Compassion or rejection? *Journal of Personality and Social Psychology, 4*(2), 203–210.

Morrison, E. F. (1990). The evolution of a concept: Aggression and violence in psychiatric settings. *Archives of Psychiatric Nursing, 8*(4), 245–253.

Murray, M. G., & Snyder, J. C. (1991). When staff are assaulted. *Journal of Psychosocial Nursing, 29*(7), 24–29.

Perloff, L. S. (1983). Perceptions to vulnerability to victimization. *Journal of Social Issues, 39*(20), 41–61.

Peterson, C., & Seligman, M. E. P. (1983). Learned helplessness and victimization. *Journal of Social Issues, 39*(2), 105–118.

Poster, E. C., & Ryan, J. A. (1989). Nurses' attitudes toward physical assaults by patients. *Archives of Psychiatric Nursing, 3*(6), 315–322.

Poster, E. C., & Ryan, J. A. (1994). A multiregional study of nurses' beliefs and attitudes about work safety and patient assault. *Hospital and Community Psychiatry, 45*(11), 1104–1108.

Roberts, S. (1991, March). Nurse abuse: A taboo subject. *The Canadian Nurse, 87*(3), 23–25.

Schepple, K. L., & Bart, P. B. (1983). Through women's eyes: Defining danger in the wake of sexual assault. *Journal of Social Sciences, 39*(2), 63–81.

Silver, R. L., Boon, C., & Stones, M. L. (1983). Searching for meaning in misfortune: Making sense of incest. *Journal of Social Issues, 39*(2), 83–103.

Silver, R. L., & Wortman, C. B. (1980). Coping with undesirable life events. In J. Garber & M. E. P. Seligman (Eds.), *Human helplessness* (pp. 279–340). New York: Academic Press.

Taylor, S. E., Wood, J. V., & Lichtman, R. R. (1983). It could be worse: Selective evaluation as a response to victimization. *Journal of Social Issues, 39*(2), 19–40.

Vox Pop. (1987). Raising the alarm. *Nursing Times, 83*(12), 46.

Walker, L. (1979). *The battered woman.* New York: Harper & Row.

Wertz, F. (1983). Method and findings in a phenomenological study of a complex life-event: Being criminally victimized. From "everyday" to psychological description: An analysis of the moments of a qualitative data analysis. *Journal of Phenomenological Psychology, 14*(2), 155–216.

Wills, T. A. (1981). Downward comparison principles in social psychology. *Psychological Bulletin, 90*(2), 245–271.

Worthington, K. (1994). Workplace hazards: The effect on nurses as women. *The American Nurse, 26*(1), 15.

Wortman, C. (1976). Causal attributions and personal control. *New Directions in Attributional Research, 1,* 123–152.

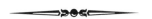

BOOKS AND ARTICLES

The following books and articles were chosen to illustrate lay and professional perspectives of verbal and physical experiences with aggressive behaviors from colleagues, patients, and patient families and friends. The paucity of information in lay literature regarding verbal and physical attacks on healthcare workers may indicate that consumers of healthcare are still unaware of the extent of the problem.

Blair, D. T. (1991). Assaultive behavior: Does provocation begin in the front office? *Journal of Psychosocial Nursing and Mental Health Services, 29*(5), 21–26.

Blair (1991) draws similarities between the "battered" nurse and the increasing rates of violence in the home and in the community. A number of trends are identified that may contribute to increased risk to healthcare providers; they include providing a less restrictive environment in the inpatient setting; decreased accessibility to hospital treatment; and deinstitutionalism. Further, a combination of risk factors interacting with the patient's psychopathology contribute to the dynamics of assault and serve to confuse the issue of preventing assaultive behavior.

Blair purports that "provocation is an important risk predictor because these issues can

be recognized, assessed, and appropriate interventions can be implemented to reduce the associated risks" (p. 22). Just what are these issues of provocation? Blair notes that the invasion of personal space, limit setting, and denial are all important elements of provocation. Denial exists on the part of the patient, the staff, and the institution. However, the author emphasizes that nursing staff are the most frequent victims of assault. Blair concludes that if poor leadership, inept treatment practice, and staff conflict are not viewed as influencing assaultive behavior, than the problem is never interrupted and the cycle continues.

Interventions should be designed to minimize issues of provocation while eliminating those that can be prevented. Institutions must promote policies and procedures designed to accommodate individualized approaches to patient care to enhance the safety of patients and staff.

Braun, K., Christle, D., Walker, D., & Tiwanak, G. (1991). Verbal abuse of nurses and nonnurses. *Nursing Management, 22*(3), 72–76.

Braun, Christle, Walker and Tiwanak (1991) examine incidents of verbal abuse directed toward nurses from physicians, patients, and patient relatives and explore incidents of verbal abuse directed toward auxiliary personnel by nurses. The investigators used the survey developed by Cox (1987) and invited 696 nurses employed at a medical center in Honolulu during June 1989 to complete the survey. Of the 327 nurses responding (a response rate of 47 percent), 264 identified themselves as staff nurses. Two months later, 125 non-nursing staff were invited to respond to a generic version of the same survey yielding a sample of 67 employees (54 percent response rate).

Patients and physicians were the most common source of verbal abuse for both nursing and non-nursing groups. Overall, nurses experienced verbal abuse from more sources than did non-nursing staff. Another interesting finding was that verbal abuse from immediate supervisors was the most common reason for resignations in both groups of healthcare providers. Both groups of healthcare workers valued their professions, although non-nurses reported feeling less valued by administrators than did nurses. Neither group of workers felt valued by physicians.

These investigators expanded their study to include medical students and found that abusive behavior in physicians is learned. Similar to abused children, medical students were as likely to get caught in the cycle of violence as the recipients of abusive behavior during their education and training programs and in turn become abusive physicians. The authors concluded that strategies designed to minimize abuse should be directed toward managers, staff, and educators. The need for collaborative practice between healthcare workers and their managers is strongly supported by the authors' findings.

Briles, J. (1994). *The Briles report on women in healthcare: Changing conflict to collaboration in a toxic workplace.* San Francisco, CA: Jossey-Bass.

Judith Briles, a business woman and founder of the Briles Group, Inc. has authored ten other books regarding the roles of women in the workplace. She lectures to clients in healthcare centers and medical associations in the United States and Canada. This particular book focuses on issues of verbal abuse, sexual harassment, and sabotaging behaviors experienced by women in healthcare.

Briles noted in earlier surveys conducted among her clients, that women felt undermined by other women more frequently than by men. To further substantiate this finding, Briles conducted a follow-up study; the results form the basis of this book. Divided into two sections, her book discusses the results of her survey and suggests tools and strategies designed to stop sabotage in healthcare settings.

Questionnaires were mailed to directors of women's centers, vice presidents for nursing, and educational centers at randomly selected hospitals. Surveys were also distributed at an annual meeting of the *National Association of Women Health Professionals* (NAWHP). Ninety eight percent of respondents were women. Of the 1,000 surveys distributed, 229 were returned for a response rate of 23 percent. The author did not note the potential for duplicate responses from these two samples nor did she note the percentage of responses from samples in the United States as compared to response rates from Canadian respondents. As many as 71 percent of the women respondents stated they had been treated unethically by another woman at work. Further, 45 percent of the women surveyed expected to be undermined in the workplace and often regretted forming friendships.

Briles found that unlike responses obtained in previous interviews and surveys she had conducted, respondents used the terms abuse and assault more openly and freely (p. xiii). Briles concluded that not only had undermining behaviors increased, but women were often the first to be affected by downsizing possessing the least authority and seniority to effect changes in the workplace.

The second section of Briles' book emphasized the differences in styles of managing conflict in the workplace and recommended strategies designed to help women resolve conflicts. She also provided examples of interactions between coworkers to illustrate ways of effectively resolving common conflicts at work. However, Briles' recommendations tended to reinforce methods of conflict resolutions historically used by male workers and neglected to consider the impact of gender and cultural biases. Conflict resolution strategies that value women's experiences were not discussed. Yet, the chapter "Cultivate Healthy Female Relationships" identifies strategies where women can be more open, honest, and supportive of each other. Overall, this book offers valuable information on the topic of violence in healthcare settings.

Burgess, A. W., Burgess, A. G., & Douglas, J. E. (1994). Examining violence in the workplace: A look at work-related fatalities. *Journal of Psychosocial Nursing and Mental Health Services, 32*(7), 11–53.

These authors examine the issue of violence in the workplace, particularly in the hospital setting. They noted that the nurse in the healthcare setting is called upon to manage both the victim and the victimizer. The violence is often influenced by the cultural backgrounds of the victims seeking care and from tensions existing in the neighborhoods. Six types of homicide are identified: authority homicide, revenge homicide, domestic homicide, felony homicide, and argument/conflict homicide. Data for this study were obtained from 132 cases identified through national wire service reporting. Particular details were obtained from telephone consultation with local law enforcement officials.

The investigators urge families of homicide victims to obtain grief assistance which provides support and counseling. Burgess, Burgess, and Douglas (1994) recommend that staff develop a safety plan for the patient/victim that is implemented during the hospital stay and continues at home and at work. Further, the safety and security of the hospital environment can be enhanced through policy development and implementation, inservice training, and consultation; and, caution that allowing violent actions or threats to go unnoticed sanctions violence.

The authors present constructive solutions to the serious issue of violence in the health-

care setting. However, in the current climate of managing costs in healthcare settings, victimized staff are often left without the necessary resources to help them cope with the sequelae of the verbal or physical attack.

Gasparis, L., & Swirsky, J. (Eds.). (1990). *Nurse abuse: Impact and resolution.* New York: Power.

This book consists of ten essays written by critical care nurses to examine experiences in healthcare settings that devalue the practice of nursing. A broad range of topics are presented: the reality of "nursework"; forms of abuse directed toward nurses; the psychology of abuse; burn-out experienced by nurses; and potential solutions to problems faced by nurses in the workplace. The authors acknowledged the social-psychological shaping of women's behavior in a paternalistic society and the ways in which this socialization perpetuates the oppression of nurses. However, several of the sweeping generalizations made by Swirsky (1990) such as the notion that "nurse abuse differs from wife abuse" (p. 175) are not supported by the literature (Chinn, 1986; Worthington, 1994). In an apparent contradiction, Swirsky (1990) notes later in the same chapter that the nurse is "subject to all of the mistreatment, harshness, inequities, deceptions . . . of other abused groups" (p. 177).

Many of the arguments seem dated and understated in terms of the current atmosphere of downsizing and consolidating of resources in healthcare institutions. Perhaps the work of professional nurses has become even more devalued in efforts to contain costs in healthcare institutions. This collection of essays was difficult to follow due to the omission of authors' names from the individual chapters. The technique of highlighting "nurse abuse" in large, bold print throughout this collection of essays was distracting to the reader.

Landau, J. (1993). The experiences of seven nurses who relate with violence-prone psychiatric in-patients. *Dissertation Abstracts International, 54*(2), 744B.

Joanna Landau a clinical instructor of psychiatric nursing students at New York University conducted a qualitative study designed to explore the experiences of psychiatric nurses working with violence-prone patients in an in-patient setting. An overview of the concepts of violence and aggression was provided followed by a review of literature concerning the prediction of violence in mentally ill individuals; management of aggressive behaviors in the mentally ill inpatient; training of staff; and staff's attitudes toward the violence-prone patient.

A sample of nurses who had worked at least three years in an inpatient psychiatric facility was chosen. The initial sample consisted of five female nurses but increased to two additional male nurses when issues of gender arose in the interviews. A profile of each nurse was developed contributing to a richer understanding of each respondent's experiences with violence-prone patients.

Landau concluded that this sample of nurses felt they had not been appropriately prepared to deal with violent behaviors in the clinical setting. Most of the aggression-management skills were learned on-the-job from more experienced staff. Although the institution had training programs in place, the nurses had mixed reactions about the efficacy of these programs. Gender biases are worth noting. Male nurses tended to consider male patients more violence-prone, while female nurses tended to think of female patients being more violence-prone. All respondents acknowledged that some staff were not psychologically prepared to deal therapeutically with the violence-prone patient.

Recommendations included incorporating into nursing curriculum more complete information on recognizing and managing violence-prone patient behaviors; providing support and opportunities for nursing staff to review violent patient incidents in a nonjudgmental environment; and conducting further studies to explore interactions that occur between the violence-prone patient and nursing staff.

This study is timely, however, in focusing on issues of education, management, and training, the investigator missed an opportunity to explore the personal toll exacted by healthcare workers dealing with violence-prone patients.

Part IV

Delivery of Healthcare
to Women

Chapter 4

Lesbian Health: Barriers to Care

Roberta Cassidy
Tonda L. Hughes

Practitioner: Are you taking any medications?
Client: No
Practitioner: What kind of birth control are you using?
Client: I'm not using any.
Practitioner: Why not?
Client: I don't need it.
Practitioner: Are you sexually active?
Client: Yes.
Practitioner: Are you trying to get pregnant?
Client: No . . .

Interactions between healthcare providers and female clients such as this one during a routine health history are common. However, such interactions represent a defining moment for women who are lesbian or bisexual. In every interaction with a healthcare provider, the lesbian or bisexual woman is confronted with a choice—to disclose or avoid disclosure of her sexual identity. If she chooses to disclose her sexual identity, the woman may be treated in a patronizing or hostile manner or she may be referred to a mental health professional (Stevens & Hall, 1988). However, if a lesbian or bisexual woman chooses to remain silent, she may receive inadequate or inappropriate care and her health may be jeopardized (Eliason, 1993).

Inadequate or inappropriate treatment also results from biases inherent in the healthcare system. Because most health-related research has focused on white, heterosexual men, information about other groups is often limited. Factors such as class, ethnicity, and able-bodiedness also affect the delivery and quality of healthcare services (Denenberg, 1992). Lesbians, like many heterosexual women, face a number of barriers to accessing quality healthcare, such as transportation, inadequate insurance or financial means, and lack of child care. Although there is no evidence to suggest that being a lesbian is itself a health hazard, lesbians may be at greater risk for health problems such as alcohol abuse and breast cancer (Haas, 1994; Hughes & Wilsnack, in press; O'Hanlan, 1995). In addition, homophobia and heterosexism, which are thoroughly entrenched in both society and in the healthcare system, create barriers to healthcare that appear to contribute significantly to health risks faced by lesbians and bisexual women.

Heterosexism, the belief that heterosexuality is the norm and is superior to other sexual identities, awards exclusive privilege and power to heterosexuals (McKee, Hayes, & Axiotis, 1994) and is manifested within the healthcare system in various ways. Heterosexism is a primary structural barrier, similar to institutional racism, in the organization and delivery of healthcare for clients who do not identify as heterosexual (Stevens, 1995). The assumption of heterosexuality and the almost exclusive focus on women's reproductive health are common examples. Homophobia, an interpersonal manifestation of heterosexism (Stevens, 1995), is the irrational fear of homosexuality that may be manifested both internally, via learned individual biases, and externally through verbal and physical acts of discrimination and violence directed at gays, lesbians, or bisexuals (O'Hanlan, 1995). Homophobia in the healthcare setting is principally manifested in the beliefs, attitudes, and practices of healthcare workers in their interactions with gay, lesbian, or bisexual clients (Booth, Mathews, Turner, & Kessler, 1986; Eliason, 1993). Homophobia is exhibited in various forms by healthcare providers in the delivery of healthcare services. Examples range from heterosexist assumptions expressed during verbal interactions to patronizing care and overt mistreatment of lesbian clients during gynecologic or other examinations. Consequently, heterosexism has a profound impact on the quality of healthcare received by the lesbian population.

The purpose of this chapter is to provide a resource for clinicians, researchers, and others interested in lesbian health. In order to include as many references and reviews as possible, abstracts are for the most part, brief, and include little or no critique. Together, the abstracts are intended to serve as an overview of issues related to lesbian health including structural and interpersonal barriers to healthcare and the potential health consequences of these barriers. We chose to focus on lesbian health because almost no research, clinical, or anecdotal information exists on the health or healthcare of bisexual and transgendered women. However, because many of the issues and concerns of lesbians are shared by bisexual and transgendered women, much of this information will be useful to healthcare practitioners who care for these populations of women as well.

The sources selected were chosen to represent as much of the diversity within the lesbian population and as broad a range of the health issues as possible. For example, articles are included that discuss the commonly reported barriers to care as well as those that address issues such as HIV, suicide, and domestic violence, areas that have only recently begun to be discussed. The interrelationships between heterosexism, classism, sexism, and racism and the impact of these systems of oppression on healthcare is an increasingly apparent theme in much of the literature related to lesbian health. Nevertheless, much of what we know about lesbian health is based on research conducted with middle class, well-educated, white lesbians. This bias remains despite strenuous attempts of many researchers to recruit more diverse samples for research studies. Although research is needed on all aspects of health and in all groups of lesbians, the most glaring gaps exist in knowledge about adolescent and older lesbians, lesbians of color, poor lesbians, and lesbians who live in rural areas. It is our hope that this chapter will serve to highlight the areas in most need of research and to encourage researchers to design and conduct studies to provide needed information to decrease health risks and barriers to care currently experienced by lesbian, bisexual, and transgendered women.

IMPLICATIONS

A number of implications for lesbian health are evident in this review. This section summarizes key findings of studies abstracted and discusses implications for research, practice, and education.

Research: Until recently, lesbians have been largely ignored in health and psychological research. Although the women's health, feminist, and gay-rights movements of the 1970s served to stimulate research focusing on lesbians, a number of gaps and limitations exist in our knowledge of this population of women. In addition to needing more research, sampling and design problems that limit previous research must also be addressed. Comparisons of health problems provides important information about similarities and differences between lesbians and heterosexual women. For example, smaller gender differences in lesbians and gay men's rates of drinking and slower and lower declines in alcohol consumption among lesbians as they age suggest that lesbians and heterosexual women may respond differently to traditional gender-role norms that influence women's drinking.

Some efforts to compare data on lesbians and heterosexual women have been made, but variations in the wording of questions and the likely inclusion of an unknown number of lesbians in general surveys of women's health limit the usefulness of such comparisons. In addition, care must be taken when selecting comparison groups. Most studies of lesbians have included women who are most visible—almost exclusively white, relatively young (under 40 years old), and college-educated women. Until strategies can be developed to obtain a broader representation of lesbians, comparison groups will need to be carefully selected and caution used in interpreting findings.

More innovative strategies are needed to ensure that adequate numbers, and more representative groups of lesbians are included in general women's health surveys as well as in research focusing specifically on lesbians. It is especially important to obtain more representative samples of older lesbians, adolescent lesbians, lesbians of color, low-income lesbians, lesbians with disabilities, and lesbians who are less open about their sexual identity. One relatively simple method of improving knowledge about lesbian health is to include questions about sexual orientation in all major surveys of women's health.

More research is needed that focuses not only on health problems for which lesbians may be at greater risk, but also on the reasons behind their higher risk status. For example, what does the high rate of drinking among lesbians say about the context in which they live their lives? What alternative methods of coping with stress do lesbians identify and use? What are the resiliency characteristics of lesbians who do not drink excessively or experience alcohol problems? More qualitative research, particularly studies that focus on the "lived experience" of lesbians, would provide valuable information to inform both theory and clinical practice.

One shortcoming of much of the research reviewed here is the emphasis placed on the healthcare provider and the healthcare system. Apart from several studies that focused on the lesbian client-provider interaction, relatively little attention is paid to the strategies lesbians use in accessing healthcare and the resulting outcomes of the care received. Although access is clearly an important issue, the health needs of lesbians must be addressed in a more wholistic manner. For marginalized and stigmatized groups, equal access does not equate with equal outcomes. While remaining focused on issues of access, we must simultaneously look at healthcare outcomes as well.

Active participation of lesbians in earlier stages of the research process (prior to data collection) could also assist in the development of a more consistent and useful definition of sexual orientation. In most of the literature to date, the meaning of "lesbian" is absent or unclear. Recognition of the need for more relevant and consistent definitions is evident in several of the articles or reports abstracted including, for example, the one definition by the National Gay and Lesbian Task Force Policy Institute (as cited in Denenberg, 1992). The definition suggested by the group takes into account the diversity of the lesbian communities, recognizes heterosexual experiences, acknowledges the discrimination encountered in all aspects of life, and emphasizes the social and political nature of sexual identity. This definition also delineates, for the healthcare professional, the importance of assessing lesbians' risk behaviors (both past and present) rather than focusing on sexual identity alone.

Education: Educating healthcare providers to the needs and concerns of gay, lesbian, and bisexual clients is a consistent recommendation of most current research. The healthcare practitioner is ideally situated to bridge the gap between a homophobic and heterosexist healthcare system and the client through provision of culturally sensitive care. However, although education of practitioners is clearly important in lessening or eliminating discrimination encountered by lesbians in the healthcare system, this focus addresses only part of the problem. The broader social and political systems that perpetuate homophobia must also be addressed.

Practice: Although it is important that healthcare providers are able to accurately assess the health needs of lesbian clients, the role of the lesbian client in her healthcare is largely unaddressed in current literature. What strategies do lesbians use in disclosing their sexual identity? What alternatives to postponing or avoiding or dreading care because of previous negative experiences do lesbians have? What sort of participation by the lesbian client, in conjunction with her healthcare provider, works best in obtaining culturally sensitive and appropriate care? Such questions are critical in addressing current barriers to healthcare for lesbians. For example, the research reviewed here emphasizes the importance of disclosure of sexual identity. However, few suggestions are made about how lesbians might anticipate responses to disclosure and what steps might be taken when disclosure is met with hostile or inappropriate responses. Strategies such as this are greatly needed to help lesbians become more active participants in their healthcare.

Also omitted in the literature reviewed here is attention to the resilience of lesbians. Most current research on lesbian health focuses on deficits, risk factors, or limitations rather than the strengths of this "vulnerable" population. Lesbians live in a largely hostile environment and, as a result, most have developed a wide range of positive coping strategies. Research aimed at identifying or exploring these coping mechanisms and resiliency in lesbians could provide important information for maximizing the resources of lesbian clients. In addition, more attention needs to be paid to lesbians' resourcefulness in developing community health services that can better meet the needs of lesbians. Examples of such services include those provided by organizations such as the Lesbian Community Cancer Project (LCCP) in Chicago, Illinois, the Whitman-Walker Clinic in Washington, DC, and the Office of Gay and Lesbian Health Concerns in New York City. The Lesbian Community Cancer Project, in addition to fostering alliances within the lesbian community, has established a relationship with the Chicago Board of Health in order to provide preventative screening services such as Pap smears and mammographies at no charge to lesbians who are unable to afford these services or prefer a lesbian-friendly environment. Other community services such as those provided by LCCP and other community agencies address issues of access encountered by many lesbians by providing childcare, transportation tokens, lesbian healthcare providers, and health services at low or no cost.

Lesbian health research is in its infancy and offers numerous and exciting opportunities for exploration and growth. This review points to the variety of opportunities to add to this knowledge base. Educators, practitioners, policy-makers, and researchers alike must build interactive and collaborative partnerships with the communities they serve in order to guarantee a healthcare foundation that meets the needs of this diverse population.

REFERENCES

Cochran, S. D., & Mays, V. M. (1988). Disclosure of sexual preference to physicians by black lesbian and bisexual women. *Western Journal of Medicine, 149,* 616–619.

Denenberg, R. (1992). Invisible women: Lesbians and health care. *Health PAC Bulletin, 22*(1), 14–21.

Eliason, M. J. (1993). Cultural diversity in nursing care: The lesbian, gay, or bisexual client. *Journal of Transcultural Nursing, 5*(1), 14–20.

Eliason, M. J. (1996). Lesbian and gay family issues. *Journal of Family Nursing, 2*(1), 10–29.

Fred Hutchinson Cancer Research Center. (1994). *Cancer and cancer risk among lesbians.* Seattle, WA: Community Liaison Program.

Gomez, J. L., & Smith, B. (1994). Taking the home out of homophobia: Black lesbian health. In E. C. White (Ed.), *The black women's health book: Speaking for ourselves* (pp. 198–213). Seattle, WA: Seal Press.

Haas, A. P. (1994). Lesbian health issues: An overview. In A. J. Dan (Ed.), *Reframing women's health* (pp. 339–356). London: Sage.

Harvey, S. M., Carr, C., & Bernheine, S. (1989). Lesbian mothers' health care experiences. *Journal of Nurse-Midwifery, 34*(3), 115–119.

Hitchcock, J. M., & Wilson, H. S. (1992). Personal risking: Lesbian self-disclosure of sexual orientation to professional health care providers. *Nursing Research, 41*(3), 178–183.

Hughes, T. L., & Wilsnack, S. C. (in press). Lesbians and alcohol: Clinical and research implications. *American Journal of Orthopsychiatry.*

Lucas, V. A. (1992). An investigation of the health care preferences of the lesbian population. *Health Care for Women International, 13*, 221–228.

Lynch, M. A. (1993). When the patient is also a lesbian. *AWHONN's Clinical Issues, 4*(2), 196–202.

Mathews, W. C., Booth, M. W., Turner, J. D., & Kessler, L. (1986). Physicians' attitudes toward homosexuality: Survey of a California County medical society. *Western Journal of Medicine, 144*, 106–110.

McKee, M. B., Hayes, S. F., & Axiotis, I. R. (1994). Challenging heterosexism in college health service delivery. *Journal of American College Health, 42*, 211–216.

O'Hanlan, K. A. (1995). Lesbian health and homophobia: Perspectives for the treating obstetrician/gynecologist. *Current Problems in Obstetrics, Gynecology and Fertility, 18*(4), 93–136.

Paroski, P. A. (1987). Health care delivery and the concerns of gay and lesbian adolescents. *Journal of Adolescent Health Care, 8*(2), 188–192.

Radecic, P. J. (1993). *Lesbian health issues and recommendations.* Unpublished manuscript.

Rankow, E. J. (1995). Lesbian health issues for the primary care provider. *Journal of Family Practice, 40*(5), 486–493.

Stevens, P. E. (1993). Lesbians and HIV: Clinical, research, and policy issues. *American Journal of Orthopsychiatry, 63*(2), 289–294.

Stevens. P. E. (1994). Lesbians' health-related experiences of care and non-care. *Western Journal of Nursing Research, 16*(6), 639–659.

Stevens, P. E. (1995). Structural and interpersonal impact of heterosexual assumptions on lesbian health care. *Nursing Research, 44*(1), 25–30.

Stevens, P. E., & Hall, J. M. (1988). Stigma, health beliefs and experiences with health care in lesbian women. *IMAGE: Journal of Nursing Scholarship, 20*(2), 69–73.

Trippet, S. E., & Bain, J. (1993). Physical health problems and concerns of lesbians. *Women & Health, 20*(2), 59–70.

Zeidenstein, L. (1990). Gynecological and childbearing needs of lesbians. *Journal of Nurse-Midwifery*, 35(1), 10–18.

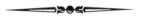

Healthcare Experiences

Cochran, S. D., & Mays, V. M. (1988). Disclosure of sexual preference to physicians by black lesbian and bisexual women. *Western Journal of Medicine*, 149, 616–619.

Although the literature on lesbian health supports the assumption that lesbians are reluctant to disclose their sexual orientation in interactions with healthcare providers, most studies have collected data from primarily white, well-educated, middle class participants. We know relatively little about black lesbians' healthcare experiences, including decisions about disclosure of sexual orientation. Based on estimated rates of disclosure between 18 percent to 49 percent among white lesbians and gay men, Cochran and Mays sought to determine whether black women are more or less likely to disclose their sexual orientation to healthcare providers. Several findings from a survey of 529 black lesbians and 65 black bisexual women are reported in this article. For example, compared with lesbians in this study, bisexual women were less likely to disclose information related to sexual orientation. As expected, bisexual women reported significantly more sexual experiences and current involvements with men than did lesbians. Most of the black lesbians in this study (91 percent) reported current or past sexual relationships with men. This finding emphasizes the inadequacy of current definitions of sexual orientation. The reality that many, if not most, lesbian-identified women have had sex with men emphasizes that sexual identity or sexual orientation encompasses much more than sexual behavior. The study findings also emphasize the need for additional research focusing on the healthcare needs and experiences of black lesbian and bisexual women.

Gomez, J. L., & Smith, B. (1994). Taking the home out of homophobia: Black lesbian health. In E. C. White (Ed.), *The black women's health book: Speaking for ourselves* (pp. 198–213). Seattle: Seal Press.

In a published conversation, Gomez and Smith define homophobia as an unhealthy condition and discuss how it affects black lesbians' health. The interrelatedness of sexism, racism, and classism are discussed and Gomez and Smith relate their own personal experiences to highlight the role these forms of oppression play in the lives of all people, but particularly in the lives of women of color.

Hitchcock, J. M., & Wilson, H. S. (1992). Personal risking: Lesbian self-disclosure of sexual orientation to professional health care providers. *Nursing Research*, 41(3), 178–183.

Most lesbian health research has focused on difficulties accessing healthcare. Only recently has research focused more specifically on the lesbian-provider relationship. Findings from this research indicate that a safe and nonjudgmental atmosphere, particularly regarding disclosure of sexual identity, is of paramount importance to lesbians' willingness to seek healthcare. This study of 33 self-identified lesbians used both questionnaire and interview data to formulate a theory describing the process of disclosing sexual identity to healthcare providers. Based on the outcomes of the study, the authors identify a two-phase process termed "personal risking" to describe the complex process involved in lesbians' decisions about self-disclosure. This description provides new and useful information about the lesbian-provider relationship and emphasizes the importance of the provision of healthcare in a physically safe and psychologically comfortable environment.

Stevens, P. E. (1994). Lesbians' health-related experiences of care and noncare. *Western Journal of Nursing Research, 16*(6), 639–659.

This multi-method feminist investigation explored lesbians' experiences of care and noncare in the healthcare setting. A diverse sample of 45 lesbians was recruited through community-based purposive sampling and snowball techniques. Lesbians in this study assessed as negative the majority of their past healthcare experiences; only 23 percent of past interactions with healthcare providers were appraised positively. Based on lesbians' reports of their experiences, Stevens describes common healthcare interactions between the client and provider among subgroups within the sample. Themes considered important to these lesbians were uniqueness, existence, emotional and bodily integrity, expression, worth, and power. A caring and noncaring example of each theme or dimension is provided. One of the most important and most disturbing findings discovered in the analysis of these stories is that almost one-half (44 percent) of the participants had nearly stopped seeking healthcare as a result of negative experiences. These findings emphasize the importance of educating healthcare providers about the health needs and concerns of lesbians.

Stevens, P. E., & Hall, J. M. (1988). Stigma, health beliefs and experiences with health care in lesbian women. *IMAGE: Journal of Nursing Scholarship, 20*(2), 69–73.

Stigmatization, a well-documented experience of lesbians in this society, has an important impact on health beliefs, healthcare experiences, and use of the healthcare system. The authors used a snowball sampling method to recruit 25 self-identified lesbians for this study. Semi-structured interviews were conducted that focused on the following areas: (1) interactions with healthcare providers; (2) lesbians' perceptions of their identifiability as a lesbian; and (3) lesbians' conceptions of health and illness. The findings suggest that, in general, lesbians are uncomfortable with their healthcare experiences; the majority of the sample reported negative experiences with

providers when their lesbian identity was apparent. Thirty-six percent of the sample reported that they terminated interactions with healthcare providers following negative responses to disclosure of sexual identity. The fact that 84 percent of the women reported reluctance to seek healthcare emphasizes the extent to which providers' negative responses (or lesbians' fear of negative responses) serve as barriers to healthcare. The majority of lesbians surveyed believed themselves to be identifiable as lesbians and that lesbians can be identified through particular ways of interaction and association. The authors speculate that identifiability may be a mediating factor influencing lesbians' health behaviors and access to healthcare. For example, the perception that one's sexual orientation is obvious may serve as stressor for some lesbians, but may act to decrease stress in other lesbians.

Additional References

Stevens, P. E. (1993). Marginalized women's access to health care: A feminist narrative analysis. *Advances in Nursing Science, 16*(2), 39–56.

Stevens, P. E. (1994). Protective strategies of lesbian clients in health care environments. *Research in Nursing & Health, 17,* 217–229.

Trippet, S. E., & Bain, J. (1992). Reasons American lesbians fail to seek traditional health care. *Health Care for Women International, 13,* 145–153.

Lesbian Health Overviews

Denenberg, R. (1994). *Report on lesbian health.* Unpublished manuscript.

Despite the American Psychiatric Association's removal of homosexuality as a mental illness from its *Diagnostic and Statistical Manual of Mental Disorders* in 1974, homophobia remains deeply ingrained in the healthcare system. Today, discrimination based on sexual orientation remains a primary barrier to adequate and appropriate healthcare for lesbians. Denenberg's report summarizes existing literature pertaining to lesbian health, discusses specific health concerns of lesbians, and develops justifications for the inclusion of lesbian health concerns within the context of women's health. Three goals are identified as necessary to correct current deficits in lesbian healthcare: (1) enhanced access to care; (2) increased utilization of services; and (3) improved health outcomes. The report emphasizes the importance of a lesbian health agenda to encourage responsiveness of the healthcare system to the needs of lesbians.

Eliason, Michele J. (1996). *Who cares? Institutional barriers to health care for lesbian, gay, and bisexual persons.* New York: NLN Press.

Lesbian, gay, and bisexual persons and healthcare professionals are often harassed, mistreated, or misunderstood in our healthcare systems. This book uncovers the roots of these problems, explores how prejudices have become institutionalized, and offers viable solutions for real change. Essential for educators, students, nurses, healthcare professionals, community activists—anyone interested in combatting prejudice.

Haas, A. P. (1994). Lesbian health issues: An overview. In A. J. Dan (Ed.), *Reframing women's health* (pp. 339–356). Thousand Oaks: Sage.

Little is known about lesbian health and even less is known about how lesbians' health may differ from the health of heterosexual women. In this comprehensive overview, the author summarizes current information related to healthcare interactions, health status, and legal and partnership issues relevant to lesbians and emphasizes potential differences between lesbians' and heterosexual women's health. Haas notes current limitations in research on lesbian health including, for example, lack of appropriate comparison groups of heterosexual women and inconsistent definitions related to sexual orientation. Strategies for healthcare providers to improve the health status of lesbian clients are discussed.

Lucas, V. A. (1992). An investigation of the health care preferences of the lesbian population. *Health Care for Women International, 13,* 221–228.

Much research to date has documented lesbians' avoidance of the traditional healthcare system due to abuses encountered while seeking care. The purpose of this study was to investigate healthcare preferences. To accomplish this, 178 self-identified lesbians who were recruited through various lesbian organizations and events completed a questionnaire assessing their healthcare preferences in the following areas: services, providers, health settings, and disclosure and documentation of sexual identity. In general, the sample identified preventative services as their foremost priority. The majority (58 percent) agreed that clinics and other outpatient healthcare agencies need to designate specific hours or days when only women are seen. In addition, female providers were the choice of the majority of study participants; 78 percent identified a female family physician as the preferred provider. Although 63 percent of the women agreed that questions relating to sexual identity should be asked during health assessments, 28 percent preferred that their sexual identity not be recorded on the chart. Based on the healthcare priorities identified by the participants, the author speculates that lesbians may be more health-oriented than treatment-oriented.

O'Hanlan, K. A. (1993, July). Lesbians in health research. In *Scientific meeting: Recruitment and retention of women in clinical studies* (Appendix 7, pp. 101–104). Bethesda, MD: National Institute of Health, Office of Research on Women's Health.

This brief report provides data from three large studies of lesbians which support the belief that important epidemiologic differences exist between lesbians and heterosexual women. O'Hanlan reviews the objectives related to research on lesbian health published by the Office of Research on Women's Health and discusses issues related to sampling and recruitment, development of research instruments, and data collection.

Radecic, P. J. (1993). *Lesbian health issues and recommendations.* Unpublished manuscript.

This report provides a succinct overview of lesbian health issues documented by the Los Angeles Lesbian Health Needs Assessment, the National Lesbian Health Care Survey, the Iowa Survey on Bisexual Women and Lesbians, and the Michigan Lesbian Health Survey. The report includes a definition of lesbian, a definition of a women's health issue, defines related terms such as heterosexism and homophobia, and outlines an action plan for lesbian health with both general and specific recommendations. In addition, a list of resources for lesbians seeking care is included.

Rankow, L. (1995). *Lesbian health bibliography.* Unpublished manuscript.

According to Marj Plumb, Director of the Office of Gay and Lesbian Health Concerns, this is the most thorough bibliography of lesbian health books, articles, and studies ever compiled. The bibliography contains close to 800 references about lesbian health issues. Among the subheadings included are cancer, HIV/AIDS, parenting, domestic violence, sex/sexuality, and substance abuse. The bibliography can be obtained by writing the National Center for Lesbian Rights (NCLR), 462 Broadway, Suite 500A, New York, NY 10013, or calling (212) 343-9589.

Trippet, S. E., & Bain, J. (1993). Physical health problems and concerns of lesbians. *Women and Health, 20*(2), 59–70.

This article reviews existing research related to lesbian health and notes that homophobia is central to concerns and healthcare decisions of lesbians. In addition, the authors report findings from a study in which they surveyed a convenience sample of 503 women (78 percent lesbian) recruited from women's cultural events. These women completed a questionnaire addressing lesbian health concerns in the following areas: (1) support systems; (2) healthcare interactions; (3) legal issues interfering with the utilization of services; and (4) health problems. The article focuses on physical health problems experienced by lesbians, participation in healthcare, and perceptions about the healthcare they received. The most frequent physical health problems for which lesbians sought healthcare were related to menstruation, sexually transmitted diseases, and other problems of the reproductive system, the bladder, kidney, musculoskeletal system, and breast. Interestingly, these problems were also those for which respondents most frequently reported that healthcare was not sought. The majority of lesbians in this study rated the care received as fair, good, or excellent. Suggestions for changes in the healthcare system identified by the participants are discussed.

Additional References

Mills, S., Garcia, D., & Martinez, T. (1993). *Health behaviors among lesbian and bisexual women: A community-based women's health survey.* San Francisco, CA: The San Francisco Department of Public Health.

Plumb, M. (1994). *Lesbian health advocacy plan.* San Francisco, CA: National Center for Lesbian Rights.

Zambrana, R. E. (1987). A research agenda on issues affecting poor and minority women: A model for understanding their health needs. *Women and Health, 12*(3–4), 137–160.

Adolescent Health

Paroski, P. A. (1987). Health care delivery and the concerns of gay and lesbian adolescents. *Journal of Adolescent Health Care, 8*(2), 188–192.

In this article, Paroski explores gay and lesbian adolescents' healthcare concerns and experiences. Participants included gay and lesbian adolescents who sought care at an urban community health center over an 18-month period. A self-administered questionnaire focusing on psychosocial health needs was completed by 121 self-identified gay and lesbian adolescents. Six areas were examined: (1) healthcare concerns and recommendations; (2) how the gay and lesbian lifestyle was discovered; (3) perceptions of gay men and lesbians; (4) the coming out process; (5) the process of acceptance of a gay or lesbian identity; and (6) coping mechanisms. Significant differences between males and females were evident in the selection of a healthcare provider; lesbians identified gender as their primary criterion in selecting a provider, whereas gay males identified the provider's sexual orientation as most important. Although the respondents reported a variety of sources of information about the lesbian/gay lifestyle, 95 percent of males obtained information through sexual encounters, whereas 88 percent of females relied on media for information. In general, both gay and lesbian adolescents ascribed to stereotypical images of the gay or lesbian person. The coming out process and acceptance of gay or lesbian identity was sequentially described by the majority of adolescents. Recommendations to healthcare providers include the elimination of heterosexist assumptions, the provision of visible gay and lesbian role models, peer support groups, relevant educational materials, and support services that address gay and lesbian adolescents' concerns and feelings related to sexual identity. A great deal more research is needed to better understand and respond to the healthcare concerns, particularly psychosocial and mental health concerns, of gay and lesbian adolescents.

Additional References

American Academy of Pediatrics Committee on Adolescence. (1993). Homosexuality and adolescence. *Pediatrics, 92*(4), 631–634.

Anderson, D. (1994). Lesbian and gay adolescents: Social and developmental considerations. *The High School Journal, 77*(1), 13–19.

Downey, J. I. (1994). Sexual orientation issues in adolescent girls. *Women's Health Issues, 4*(2), 67–70, 117–121.

Humm, A., & Kunreuther, F. (1991). The invisible epidemic: Teenagers and AIDS. *Social Policy, 21*(4), 40–46.

Igra, V., & Millstein, S. G. (1993). Current status and approaches to improving preventative services for adolescents. *Journal of the American Medical Association, 269*(11), 1408–1412.

Aging

Kehoe, M. (1986). Lesbians over 65: A triple invisible minority. *Journal of Homosexuality, 12*(3/4), 139–152.

Older lesbian women remain invisible both within the lesbian community and in the larger society. Although this study represents an important step in increasing our understanding about older lesbians, it includes relatively little information about the health status or health needs of this group of women. Fifty women (43 lesbian and 7 bisexual) completed a questionnaire designed to explore present needs, expectations for the future, and attitudes toward relationships. The participants were recruited using snowball sampling from a variety of sources including feminist, gay, and lesbian organizations. Study findings related to (1) personal and psychosocial concerns, (2) economic and occupational status, (3) physical and mental health, and (4) sexual attitudes and behavior are summarized. Study participants ranged in age from 65 to 85 years old. Although one-half of the women had been in a heterosexual marriage at some time in the past, the majority were childless. Thirty-five of the women were college graduates, 25 of whom held graduate degrees. The majority of the sample viewed their lesbian identification positively; 44 percent viewed themselves as "well adjusted." The majority of women reported that they owned their own homes and most had gross incomes ranging from $10,000 to $20,000 per year. Two-thirds had made arrangements for getting older such as having supplemental health insurance. Most of the women reported having arthritis and 12 women reported having a disabling physical handicap. Although only five women reported having a drinking problem, this rate (10 percent) is significantly higher than rates reported by women in the general population. One-half of the women described themselves as "unattached" and many reported that they had been celibate for a long period of time (3 months to 66 years). Aging, finances, loneliness, health, and isolation were identified as the areas of greatest concern. These findings emphasize the fact that older lesbians are a hidden population in which further research is greatly needed.

Quam, J. K., & Whitford, G. S. (1992). Adaptation and age-related expectations of older gay and lesbian adults. *The Gerontologist, 32,* 367–374.

These authors begin by noting that the lack of research on lesbians and gay men has helped to perpetuate myths and stereotypes about this group—stereotypes that are held by many healthcare providers. To counter such stereotypes, results of a study of 39 lesbian and 41 gay men whose ages ranged from 50 to 73 years are described. For example, the lesbians and gay men in this study reported high levels of life satisfaction, current health, and acceptance of their aging process. Although a few of the respondents reported the belief that their sexual orientation hindered their aging process (e.g., increased loneliness, difficulty forming long-lasting relationships, fear of discrimination in the healthcare system), the majority (86 percent) believed that being lesbian or gay helps in the aging process. Reasons given for this belief include: (1) lesbian/gay identity increases acceptance of self; (2) the lesbian/gay community provides an accepting and reinforcing environment; (3) the stress of being a sexual and social minority enhances psychological and spiritual dimensions of life; and (4) minority status forces one to plan carefully for the economic problems associated with aging.

The authors conclude with appropriate cautions in generalizing these findings to all lesbians and gay men. Like most research on this population, respondents in this study tended to be white, well-educated, and relatively well-integrated into the gay and lesbian community. Nevertheless, the findings of this study, as well as findings from other studies reviewed in the article, are important for all healthcare and social service providers. Of particular concern to healthcare providers should be the repeated reference by many of the respondents to fears of discrimination as encounters with the healthcare system increase.

Additional References

Deevy, S. (1990). Older lesbian women: An invisible minority. *Journal of Gerontological Nursing, 16*(5), 35–39.

Sang, B., Warshow, J., & Smith, A. (1991). *Lesbians at midlife: The creative transition.* San Francisco, CA: Spinsters.

Alternative Insemination, Childbearing, and Parenting Issues

Eliason, M. J. (1996). Lesbian and gay family issues. *Journal of Family Nursing, 2*(1), 10–29.

Addressing nurses' daily interactions with families, Eliason notes that nurses, like most members of the general population, are likely to hold negative attitudes toward lesbian and gay parents and families. Consequently, in addition to the negative attitudes that gays and lesbians face in their daily lives, negative attitudes and beliefs of nurses may serve as an additional barrier for the gay or lesbian client in accessing healthcare. The author provides an overview of current information about gay and lesbian headed (or parented) families, explores the attitudes of nurses regarding gay and lesbian clients, and offers suggestions and strategies for nurses when working with gay or lesbian families.

Harvey, S. M., Carr, C., & Bernheine, S. (1989). Lesbian mothers' health care experiences. *Journal of Nurse-Midwifery, 34*(3), 115–119.

Lesbians are increasingly choosing to become mothers. However, there is little information available that addresses the healthcare needs and experiences of lesbian parents. Thirty-five self-identified lesbians completed a self-administered questionnaire which collected information in the following areas: demographics; support systems during pregnancy and childbirth; parenting and co-parenting issues; conception method; and utilization of obstetrical care. The method of conception used by the majority of the participants was alternative insemination in which the medical care system was accessed for assistance. Although physicians provided services for 52 percent of the participants, midwives (nurse midwives and lay midwives) provided services for all of the other women. Overall, 83 percent of the study participants reported that they felt comfortable with their providers; 91 percent disclosed their lesbianism to their provider and 79 percent reported that the provider was supportive. Most rated the quality of care as ranging from adequate to excellent. Nonetheless, practitioners were rated as inadequate to poor in terms of their awareness of homophobia and their knowledge about and sensitivity to the health concerns of lesbians. The authors suggest that the high rate of disclosure among this group of lesbians may have led to more positive experiences in their obstetrical care. However, it is also likely that participants had more positive experiences because they were predominately white, well-educated, and privately insured. Further research with a more diverse group of lesbians is needed. In addition, it is important to note that despite the positive obstetrical experiences reported in this study, providers' assumption of heterosexuality and lack of knowledge specific to the needs of lesbian mothers remained a primary criticism of the participants.

Zeidenstein, L. (1990). Gynecological and childbearing needs of lesbians. *Journal of Nurse-Midwifery, 35*(1), 10–18.

Literature pertaining to the gynecological and childbearing needs of lesbians is sparse. Homophobia and heterosexism are two factors that compound the lack of obstetric and gynecologic services for lesbians. In this study, 20 interviews were conducted to examine the gynecological and childbearing experiences of self-identified lesbians. Questions explored lesbians' disclosure of their sexual orientation in various settings such as among friends, family, and healthcare professionals; demographic information; coming-out decisions; utilization of gynecological services; and parenting issues. Patterns of disclosure to healthcare providers varied depending on the sex and sexual orientation of the provider. Full disclosure for those participants who sought the services of a lesbian provider were noted while disclosure rates were the lowest when the provider was a heterosexual man. Nurse-practitioners were chosen as the providers of obstetric and gynecologic care by the majority of participants. One-half of the participants reported having gynecologic exams annually; frequency of exams for the other one-half ranged from never to every three to five years. The majority of the interviewees were childless (65 percent). Seventy percent of the participants expressed a desire to have children. Alternative insemination was an acceptable conception method for this sample. Level of comfort in discussing lesbian parenting with providers varied with the majority reporting that they were "somewhat comfortable." Specific services related to the gynecologic and childbearing needs of lesbians need further development. Current services must be redesigned to lessen the existing heterosexist bias that limits use of these services by lesbians. Because many lesbians may choose to have their babies at home, midwives are in an excellent position to advocate for the needs of lesbians and their families.

Additional References

Chiasson, M. A., Stoneburner, R. L., & Joseph, S. C. (1990). Human immunodeficiency virus transmission through artificial insemination. *Journal of Acquired Immune Deficiency Syndromes, 3*(1), 69–72.

Kenney, J. W., & Tash, D. T. (1992). Lesbian childbearing couples' dilemmas and decisions. *Health Care for Women International, 13*(2), 209–219.

Cancer

Fred Hutchinson Cancer Research Center. (1994). *Cancer and cancer risk among lesbians.* Seattle, WA: Community Liaison Program.

This report on cancer risk among lesbians is the result of an interactive conference between the lesbian community and the Fred Hutchinson Cancer Research Center. Cancer risk among lesbians is believed to be the result of a coalescence of associated risk factors such as never having been pregnant, obesity, and alcohol consumption that are more common among lesbians than among women in the general population. This risk is compounded by lesbians' lower access to and utilization of healthcare services. The report concludes with the results of community discussion groups held at the conference that addressed concerns of the lesbian community and future research needs.

Additional References

Bowen, D. (1991). *Counseling lesbians on breast cancer risk.* Seattle, WA: Fred Hutchinson Cancer Research Center.

Mautner Project for Lesbians with Cancer (technical assistance manual for developing feminist/lesbian cancer projects). Available from 1707 L. Street, NW, Suite 1060, Washington, DC 20036. Telephone number (202) 332-5536.

Rankow, E. J. (1994). *Breast and cervical cancer among lesbians and women who partner with women.* Washington, DC: National Gay and Lesbian Task Force.

Winnow, J. (1992). Lesbians evolving health care: Cancer and AIDS. *Feminist Review, 41,* 68–76.

Mental Health

Greene, B. (1994). Lesbian women of color: Triple jeopardy. In L. Comas-Diaz & B. Greene (Eds.), *Women of color: Integrating ethnic and gender identities in psychotherapy* (pp. 389–427). New York: Guilford Press.

In this comprehensive chapter, Beverly Greene describes how lesbians of color exist within a tangle of multiply devalued identities surrounded by the oppression and discrimination that accompany institutionalized racism, sexism, and heterosexism. She states that the aim of this chapter is to assist in sensitizing mental health and other practitioners to cultural factors that impact the ways in which lesbians of color perceive the world and the unique tasks and stressors they must manage on a routine basis. Green provides relatively indepth information about African American, Native American, Asian American, Indian and Southeast Asian American, and Latina lesbians. Among the important issues discussed are reasons for immigration, language, and family and gender roles. For example, the difficult process of negotiating a lesbian identity within the family and ethnic community is complicated by strong ties to family and ethnic identity. However, Greene points out that although the stressors experienced by lesbians of color, particularly those related to coming out, are intense, we must also recognize that these women bring unique resources and resiliences to this task. That is, they have often been forced to learn useful coping mechanisms against racism and discrimination long before they realized that they were lesbian.

This chapter provides health practitioners a valuable framework from which to begin looking at lesbians and women of color from a more diverse perspective and at lesbians of color with greater cultural sensitivity.

Research issues in suicide and sexual orientation [Special issue]. (1995). *Suicide and Life-Threatening Behavior, 25* (Suppl.), 1–91.

This special issue of *Suicide and Life-Threatening Behavior* includes most of the papers from a Workshop on Research Issues in Suicide and Sexual Orientation held by the American Association of Suicidology. The papers fall generally into four categories based on working groups organized around four themes: (1) conceptual foundations for studies of suicide and sexual orientation, (2) research design for the study of suicide and sexual orientation, (3) measurement and sampling issues, and (4) research ethics.

The following general principles were developed by the working groups as guidelines for all research on suicide and sexual orientation: (1) the fundamental question is whether or not there is a relationship between sexual orientation and suicidality; (2) adherence to rigorous standards of research design is essential in studies of suicide and sexual orientation; (3) researchers must know the community they are studying; (4) research should be sensitive to the dynamic processes involved in the development of sexual orientation; (5) research should be conducted on what makes particular individuals resilient (i.e., unlikely to engage in suicidal behaviors despite otherwise high risk), and on factors that protect against suicide behavior; (6) more studies are needed, not only in the area of suicide and sexual orientation, but also in health and health-related behaviors of gay, lesbian, bisexual, and transsexual (GLBT) populations; and (7) even if future studies should yield evidence that GLBT persons do not have higher rates of suicidal behavior than do heterosexual persons, legitimate research questions remain regarding the health effects of prejudice, hostility, and violence directed against them. This special issue provides valuable information for all researchers and advocates interested in the health of GLBT persons.

Rothblum, E. D. (1990). Depression among lesbians: An invisible and unresearched phenomenon. *Journal of Gay and Lesbian Psychotherapy, 1*(3), 67–87.

The subtitle of this article, "An invisible and unresearched phenomenon," could be used to describe most, if not all, issues related to lesbians' mental health. Although depression among women in the general population has received a great deal of research attention, very little is known about lesbians' experience of depression—even though homophobia, discrimination, and overall invisibility in society present clear mental health risks. In this review article, Rothblum draws from research on factors believed to influence depression in heterosexual women, as well as from the limited research on lesbians, to piece together a picture of overall risk and protective factors related to depression among lesbians. Among the factors shared by both lesbians and heterosexual women are social support, partner relationships, children, and employment. Factors believed to influence risk of depression that are unique to lesbians are invisibility and alienation by heterosexual society, coming out, and integration into the lesbian community. Rothblum briefly reviews several mental health problems related to depression including suicide, alcohol abuse, and sexual and physical abuse.

Like other authors writing about lesbian health, Rothblum notes the limited focus of much existing research on lesbians; lesbians who are nonwhite, adolescent or older, or those in prison are likely to be at greater risk for mental health problems, yet we know very little about their experiences. The review concludes with a discussion of implications for treatment of lesbians who are depressed.

Additional References

Bradford, J., Ryan, C., & Rothblum, E. D. (1994). National lesbian health care survey: Implications for mental health care. *Journal of Consulting and Clinical Psychology, 62*(2), 228–242.

Erwin, K. (1993). Interpreting the evidence: Competing paradigms and the emergence of lesbian and gay suicide as a "social fact." *International Journal of Health Services, 23*(3), 437–453.

Greene, B. (1994). Lesbian and gay sexual orientations. In B. Greene & G. M. Herek (Eds.), *Lesbian and gay psychology: Theory, research, and clinical applications* (Vol. 1, pp. 1–24). Thousand Oaks: Sage.

Peplau, L. A. (1993). Lesbian and gay relationships. In L. D. Garnets & D. C. Kummel (Eds.), *Psychological perspectives on lesbian and gay male experience* (pp. 395–419). New York: Columbia University Press.

Peters, D. K., & Cantrell, P. J. (1993). Gender roles and role conflict in feminist lesbian and heterosexual women. *Sex Roles, 28*(7/8), 379–392.

Ross, M. W., Paulsen, J. A., & Stalstrom, O. W. (1988). Homosexuality and mental health: A cross-cultural review. *Journal of Homosexuality, 15*, 131–152.

Rothblum, E. D. (1994). I only read about myself on bathroom walls: The need for research on the mental health of lesbians and gay men. *Journal of Counseling and Clinical Psychology, 62*(2), 213–220.

Saunders, J. M., & Valente, S. M. (1987). Suicide risk among gay men and lesbians: A review. *Death Studies, 11*(1), 1–23.

Substance Use and Abuse

Hughes, T. L., & Wilsnack, S. C. (in press). Lesbians and alcohol: Research and clinical implications. *American Journal of Orthopsychiatry.*

Although the AIDS crisis has precipitated an increased interest in substance abuse among gay men, relatively little research has been done to systematically explore lesbians' use of alcohol and other drugs. This is of particular concern given persistent claims in the literature over the past two decades that as many as one-third of all women who identify as lesbian drink excessively or experience alcohol problems. This article reviews research on lesbians' use of alcohol as well as on alcohol use and abuse among women in the general population to identify potential risk and protective factors associated with alcohol abuse among lesbians.

Despite numerous limitations in the research on lesbians and alcohol, several findings are surprisingly consistent. The most notable include the following: (1) fewer lesbians than heterosexual women abstain from alcohol; (2) although rates of heavy drinking among lesbians and heterosexual women are reasonably comparable, lesbians' rates of problem drinking are higher than those of heterosexual women; and (3) the relationships between some demographic characteristics and drinking behaviors differ for lesbians and heterosexual women. This difference is particularly striking in relation to age: in contrast to heterosexual women, lesbians' rates of drinking, heavy drinking, and problem drinking do not appear to decrease with age. This finding suggests a positive relationship between age and more frequent drinking. However, an alternative explanation based on cohort or generational differences is also plausible; that is, that younger cohorts of lesbians may be drinking less than older ones.

The authors explore potential influences on drinking that may help explain lesbians' possible higher risk status. They note that despite some gains in knowledge about lesbians' drinking in recent years, there are still major gaps in this area of research. There is a clear and pressing need for studies that will more accurately document alcohol use patterns and problems as well as help to identify specific risk factors that contribute to alcohol problems among lesbians.

Additional References

Bloomfield, K. (1993). A comparison of alcohol consumption between lesbians and heterosexual women in an urban population. *Drug and Alcohol Dependence, 33*, 257–269.

Bushway, D. J. (1991). Chemical dependency treatment for lesbians and their families: The feminist challenge. In C. Bepko (Ed.), *Feminism and addiction* (pp. 161–172). New York: Haworth Press.

Hall, J. M. (1994a). The experience of lesbians in Alcoholics Anonymous. *Western Journal of Nursing Research, 16*(5), 556–576.

Hall, J. M. (1994b). How lesbians recognize and respond to alcohol problems: A theoretical model of problematization. *Advances in Nursing Science, 16*(3), 46–63.

McNally, E. B., & Finnegan, D. G. (1992). Lesbian recovering alcoholics: A qualitative study of identity transformation—A report on research and applications to treatment. *Journal of Chemical Dependency, 5*(1), 93–103.

Norris, J., & Hughes, T. L. (in press). Alcohol consumption and female sexuality. In *Women and alcohol: Prevention throughout the lifespan* (U.S. Department of Health and Human Services, National Institute on Alcohol Abuse and Alcoholism (NIAAA), Research Monograph Series). Washington, DC: U.S. Government Printing Office.

Skinner, W. F. (1994). The prevalence and demographic predictors of illicit and licit drug use among lesbians and gay men. *American Journal of Public Health, 84*(8), 1307–1310.

Underhill, B. L., & Wolverton, T. (1993). *Creating visibility: Providing lesbian-sensitive and lesbian specific alcoholism recovery services.* Los Angeles: Alcoholism Center for Women.

Violence/Abuse

Renzetti, C. M. (1993). Violence in lesbian relationships. In M. Hansen & M. Harway (Eds.), *Battering and family therapy: A feminist perspective* (pp. 188–199). Newbury Park: Sage.

Despite the fact that it is not possible to reliably estimate the incidence of violence and abuse in lesbian couples, the little existing research on this topic clearly demonstrates that lesbian relationships are not immune from these problems. In this chapter, Renzetti presents a comprehensive review of existing research (including her own) on abuse in lesbian relationships and discusses some of the most important correlates of abuse by lesbians. For example, abusers appear to be excessively dependent on their partners for emotional or financial support. Often abuse occurs in relationships in which one partner has greater resources than the other.

Renzetti suggests a number of strategies to help healthcare and social service providers respond to the needs of lesbian victims of battering. Renzetti reports that in her own and other's research, lesbians typically do not seek help for battering from traditional sources such as police, attorneys, physicians, hotlines, or battered women's shelters. Lesbians who have attempted to use these sources of support typically report negative responses to their request for help. Furthermore, lesbians in abusive relationships who seek help from the lesbian community are also often met with denial or minimization of the problem. Renzetti notes that there are compelling reasons for the lesbian community to overlook or deny battering among its members. For example, it is feared that exposure of the problem will increase already existing homophobia or that it will threaten the image of lesbian relationships as egalitarian and safe.

Renzetti ends by addressing strategies that providers can take to more effectively assist lesbians who are involved in battering relationships. She emphasizes the importance of heterosexual help providers confronting and overcoming their homophobia. Before lesbian battering can be acknowledged, providers must first acknowledge lesbian relationships. At the same time, the gay or lesbian healthcare provider must recognize that battering does exist in lesbian relationships and that it should not be minimized.

Additional References

Hughes, T. L., & Norris, J. (1995). Sexuality, sexual orientation, and violence: Pieces in the puzzle of women's use and abuse of alcohol. In B. J. McElmurry & R. S. Parker (Eds.), *Annual review of women's health* (Vol. 2, pp. 285–317). New York: NLN Press.

Neisen, J. H., & Sandall, H. (1990). Alcohol and other drug abuse in gay/lesbian populations:

Related to victimization? *Journal of Psychology and Human Sexuality, 3*(1), 151–168.

Renzetti, C. M. (1992). *Violent betrayal: Partner abuse in lesbian relationships.* New York: Sage.

Schilit, R., Lie, G., & Montagne, M. (1990). Substance abuse as a correlate of violence in intimate lesbian relationships. *Journal of Homosexuality, 19*(3), 51–65.

HIV

Stevens, P. E. (1993). Lesbians and HIV: Clinical, research, and policy issues. *American Journal of Orthopsychiatry, 63*(2), 289–294.

The fastest growing HIV-infected group is women. Lesbians with HIV, whose needs differ from other populations, remain invisible within this population. This invisibility is demonstrated by the failure, until recently, of the Centers for Disease Control (CDC) to include lesbians in their documentation of affected groups. This omission, as well as the lack of information about HIV in women generally, has contributed to the failure to develop adequate healthcare services specific to the needs of lesbians and has increased the potential for abuse of lesbians who are HIV-positive or who have AIDS. Stevens' review focuses on two major areas concerning lesbians and HIV: risks and sources of HIV infection and barriers to care. She concludes by summarizing some of the issues related to research, practice, and policy and suggests strategies for prevention and treatment.

Additional References

Brain, N. (1994). An activist's perspective on AIDS and the lesbian community. *Focus: A Guide to AIDS Research and Counseling, 8*(9), 5–8.

Chu, S. Y., Buehler, J. W., Flemming, P. L., & Berkelman, R. L. (1990). Epidemiology of reported cases of AIDS in lesbians, United States 1980–1989. *American Journal of Public Health, 80*(11), 1380–1381.

Hollibaugh, A. (1992). Lesbianism is not a condom. In *LAP Information Packet* (pp. 1–3). New York: Lesbian AIDS Project/Gay Men's Health Crisis.

Hollibaugh, A., & Vasquez, C. (1994). The myth of invulnerability: Lesbians and HIV disease. *Focus: A Guide to AIDS Research and Counseling, 8*(9), 1–4.

Maldono, M. (1991). Latinas and HIV/AIDS: Implications for the 90's. *SEICUS, 19*(2), 11–15.

Office of Gay and Lesbian Health Concerns, Bureau of HIV Program Services. (1995). *Lesbians and HIV/AIDS: Female to female transmission* (Resource Packet). New York: New York City Department of Health.

Healthcare Providers

Eliason, M. J. (1993). Cultural diversity in nursing care: The lesbian, gay, or bisexual client. *Journal of Transcultural Nursing, 5*(1), 14–20.

Homophobia remains deeply ingrained within our society and is perpetuated by traditional gender-role socialization in the dominant American culture. Nurses, like most people from the general population, are socialized to negatively view gay men, lesbians, and bisexual women and men. The author briefly discusses values and beliefs of the dominant American culture about same-sex relationships and examines the effects of heterosexism and homophobia in the healthcare system. The gay, lesbian, and bisexual subculture is examined in relation to the healthcare system and its consequent impact on access and utilization of the services. The author acknowledges that nursing education currently addresses racial and ethnic diversity yet fails to include gender, religion, able-bodiedness, and sexual identity and how these factors also impact the healthcare of the diverse and complex individuals nurses serve. Because all nurses inevitably encounter gay, lesbian, and bisexual coworkers and clients, it is imperative that they be educated about these groups, particularly as to how the present system effects healthcare for these clients.

Lynch, M. A. (1993). When the patient is also a lesbian. *AWHONN'S Clinical Issues, 4*(2), 196–202.

Stigmatization clearly impacts the quality of healthcare that lesbians receive. In this article, Lynch focuses on how health assessments can be conducted with lesbians in a manner that is both nonthreatening and conducive to obtaining useful and necessary information. The author discusses the impact of homophobia and identifies the stages of the coming out process. Several clinical situations are described as examples of how lesbian-specific concerns can be identified and addressed. Such nonjudgemental approaches to the delivery of healthcare increases the likelihood of future utilization of health services by the lesbian client.

O'Hanlan, K. A. (1995). Lesbian health and homophobia: Perspectives for the treating obstetrician/gynecologist. *Current Problems in Obstetrics, Gynecology and Fertility, 18*(4), 93–136.

O'Hanlan, in this special journal issue devoted to lesbian health and homophobia, frames homophobia as a health hazard warranting medical attention. The author begins with a discussion of the meaning of the term lesbian and proceeds to describe several theories on the formation of sexual orientation. In addition to a penetrating analysis of the effects of homophobia on the lesbian-provider relationship, O'Hanlan provides an overview of current information about lesbian health including lesbian-specific obstetrical and gynecological issues. Current information about adolescent and aging lesbians, lesbian families and family of origin issues is also summarized. Finally, strategies to combat homophobia at the micro- and macrolevels are offered. O'Hanlan notes that failure to recognize the homophobia as a clear health hazard for lesbians and gay men is a failure to recognize the opportunity to improve the health outcomes of all people.

Rankow, E. J. (1995). Lesbian health issues for the primary care provider. *The Journal of Family Practice, 40*(5), 486–493.

Marginalization and stigmatization of the lesbian-, bisexual-, or transgendered-identified person serves as barriers to accessing healthcare. The author examines the barriers to care experienced by lesbians as a result of their marginalized status as well as barriers stemming from the heterosexist assumptions of the healthcare system. In addition to barriers to healthcare experienced by all women generally (e.g., child care, transportation, economics), lesbians must also contend with discrimination, myth, and stereotypes (e.g., lesbians are immune to particular cancers, HIV infection, or sexually transmitted diseases). Personal and professional responsibility on behalf of healthcare providers to examine their own biases and to work toward elimination of attitudes and beliefs that interfere with the delivery of healthcare is emphasized.

Additional References

Buenting, J. A. (1992). Health lifestyles of lesbian and heterosexual women. *Health Care for Women International, 13,* 165–171.

Gentry, S. E. (1992). Caring for lesbians in a homophobic society. *Health Care for Women International, 13,* 173–180.

Roberts, S. J., & Sorensen, L. (1995). Lesbian health care: A review and recommendations for health promotion in primary care settings. *Nurse Practitioner, 20*(6), 42–47.

Rosser, S. V. (1993). Ignored, overlooked, or subsumed: Research on lesbian health and health care. *National Women's Studies Association Journal, 5*(2), 183–203.

Sang, B. E. (1989). New directions in lesbian research, theory, and education. *Journal of Counseling & Development, 68,* 92–96.

Stevens, P. E. (1992). Lesbian health care research: A review of the literature from 1970 to 1990. *Health Care for Women International, 13*(2), 91–120.

Lesbian Health Resources

Community Clinics

Community Health Project Women's program
The Lesbian and Gay Community
   Services Center
208 West 13th Street
New York, NY 10011
(212) 675-3559

Fenway Community Health Project
40 Trinity Place
Boston, MA
(617) 267-0900 x287

Lyon-Martin Clinic
1748 Market Street
San Francisco, CA 94102
(415) 565-7667

Whitman Walker Clinic
1407 S. Street, NW
Washington, DC 20009
(202) 797-3500

HIV/AIDS

ACT-UP Women's Safer Sex Working Group
ACT-UP Workspace
135 West 29th Street
New York, NY 10010
(212) 564-AIDS

Lesbian AIDS Project
129 West 20th Street
New York, NY 10011
(212) 807-6664

Lesbian's Educational AIDS Resource
Network
14002 Club House Circle #205
Tampa, FL 33524
(813) 362-7543

Cancer

Lesbian Community Cancer Project
4753 North Broadway, Suite 602
Chicago, IL 60640-4907
(312) 561-4662

Mautner Project for Lesbians with Cancer
P.O. Box 90437
Washington, DC 20090
(202) 332-5536

Women's Cancer Resource Center
3023 Shattuck Avenue
Berkeley, CA 94705
(415) 548-WCRC

Policy

Office of Gay and Lesbian Health Concerns
New York City Department of Health
125 Worth Street, Box 67
New York, NY 10013
(212) 566-4995

Lesbian Research Network.

Currently under development by Judy Bradford and Caitlin Ryan. Activities of the network will include: developing a communications system, formalizing a network of mentors, and providing access to technical assistance. For more information contact Caitlin Ryan, (202)232-0188, Caitlinon@aol.com.

Lesbian Health Newsletters

Lesbian Health News
P.O. Box 12121
Columbus, Ohio 43212
(614) 481-7656

Lesbian Health Issues Newsletter

National Center for Lesbian Rights
870 Market Street, #570
San Francisco, CA 94102
(415) 392-6257; FAX (415) 392-8442;
Leshealth@aol.com

Part V

Health and Work

Chapter 5

Latex Allergy: Environmental Health Threats for Women

Joan N. Martellotto

S ince the 1930s, physicians have recognized that contact with rubber products causes localized allergic dermatitis because residual chemicals used during the manufacturing process are sensitizing agents (Granady & Slater, 1995; Hamann, 1993). Within the past 20 years, a serious "new" type of rubber allergy has emerged that is capable of causing severe systemic allergic reactions and even death. Termed *latex allergy*, this condition involves a hypersensitization to proteins in natural rubber latex, the substance from which natural rubber products are manufactured. Latex allergy is an international health problem affecting a growing number of people, many of whom are women and children (Kelly, 1995a; Slater, 1994; Turjanmaa, 1994). This allergy is causing chronic illness, career loss, and hardship for persons with advanced sensitization. And, it is generating important economic, technical, legal, and safety issues for manufacturers, regulatory agencies, employers, healthcare providers, and consumers.

Since latex allergy affects women's health from several different perspectives, this chapter provides information that women can use to understand the disease and reduce risk for themselves, their families, and persons with whom they associate in other roles. The initial discussion explains latex and the outbreak of latex allergy, then describes how sensitization develops, who is at risk, how the disease is diagnosed and managed, and glove issues that affect the risk of sensitization. Following the discussion, abstracts describe research concerning allergens in latex gloves. The chapter concludes with implications for education, practice, research, and health policy.

NATURAL RUBBER LATEX

Natural rubber latex is the liquid portion of cell cytoplasm in numerous species of plants (Truscott, 1995). Many people recognize latex as the milky fluid that appears when they remove a poinsettia leaf, prune a ficus houseplant, or snap a dandelion root. Latex is also a generic term that includes synthetic emulsions such as latex paint, but synthetic latex does not apply to latex allergy (Slater, 1992).

The source of latex for rubber manufacturing is the rubber tree, *Heavea brasiliensis,* native to the Amazon rainforest and cultivated on commercial plantations mainly in southeast Asia. Raw latex consists of molecules of rubber hydrocarbon that are surrounded by proteins and lipids and suspended in an aqueous serum. When latex is processed and reacted with various chemicals, the rubber molecules link into a network that is strong, elastic, durable, and relatively insoluble (Truscott, 1995). These characteristics make latex highly desirable for heavy-duty rubber products, as well as for medical devices and consumer products that require flexibility, durability, and good tactile and barrier properties. Over 40,000 products are made from latex (Stapleton, 1993).

HISTORY OF LATEX ALLERGY

Allergy to proteins in natural rubber products became an important issue only within the past 20 years. Before that, the disease was practically unrecognized. In 1927, systemic allergy to rubber appeared in two case reports in Germany, then disappeared from the medical literature for over 30 years except for two unconfirmed cases in 1954 and 1960 in Europe and brief mention in 1957 in a German textbook of allergy (Fuchs, 1994; Hamann, 1993).

In 1979, Nutter confirmed latex allergy in a 34-year-old English housewife who developed intense itching and hives on her hands from wearing household gloves, and had long-standing dermatitis mainly involving her hands (Nutter, 1979). Soon, case reports from other European countries described systemic allergic reactions to latex gloves. And in 1987, Turjanmaa in Finland published the first research report showing the incidence of systemic allergy to latex gloves in hospital personnel (Turjanmaa, 1987).

In the United States, latex allergy erupted late in 1987, shortly after the Centers for Disease Control announced universal precautions to prevent transmission of bloodborne pathogens in healthcare settings. By September 1992, the Food and Drug Administration (FDA) received reports of 1,133 serious allergic reactions occurring to patients and healthcare workers mostly from medical gloves and barium enema catheters. Fifteen patients died (Dillard & MacCollum, 1992). The FDA estimated that these figures represented only 1 percent of actual cases (Levy, 1993). During that same period, many children with spina bifida who underwent anesthesia and surgery developed anaphylactic shock from latex medical devices (Slater, 1992).

In 1991, the FDA advised healthcare providers to identify latex-allergic patients, notified manufacturers to correct deficiencies in manufacturing processes, and issued regulations to improve sampling and testing gloves for leakage. In 1992, the agency convened an international latex allergy conference. Subsequently the FDA announced it would develop regulations to label the latex content of medical devices, and change confusing "hypoallergenic" labeling [Food and Drug Administration (FDA), 1993].

Researchers have proposed multiple causes for the latex allergy outbreak. Among these are: (a) increased exposure to latex caused by universal precautions; (b) alterations in latex proteins due to changes in latex source, cultivation, harvesting, and aging; (c) changes in manufacturers' processes; (d) the action of glove powder to absorb and bind proteins from latex gloves; (e) glove wearers' use of handcare products; (f) immunological cross-reactions between latex proteins and other allergens; and (g) improved recognition of latex allergy (Charous, 1994; Truscott, 1995).

LATEX SENSITIZATION

Allergies are responses in which the immune system reacts strongly to foreign substances, or allergens, that normally are inoffensive (Lichtenstein, 1993). Latex, which had seemed to be an inoffensive substance, contains over 200 protein fragments, and many of them induce allergy (Alenius, Makinen-Kiljunen, Turjanmaa, Palosuo, & Reunala, 1994). Persons become allergic to latex by repeated exposures to rubber products through an intricate process in the immune system called *sensitization*. Latex sensitization begins when the allergen enters the body, and continues silently for weeks or months before the individual experiences allergic symptoms. The routes of allergen entry are through skin or mucous membrane, inhalation, inoculation of surgical wounds, injection, or ingestion (Kelly, 1995a; Schwartz, 1995).

During sensitization, the immune system produces antibodies, known as antilatex IgE, that identify and bind the latex allergens. After repeated contact with allergens in rubber products, a critical level of latex-specific IgE develops, and subsequent latex exposures trigger allergic reactions (Lichtenstein, 1993). The amount of allergen and the time necessary to develop latex allergy are unknown (Kelly, 1995b), and persons differ according to the various combinations of latex proteins to which they become sensitized (Alenius et al., 1994).

Symptoms of latex allergic reactions include dermatitis, flushing, burning and itching skin, localized or generalized hives, facial swelling, nasal congestion, tearing eyes, cough, asthma, abdominal cramping, diarrhea, hoarseness, laryngeal swelling, hypotension, cardiopulmonary collapse, and sometimes death (Hamann, 1993; Kelly, 1995a; Moneret-Vautrin et al., 1993; Slater, 1994). Symptom onset may be mild with gradual progression, although some individuals skip this progression and experience an abrupt onset of anaphylaxis, a multi-system response which can be life-threatening (Kelly, 1995a). The severity of the allergic reaction does not necessarily correlate with an individual's level of antilatex IgE (Charous, Hamilton, & Yunginger, 1994; Kwittken, Sweinberg, Campbell, & Pawlowski, 1995). Persons with latex allergy can react to very low levels of allergens and have an unusual propensity to develop asthma and anaphylaxis (Kelly, 1995a, 1995b).

VULNERABLE POPULATIONS

Although anyone can become sensitized to latex, persons at most risk are those with a genetic tendency to develop allergies who also have frequent exposure to rubber products (Kelly, 1995a; Kwittken, Sweinberg, Campbell, & Pawlowski, 1995; Moneret-Vautrin et al., 1993). The highest risk groups are healthcare workers and others with occupational exposure to latex, persons with multiple surgical procedures, and children with spina bifida or urogenital disorders (Kelly, 1995a; Slater, 1994; Turjanmaa, 1994).

Risk increases for individuals with allergies to fruits and vegetables containing proteins similar to latex proteins, but it is not clear whether allergy to latex or food appears first (Moneret-Vautrin et al., 1993). Cross-reacting foods include avocado, potato, banana, tomato, chestnut, and kiwi (Beezhold, Sussman, Liss, & Chang, 1996), conduirango, an ingredient in some herbal teas (Justicia, Munoz, Sequardo, & Barcelo, 1996), and papain, a fruit enzyme used in meat tenderizers, beer, chewing gum, and in non-food items (e.g., douche powder, cosmetics, and more), (Bauer, Chen, Rozynek, Duser, & Raulf-Heimsoth, 1995; Niimaki, Reijula, Pirila, & Koistinen, 1993). Other foods also may cross-react with latex proteins.

The exact prevalence of latex allergy is unknown, and broad based epidemiological studies are urgently needed (Charous, 1995). Researchers identified latex sensitization in 6.5 percent of blood donors in southeastern

Michigan (Ownby, Ownby, McCullough, & Shafer, 1994), in 14 percent of blood donors and 26 percent of asthmatics in Los Angeles (LeBerthon, Glovsky, Miguel, Weiss, & Cass, 1996), and in 4.5 percent of patients in an adult allergy clinic in Canada (Hadjiliadis, Khan, & Tarlo, 1995).

OCCUPATIONALLY INDUCED LATEX ALLERGY

Concerning occupationally induced latex allergy, numerous small studies in healthcare institutions have shown that between 8 percent and 17 percent of healthcare workers in all disciplines are sensitized to latex (Charous, 1995). However, many studies are biased by selective sampling techniques.

Latex gloves contribute significant allergen exposure among healthcare workers (Kelly, 1995a) and are the most important cause of symptoms (Turjanmaa, 1994). Protein allergens are loosely bound to glove surfaces, readily transfer to the skin of glove wearers and patients, and are absorbed through skin (Beezhold, Kostyal, & Wiseman, 1994). The exact mechanism of skin penetration is not understood (Turjanmaa, 1994). Hand dermatitis increases risk of latex sensitization among glove users by enhancing allergen absorption through injured skin (Turjanmaa, 1994). Hand cream increases the amount of protein that transfers from gloves to wearers' hands (Beezhold, Kostyal, & Wiseman, 1994). Oil-based handcare products (e.g., lanolin, jojoba, cocoa butter, palm oil, mineral oil, petrolatum, or other petroleum products) worn with latex gloves degrade latex, damage the glove barrier, and release additional allergens to the skin (Truscott & Roley, 1995).

Cornstarch glove powder, which is the approved donning powder in the United States, absorbs and binds protein allergens from gloves and deposits them on glove wearers' hands, and also transfers by touch to other persons and objects (e.g., telephones, medical records, door knobs) immediately upon contact. Protein transfer is higher with powdered gloves than powder-free gloves. Glove wearers who do not wash their hands thoroughly after removing gloves increase their personal allergen exposure and also contaminate the environment. In surgery, wiping surgical gloves with saline-soaked sponges is inadequate to remove powder or latex protein, which subsequently innoculate surgical wounds (Beezhold, Kostyal, & Wiseman, 1994). Additionally, glove powder binds and aerosolizes latex allergens, is inhaled by persons in the vicinity, contaminates surfaces and enters ventilating systems (Beezhold, Kostyal, & Wiseman, 1994; Swanson et al., 1994). Cornstarch glove powder in itself is not an allergen, as glove users commonly believe it to be, but instead absorbs and transfers glove allergens (Turjanmaa, 1994).

In occupations other than healthcare, research has shown that latex allergy is prevalent in 11 percent of latex glove factory workers (Tarlo, Wong, Roos, & Booth, 1990), 9 percent of doll manufacturing plant workers (Orfan, Reed, Dykewicz, Ganz, & Kolski, 1994), and 5 percent of greenhouse workers (Carrillo et al., 1995). Latex-sensitization occurs among beauticians, dairy workers, kitchen workers, cleaners, textile workers, day care workers, cashiers, farmers' wives, artists, rubber band factory workers, and others (Hadjiliadis, Khan, & Tarlo, 1995; Taylor, 1996; Turjanmaa, 1994).

WOMEN AND LATEX ALLERGY

Women predominate in all published studies reporting latex allergy among glove users, but this sex preponderance is not clear among physicians, and does not prevail among persons with spina bifida (Kelly, 1995a; Turjanmaa, 1994). Most women working in healthcare wear ambidextrous nonsterile examination gloves, which generally contain more allergens than surgical gloves (Kelly, 1995b). Non-medical gloves worn by workers in food service, hairdressing, and other female-dominated occupations are a low quality that fails to meet FDA standards for medical use (FDA, 1993). Latex-sensitized women have experienced anaphylaxis while wearing household gloves (Morales, Basomba, Carriera, & Sastre, 1989) or medical gloves, during vaginal examination, childbirth, anesthesia and surgery, after dental work, after sexual intercourse, and after a squash game (Granady & Slater, 1995).

CHILDREN AND LATEX ALLERGY

Between 18 percent and 67 percent of persons with spina bifida have developed latex-specific antibodies, although not all are symptomatic (Kelly, 1995a). The sources of latex exposure for these persons are multiple surgical procedures and removal of fecal impactions with latex gloves, and frequent urinary catheterization. Children with urinary-genital abnormalities are also at risk from multiple surgeries and frequent instrumentation with latex gloves and catheters. It is essential that persons with spina bifida or urinary-genital abnormalities avoid contact with latex in medical care and personal life because of their high risk for latex sensitization (American Academy of Allergy and Immunology, 1993; Kelly, 1995a).

Multiple surgical procedures, particularly at an early age, constitute an independent risk factor (Moneret-Vautrin et al., 1993). Researchers at the Children's Hospital of Pennsylvania reported that 40 percent of latex-sensitized children did not have spina bifida or urinary-genital abnormalities, although multiple surgeries or multiple hospitalizations were common (Kwittken et al., 1995). The role of intense latex exposure early in life leading to latex sensitization is not yet understood (Kelly, 1995a).

DIAGNOSIS

Early diagnosis of latex allergy is essential to prevent advanced sensitization and chronic illness, and also to eliminate unnecessary concern for persons whose allergic symptoms are not caused by latex. Persons who have symptoms suggestive of latex allergy are advised to consult a board-certified allergist who is knowledgeable about the disease. Examples of symptoms requiring further evaluation are: (a) reddened, itching, or burning skin, hives, nasal congestion, or asthma after contact with rubber products (e.g., balloons, nipples, pacifiers, gloves, handle grips, elastic, wrist straps, adhesives, shoes, stretch textiles, sports equipment); (b) itching or swelling after contact with condoms; (c) swollen lips or tongue after dental care; (d) hand dermatitis, hives, nasal congestion, or asthma associated with latex exposure at work; (e) unexplained hives or anaphylaxis associated with surgery, medical care, or everyday activities; (f) oral itching or abdominal cramps after eating fruits or vegetables, or food handled with latex gloves; (g) hand dermatitis associated with rubber; or (h) pain, burning, swelling, or difficulty urinating after catheterization (Moneret-Vautrin et al., 1993; Schwartz, 1995; Sussman & Beezhold, 1995; Turjanmaa, 1994). A history of allergic symptoms is not diagnostic of latex allergy and requires further evaluation.

Diagnostic testing consists of skin prick, serum, or wear tests. Skin prick testing, the most accurate diagnostic method, is not generally available in the United States because of lack of a standardized extract and latex glove extracts developed in research centers have caused anaphylaxis. Testing of a new extract is progressing (Kelly, 1995a), and extracts are being used safely in Canada and Europe.

Serum studies for antilatex antibodies are the ELISA and RAST tests, which have great variability among laboratories, and may lack sensitivity because of the different antigen sources (Kelly, 1995a; Turjanmaa, 1994). In 1995, the FDA approved the AlaSTAT® test for antilatex IgE (Diagnostic Products Corporation, Los Angeles, CA), and it is available at many reference laboratories throughout the country.

Individuals who have a compelling history but a negative serum test require further evaluation by a wear or use test. The use test is performed by placing a moistened glove finger on the patient's index finger for 15 minutes with adequate resuscitation and medical support services available in case anaphylaxis occurs. Immediate itching, redness, or hives indicate a positive test. If the finger test is negative, the use test continues with a whole latex glove on the wetted hand and a vinyl glove on the other hand as a control. If the whole hand test is negative, the use test may continue for up to a week (Kelly, 1995a; Turjanmaa, 1994).

Persons with hand dermatitis related to rubber require early differential diagnosis from a board-certified dermatologist who is knowledgeable about glove-associated dermatitis and latex allergy. Early diagnosis and treatment are essential to prevent advanced latex sensitization, chronic skin disease, and secondary infections. Evaluation consists of patch testing for rubber chemicals and also testing for latex allergy because the two conditions can occur concurrently (Moneret-Vautrin et al., 1993; Taylor, 1996; Turjanmaa, 1994).

PATIENT SELF-CARE

There is no treatment for latex allergy except complete avoidance of latex, although immunotherapy may become available when the allergens are fully identified. Sensitized persons and parents of sensitized children need to implement the following self-care measures: (a) avoid all contact with rubber by any route of exposure, (b) wear a Medic Alert® bracelet to provide emergency information, (c) carry auto-injectable epinephrine and avoid using beta blockers that will potentiate anaphylaxis (Selner & Kopke, undated), (d) carry synthetic medical gloves and tourniquet, and emergency orders, (e) negotiate latex-safe healthcare, emergency services, and dental care with healthcare providers and hospitals; and (f) inform family, friends, teachers, employers, and colleagues about latex allergy (American Academy of Allergy and Immunology, 1993; Kelly, 1995a; Kwittken et al., 1995). Latex-sensitized persons must *never* wear latex gloves (Gehring, Fink, & Kelly, 1996) and must not be in the vicinity of persons wearing powdered latex gloves because of aerosolized allergens bound to glove powder (Truscott & Roley, 1995). Individuals who have developed asthma need to be well-informed about appropriate management to prevent progression and emergencies. It is inadvisable for sensitized individuals to remain in contact with latex and medicate with antihistamines to reduce allergic symptoms because antihistamines are not known to block IgE production, and sensitization may increase.

Anecdotal information from allergists and support groups indicates that many newly diagnosed persons with advanced sensitization experience an initial period of severe crisis. While coping with illness and frightening acute allergic reactions, they are disbelieved (Hospital Employee Health, 1994). They must identify and eliminate direct contact with natural rubber products, which are ubiquitous and generally unlabeled, and find nonlatex alternatives for their workplaces, healthcare, homes, clothing, recreation, and everyday activities. And some persons cannot continue working because of reactions to latex contamination in the workplace. The transition for otherwise healthy, stable individuals can be shocking, costly, and time-consuming. Finances and relationships become strained, and uninformed employers, healthcare providers, and associates compound patients' difficulties in regaining physical, emotional, and financial stability (Gehring, 1994; Hospital Employee Health, 1994; Martellotto, 1994).

Importantly, Sussman and Beezhold (1996) observe that *rubber phobia*, a morbid fear of all products potentially containing rubber, has emerged in response to latex allergy. Thus, sensitized individuals need to know that various products made from natural rubber latex vary in their allergenic potential, and healthcare providers must calm the hysteria that develops with increasing problems with latex.

Many individuals with advanced latex sensitization report making successful transitions with psychological counseling to cope with depression and identity issues, legal counsel to deal with employment issues, and support group affiliation to learn practical aspects of living with latex allergy. Information and support is available from A.L.E.R.T., Inc. (Milwaukee, WI), Latex Allergy Information Service, and the ELASTIC Support Network (Torrington, CT), the Canadian Latex Allergy Association (Port Hope, Ontario), the Spina Bifida Association of America (Washington, DC), and the Spina Bifida Association of Canada (Winnipeg).

HEALTHCARE SETTINGS

Hospitals and other healthcare and dental care settings have the dual challenge of providing latex-safe care for sensitized and high risk patients, and providing a safe workplace for all employees. Hospitals can accomplish this mission by forming a multidisciplinary latex allergy taskforce to set standards and establish policies and procedures for all inpatient and outpatient care and for employee health (Kelly, 1995a). Disciplines essential to the taskforce include administration, risk management, nursing, allergy-immunology, dermatology, pediatrics, anesthesiology, operating room, intensive care, respiratory therapy, emergency services, pharmacy, materials management, central supply, housekeeping, and dietary services.

Patient Care

Standards of care for patients with latex allergy should identify high risk and sensitized patients, provide patient education and referrals, and deliver care with nonlatex medical devices. The FDA expects to publish new regulations requiring manufacturers to label the latex content of medical devices during 1997 (FDA, 1996). But until latex is labeled, healthcare facilities must develop an inventory of latex-free medical devices by obtaining manufacturers' written verification of the material content of each medical device. Examples of latex-containing items that require nonlatex alternatives include gloves, stethoscopes, blood pressure equipment, tourniquets, IV sets, Heparin lock devices, band aids, adhesive tape, elastic wraps, syringe plungers, medication vial tops, prefilled syringes, tubings, anesthesia and resuscitation equipment, electrode pads, drains, occlusive dressings, straps, heating/cooling blankets, nipples and pacifiers, and more.

Employee Health

Employee health standards should be proactive, providing a safe workplace that is free of latex contamination to reduce employees' risk of sensitization and accommodate sensitized workers (Culver, 1995). Failure to address latex sensitization in the workplace generates significant costs for employers in the forms of sick time, medical diagnosis, worker retraining, worker replacement, disability, workers' compensation, and vocational rehabilitation. A risk reduction program for employee health includes policies and procedures that: (a) minimize latex exposure by cleaning contaminated environments and ensuring that all gloves are powder-free and low in latex and chemical allergens, (b) ensure that employees wear gloves that are suitable for their tasks, (c) inform employees of the risk of occupational latex sensitization, (d) provide staff orientation and inservice education regarding safe glove use practices and latex allergy, (e) accomplish early detection and treatment of hand dermatitis, and (f) provide early identification and accommodation of latex-sensitized personnel.

Policies regarding hand care can ensure that employees with dermatitis do not wear latex gloves or work in situations where risk is high for exposure to bloodborne pathogens until the skin heals. The employee's medical diagnosis should direct glove selection (Hamann, 1993). Employers must provide synthetic gloves for latex-allergic employees, and gloves free of offending chemicals for workers with glove-associated chemical contact dermatitis (Occupational Safety and Health Administration, 1991). Latex-allergic staff and patients must *never* have contact with so-called "hypoallergenic" latex gloves. The term "hypoallergenic," which refers to reduced sensitizing chemicals, does not have uniform meaning among manufacturers and will be discontinued under the new FDA labelling regulations (FDA, 1996). Personnel responsible for glove purchases may obtain additional information from a comprehensive list of gloves classified according to sensitizing chemicals and latex and synthetic material content developed by Hamann and Kick (1994). Newer information is available from manufacturers' representatives.

Concerning latex allergens in gloves, many manufacturers have improved processes to remove allergens, but progress is not uniform among all manufacturers (Kelly, 1995b). The FDA has not limited the allowable allergen content of medical devices because there is no standard test method for protein allergens. As an interim measure, the FDA is allowing manufacturers the option of labelling medical gloves according to their extractable protein level determined by the modified Lowry Method (FDA, 1995). The agency expects that buyers who choose gloves with lower extractable protein content generally will get a lower concentration of allergens (V. Tomazic, personal communication, April 26, 1996), which will slow the rate of sensitization (Truscott, 1995).

Considering the seriousness of latex allergy, it is imperative that persons who buy gloves make informed choices that reduce the risk of latex and chemical sensitization while providing a durable barrier against pathogens. Concerning barrier quality, latex remains the material of choice because of its durability and capacity to seal pin holes. However, healthcare facilities can reduce latex exposure by substituting synthetic gloves for latex in selected situations. Vinyl tears easily, but is acceptable for brief use in situations that do not stress the material (Korniewicz, 1995). Improved vinyls and new synthetic materials show promise, and their efficacy in various clinical situations will be defined by further research.

RISK REDUCTION IN OTHER SETTINGS

Workers in all occupations where there is latex exposure can request workplace risk evaluations from local offices of the Occupational Safety and Health Administration (OSHA) and the National Institute of Occupational Safety and Health (NIOSH, phone [800]-356-4674). Both agencies regard latex allergy as a high-priority issue and are preparing advisory statements.

It is inadvisable to use latex gloves unnecessarily in situations where synthetic gloves or lined utility gloves would be more appropriate. Cleaners, food industry workers, beauticians, cashiers, and others wearing latex medical-type gloves need to know that nonmedical latex gloves are an inferior quality that fails FDA standards for medical gloves (FDA, 1993). They may provide unnecessary exposure to latex allergens and may not be reliable barriers against microorganisms. Additionally, when these gloves are used with detergents or chemicals, they degrade in minutes and increase wearers' exposure to latex allergens (Truscott & Roley, 1995). Furthermore, allergens transfer from latex gloves onto objects and food, and can produce allergic reactions in latex-sensitized people who touch the objects or eat the food (Beezhold, Kostyal, & Wiseman, 1994; Schwartz, 1995).

IMPLICATIONS OF LATEX ALLERGY

The implications generated by latex allergy for education, practice, research, and health policy are numerous and overlapping. Although latex allergy is a serious and growing international health problem, the healthcare community and public generally are unaware of this disease, and practice, research, and policy areas have been slow to evolve. Therefore, education is urgently needed within the healthcare community and health professions schools to emphasize prevention, and to diagnose and treat sensitized individuals. Since the FDA has not regulated the allergen content of medical gloves, primary prevention requires personnel who purchase medical gloves to be well-informed about glove materials, allergens, FDA regulatory requirements, and methods of glove evaluation. In turn, glove wearers must be knowledgeable about glove use practices that affect the risk of latex sensitization, and should avoid wearing high-allergen or powdered latex gloves.

In occupations where workers wear protective gloves such as cleaning, food service, hairdressing, workers need education about the unnecessary risk they assume by using latex gloves when other materials are more appropriate for their tasks. Educational needs are particularly apparent in food service industries (e.g., restaurants, grocery stores, food processing plants) where latex gloves can harm workers and latex-sensitized consumers.

In healthcare, workers who wear gloves can reduce risk for patients and staff by requiring employers to provide low allergen powder-free gloves for situations where a latex barrier is necessary to prevent transmission of bloodborne pathogens, and synthetic materials in situations where bloodborne pathogen exposure is a low risk. Practice guidelines are needed to define appropriate clinical uses of latex and synthetic gloves. Concerning workplace safety, employers and workers may request assistance from NIOSH and OSHA to resolve problems with latex contamination in the workplace.

Women may decide to reduce unnecessary latex exposures for themselves and their families by ensuring that their health and dental care providers treat them with low allergen gloves. Women also can reduce exposure by selecting nonlatex products for household gloves, condoms, balloons, nipples, pacifiers, teething rings, and other consumer products.

Concerning research, epidemiological studies are needed to measure the prevalence of latex allergy and refine knowledge of risk factors, including studies of latex contamination in workplaces. Urgent priorities in immunological research are to develop a commercial latex extract for skin testing, identify the major latex allergens and characterize their molecular structure, and develop immunotherapy for sensitized patients. Additionally since many glove manufacturers are able to produce gloves that are low in latex and chemical allergens, immunological research is necessary to standardize a method to assay extractable allergens that will guide glove selection. Furthermore, research is required to develop synthetic glove materials as alternatives to latex, and to define their functional scope in clinical applications.

Health policy implications of latex allergy are numerous and challenging. On the federal level, the FDA, OSHA, and NIOSH must notify healthcare workers of the risk of latex sensitization. Additionally, OSHA and NIOSH expertise is needed to develop standards for latex safety in the workplace, monitor progress, and require employers to announce this hazard annually as specified by OSHA regulations. Standards defining acceptable levels of latex aeroallergens in healthcare settings are needed to prevent sensitization and accommodate latex-allergic patients and workers. When reasonable accommodation in the workplace is not possible, but workers are not totally disabled, policy is needed to develop latex-safe vocational alternatives for this unique population.

FDA labeling regulations specifying material content and the presence of sensitizing chemicals are necessary to ensure the safety of patients and staff and relieve the costly replication of effort that healthcare providers expend to obtain this information. Relatedly, FDA regulations are needed to define maximal allowable levels of extractable allergens in medical devices, and to specify a standardized method of measuring allergens, and to standardize the definition of powder-free gloves.

Additionally, clinical practice guidelines for prevention, evaluation, and management of latex allergy with a companion consumer's guide are needed to enhance the quality of healthcare services for latex-sensitized individuals and prevent costly duplication of effort among healthcare institutions. Input for these guides should incorporate the expertise of all concerned disciplines including the sensitized healthcare worker population and parents of sensitized children.

The outbreak of latex allergy is a complex challenge with many implications for women and their families. Effective prevention of latex allergy and treatment of latex-allergic patients requires immediate, intensive cooperation between government agencies, the rubber industry, manufacturers, researchers, clinicians, healthcare facilities, and the growing population of sensitized patients. Women can participate in this collaboration by acting within their many roles to stop the threat of latex sensitization for themselves and their families.

REFERENCES

Alenius, H., Kurup, V., Kelly, K., Palosuo, T., Turjanmaa, K., & Fink, J. (1994). Latex allergy: Frequent occurrence of IgE antibodies to a cluster of 11 latex proteins in patients with spina bifida and histories of anaphylaxis. *Journal of Laboratory and Clinical Medicine, 125,* 712–720.

American Academy of Allergy and Immunology. (1993). Task Force on Allergic Reactions to Latex: Committee report. *Journal of Allergy and Clinical Immunology, 92,* 16–18.

Bauer, X., Chen, Z., Rozynek, P., Duser, P., & Raulf-Heimsoth, M. (1995). Cross-reacting antibodies recognizing latex allergens, including Hev b I, as well as papain. *Allergy, 50,* 604–609.

Beezhold, D. H., Kostyal, D. A., & Wiseman, J. (1994). The transfer of protein allergens from latex gloves: A study of influencing factors. *AORN Journal, 59,* 605, 607–608, 610, 612–613.

Beezhold, D. H., Sussman, G. L., Liss, G. M., & Chang, N. S. (1996). Latex allergy can induce clinical reactions to specific foods. *Clinical and Experimental Allergy, 26,* 416–422.

Carrillo, T., Blanco, C., Quiralte, J., Castillo, R., Cuevas, M., & de Castro, F. (1995). Prevalence of latex allergy among greenhouse workers. *Journal of Allergy and Clinical Immunology, 96,* 699–701.

Charous, B. L. (1994). The puzzle of latex allergy: Some answers, still more questions. *Annals of Allergy, 73,* 277–281.

Charous, B. L. (1995). American College of Allergy, Asthma and Immunology position statement: Latex allergy—an emerging healthcare problem. *Annals of Allergy, Asthma, and Immunology, 75,* 19–21.

Charous, B. L., Hamilton, R. G., & Yunginger, J. W. (1994). Occupational latex exposure: Characteristics of contact and systemic reactions in 47 workers. *Journal of Allergy and Clinical Immunology, 94,* 12-18.

Culver, J. B. (1995). Latex sensitivity in health care workers: Part 2: A risk reduction model. *Journal of Hospital Occupational Health, 15*(3), 1, 6–10.

Dillard, S. F., & MacCollum, M. A. (1992, November). Reports to the FDA: Allergic reactions to latex-containing medical devices. In *Program and Proceedings of the International Latex Conference: Sensitivity to Latex in Medical Devices* (p. 23). Baltimore, MD: Food and Drug Administration, Center for Devices and Radiological Health.

Food and Drug Administration, Center for Devices and Radiological Health. (1993). *Regulatory requirements for medical gloves: A workshop manual* (HHS Publication No. FDA 93-4257). Washington, DC: U.S. Government Printing Office.

Food and Drug Administration, Center for Devices and Radiological Health. (1995, March). *Interim guidance on protein content labeling claim for latex medical gloves.* Rockville, MD: Author.

Food and Drug Administration. (1996, June 24). Latex-containing devices; User labeling; Proposed rule. *Federal Register, 61*(122), 32618–32621.

Fuchs, T. (1994). Latex allergy. *Journal of Allergy and Clinical Immunology, 93*, 951–952.

Gehring, L. L. (1994). Support for healthcare workers with latex allergy. *Source to Surgery, 2*(2), 1, 4. (Available from AnsellCares, P. O. Box 537, Hartland, WI 53029)

Gehring, L. L., Fink, J. N., & Kelly, K. J. (1996). Evaluation of low allergenic gloves in latex sensitive patients. *Journal of Allergy and Clinical Immunology, 97*, 186. (Abstract No. 13)

Granady, L., & Slater, J. E. (1995). The history and diagnosis of latex allergy. *Immunology and Allergy Clinics of North America, 15*(1), 21–29.

Hadjiliadis, D., Khan, K., & Tarlo, S. M. (1995). Skin test responses to latex in an allergy and asthma clinic. *Journal of Allergy and Clinical Immunology, 96*, 431–432.

Hamann, C. P. (1993). Natural rubber latex protein sensitivity in review. *American Journal of Contact Dermatitis, 4*(1), 4–21.

Hamann, C. P., & Kick, S. A. (1994). Diagnosis-driven management of natural rubber latex glove sensitivity. In G. A. Mellstrom, J. E. Wahlberg, & H. I. Maibach (Eds.), *Protective gloves for occupational use* (pp. 131–156). Boca Raton, FL: CRC Press.

Hospital Employee Health. (1994). Latex allergy suffers fight uphill battle to collect worker's compensation. *Hospital Employee Health, 13*(2), pp. 1, 14–18.

Justicia, J. L., Munoz, M. A., Sequardo, E., & Barcelo, M. (1996). Cross-reactivity between latex and a medicinal plant: Martadenia conduirango. *Journal of Allergy and Clinical Immunology, 97*, 322. (Abstract No. 557)

Kelly, K. J. (1995a). Management of the latex-allergic patient. *Immunology and Allergy Clinics of North America, 15*(1), 139–157.

Kelly, K. J. (1995b). Stop the sensitization. *Source to Surgery, 3*(1), 1, 6–7, 12. (Available from AnsellCares, P. O. Box 537, Hartland, WI 53029)

Korniewicz, D. M. (1995). Barrier protection of latex. *Immunology and Allergy Clinics of North America, 15*, 123–137.

Kwittken, P. L., Sweinberg, S. K., Campbell, D. E., & Pawlowski, N. A. (1995). Latex hypersensitivity in children: Clinical presentation and detection of latex-specific immunoglobulin E. *Pediatrics, 95*, 693–699.

LeBerthon, B., Glovsky, M. M., Miguel, A., Weiss, J., & Cass, G. (1996). Latex antibody in asthmatics and blood donors and latex allergens in paved road dust and airborne particles in Los Angeles. *Journal of Allergy and Clinical Immunology, 97*, 324. (Abstract No. 567)

Levy, D. A. (1993). Report on the International Latex Conference: Sensitivity to latex in medical devices. *Allergy, 48*(4, Suppl. 1–9).

Lichtenstein, L. M. (1993, September). Allergy and the immune system. *Scientific American,* 117–124.

Martellotto, J. N. (1994). Experiences of latex-allergic hospital employees. *Source to Surgery, 2*(2), 3–4. (Available from AnsellCares, P. O. Box 537, Hartland, WI 53029)

Moneret-Vautrin, D. -A., Beaudouin, E., Widmer, S., Mouton, C., Kanny, G., Prestat, F., Kohler, C., & Feldmann, L. (1993). Prospective study of risk factors in natural rubber latex hypersensitivity. *Journal of Allergy and Clinical Immunology, 92,* 668–699.

Morales, C., Basomba, A., Carriera, J., & Sastre, A. (1989). Anaphylaxis produced by rubber glove contact. Case reports and immunological identification of antigens involved. *Clinical and Experimental Allergy, 19,* 425–430.

Niimaki, A., Reijula, K., Pirila, T., & Koistinen, A. M. (1993). Papain-induced allergic rhinoconjunctivitis in a cosmetologist. *Journal of Allergy and Clinical Immunology, 92,* 492–493.

Nutter, A. F. (1979). Contact urticaria to rubber. *British Journal of Dermatology, 101,* 597–598.

Occupational Safety and Health Administration. (1994, April 6). Occupational exposure to bloodborne pathogens: Final rule, 29 CFR Part 1910.1030. *Federal Register, 56,* 64175–64182.

Orfan, N. A., Reed, R., Dykewicz, M. S., Ganz, M., & Kolski, G. B. (1994). Occupational asthma in a latex doll manufacturing plant. *Journal of Allergy and Clinical Immunology, 94,* 826–830.

Ownby, D. R., Ownby, H. E., McCullough, J. A., & Shafer, A. W. (1994). The prevalence of anti-latex IgE antibodies in 1000 volunteer blood donors. *Journal of Allergy and Clinical Immunology, 95,* 282. (Abstract No. 717)

Schwartz, H. J. (1995). Latex: A potential hidden "food" allergen in fast food restaurants. *Journal of Allergy and Clinical Immunology, 95,* 139–140.

Selner, J. C., & Koepke, J. W. (undated). *Beta blockers and potentiation of anaphylaxis.* Denver: Allergy Respiratory Institute of Colorado.

Slater, J. E. (1992). Allergic reactions to natural rubber. *Annals of Allergy, 69,* 203–209.

Slater, J. E. (1994). Latex allergy. *Journal of Allergy and Clinical Immunology, 94,* 139–150.

Stapleton, C. (1993, February 2). The latex scare. *Woman's Day,* 74–75.

Sussman, G. L., & Beezhold, D. H. (1995). Allergy to latex rubber. *Annals of Internal Medicine, 122,* 43–46.

Sussman, G. L., & Beezhold, D. H. (1996). Safe use of natural rubber latex (editorial). *Allergy and Asthma Proceedings, 17*(2), 101–102.

Sussman, G. L., Lem, D., Liss, G., & Beezhold, D. (1995). Latex allergy in housekeeping personnel. *Annals of Allergy, Asthma and Immunology, 74,* 415–418.

Swanson, M. C., Bubak, M. E., Hunt, L. W., Yunginger, J. W., Warner, M. A., & Reed, C. E. (1994). Quantification of occupational latex aeroallergens in a medical center. *Journal of Allergy and Clinical Immunology, 94,* 445–451.

Tarlo, S. M., Wong, L., Roos, J., & Booth, N. (1990). Occupational asthma caused by latex in a surgical glove manufacturing plant. *Journal of Allergy and Clinical Immunology, 85,* 626–631.

Taylor, J. S. (1996). Latex allergy: Review of 44 cases including outcome and frequent association with allergic hand eczema. *Archives of Dermatology, 132,* 265–271.

Truscott, W. (1995). The industry perspective on latex. *Allergy and Immunology Clinics of North America, 15*(1), 89–121.

Truscott, W., & Roley, L. (1995). Glove-associated reactions: Addressing an increasing concern. *Dermatology Nursing, 7,* 283–292, 303.

Turjanmaa, K. (1987). Incidence of immediate allergy to latex gloves in hospital personnel. *Contact Dermatitis, 17,* 270–275.

Turjanmaa, K. (1994). Contact urticaria from latex gloves. In G. A. Mellstrom, J. E. Wahlberg, & H. I. Maibach (Eds.), *Protective gloves for occupational use* (pp. 241–254). Boca Raton, FL: CRC Press.

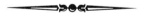

Research Review

The following six studies conducted by researchers at centers in North America and Europe demonstrate that highly allergenic medical gloves and household gloves are being marketed even though the serious effects of latex allergy are well-publicized. In general, powdered gloves contain more extractable allergen than powder-free gloves, and examination gloves are more allergenic than surgical gloves. There is no consensus on the value of total protein as an indicant of glove allergenicity.

Abbosh, J., Ownby, D., & McCullough, J. (1996). Quantification of airborne latex allergens produced by bursting and snapping of latex gloves. *Journal of Allergy and Clinical Immunology, 97,* 429 (Abstract No. 985).

Researchers in Detroit measured airborne latex allergens produced by stretching high-allergen powdered gloves and allowing them to snap back or bursting them by air pressure in a sampling chamber connected to a high flow air sampler. Allergen was measured by the AlaSTAT test for anti-latex IgE and a pool of sera from latex-allergic patients. The average allergen content of the gloves was 23,545 ± 6715 AU/glove. The amount released by bursting the same gloves was 646 ± 569 AU/glove, and by snapping the same gloves 33.1 ± 10 AU/glove. Nonpowdered gloves produced no detectable airborne allergen.

Alenius, H., Makinen-Kiljunen, S., Turjan-maa, K., Palosuo, T., & Reunala, T. (1994). Allergen and protein content of latex gloves. *Annals of Allergy, 73*, 315–320.

Researchers in Finland measured total protein content and allergen content in six brands of surgical gloves and one household glove. Allergen content was measured by IgE immunoblotting, immunoelectrophoretic, and immunospot methods and by skin prick testing 35 latex allergic patients with glove extracts. Extracts from four brands of surgical gloves and the household glove caused positive skin prick tests. The household glove showed the highest allergenicity by skin prick test.

Total protein content was measured by the Bradford and Lowry methods. Total protein varied from 3 to 337μg/g and did not always correlate with glove allergenicity in immunoblots or skin prick tests. Researchers concluded that total protein content is not a sufficient measurement of the allergenic properties of gloves.

Jones, R. T., Scheppman, D. L., Heilman, D. K., & Yunginger, J. W. (1994). Prospective study of extractable latex allergen contents of disposable medical gloves. *Annals of Allergy, 73,* 321–325.

In a follow-up study at Mayo Medical Center, researchers used the same techniques as in the previous study to measure extractable latex allergens in examination and surgical gloves stocked in inventory in July 1993, along with 10 "best-selling" brands of examination gloves purchased for the study, and 2 brands of utility (household) gloves. Among 9 lots of examination gloves from 8 different manufacturers, allergen levels varied more than 500-fold (< 10 to 5,500 AU/ml). Allergen levels in 2 "private label" brands produced and packaged under contract with another manufacturer were more variable (6 to 40-fold) than in the other 8 brands of examination gloves. Among 13 lots of surgical gloves from 8 different manufacturers, allergen levels also varied more than 500-fold (< 10 to 2,300 AU/ml), and 9 gloves had undetectable levels. Allergen levels in the 2 utility (household) gloves were markedly different (20 to 1,000 AU/ml). Mayo Medical Center phased out the purchase of high allergen gloves, increased its use of synthetic gloves, and continues to monitor allergens in gloves being purchased.

Siu, S. R., Smith, G. L., Sussman, G. L., Swanson, M. C., Yunginger, J., Cividino, M. P., Broen, S. A., & Beezhold, D. (1996). Reduction in airborne latex protein exposure by use of low protein powder-free gloves. *Journal of Allergy and Clinical Immunology, 97,* 325 (Abstract No. 569).

Researchers in Canada compared airborne allergen exposure levels during the use of regular powdered latex gloves and low protein, powder-free latex gloves. Personal breathing zone samples and area samples were collected on wards and in 2 operating rooms during summer and winter. Latex allergens were quantified by a latex-specific IgE immunoassay. Twelve samples of allergens in personal breathing zones from regular powdered gloves ranged between 5 to 616 ng/m^3 with a mean of 119 ng/m^3, and were undetectable for 14 personal samples when low protein, powder-free gloves were used. Area samples showed similar results but were of lower concentrations. Researchers concluded that airborne latex allergen exposure is reduced by the use of low protein powder-free gloves.

Sussman, G., Pugh, B., & Beezhold, D. (1996). Latex allergen levels in disposable medical gloves. *Journal of Allergy and Clinical Immunology, 97,* 326 (Abstract No. 573).

Researchers in Canada studied 7 brands of gloves to differentiate immunologically between gloves manufactured by the regular powdered process and gloves manufactured using chlorination or polymer processing to reduce allergenicity. Gloves were analyzed for total protein by the Lowry method, for latex antigens by the LEAP, and for latex allergens by skin prick testing 39 latex-allergic individuals. Powdered gloves had measurable levels of latex allergens and powder-free glove proteins were below detection and low in allergens. No difference in allergens was measured between chlorinated powder-free gloves and polycoated gloves. The Lowry protein measurements correlated with skin prick tests but did not detect protein levels below 50μg/gm, while the LEAP assay was more sensitive to gloves testing below 2μg/gm.

The next four studies demonstrate that allergens are aerosolized by powdered gloves, and are undetectable or greatly reduced when powder-free gloves are used.

Swanson, M. C., Bubak, M. E., Hunt, L. W., Yunginger, J. W., Warner, M. A., & Reed, C. E. (1994). Quantification of occupational latex aeroallergens in a medical center. *Journal of Allergy and Clinical Immunology, 94,* 445–451.

Researchers at Mayo Medical Center in Minnesota collected air samples from 11 areas with extensive glove use, 4 areas with minimal glove use, personal breathing zones, lab coats and scrub suits. Latex aeroallergens were measured by an inhibition assay with IgE antibodies from 3 latex-sensitized persons and by immunoblotting. Airborne allergen concentrations in 11 areas with high glove use ranged from 13 to 121 ng/m^3. Personal breathing zone samples for workers in areas with high glove use ranged from 8 to 978 ng/m^3. Individual personal breathing zone samples from personnel in operating rooms varied 100-fold. Allergens recovered from used scrub suits measured 200 μg. In 4 areas where glove use was minimal, or vinyl or powder-free gloves were used, allergen levels varied from 0.3 to 1.8 ng/m^3. Allergens recovered from a lab coat used for 1 week were in excess of 1 mg. Researchers concluded that most of the allergen was aerosolized when gloves were donned and removed. Most particles were 7μg or larger, but 20 percent were small enough to be inhaled and cause asthma.

Tarlo, S. M., Sussman, G., Contala, A., & Swanson, M. C. (1994). Control of airborne latex by use of powder-free latex gloves. *Journal of Allergy and Clinical Immunology, 93,* 985–989.

Researchers in Canada sampled air in a laboratory where an empirical trial of powder-free latex gloves was conducted to accommodate a latex-sensitized laboratory technician with occupational asthma and recurrent anaphylaxis. The technician was able to return to work successfully when co-workers stopped using powdered gloves. Area air samples were collected 6 hours per day for 5 consecutive days in the laboratory where staff used one type of powder-free glove and in another laboratory where staff wore powdered gloves. Air samples were assayed for latex aeroallergens by an immunochemical inhibition technique. Latex levels in air from the powder-free laboratory were less than 0.02 ng/m^3. And samples in the laboratory with powdered gloves ranged from 39 to 311 ng/m^3.

Turjanmaa, K., Makinen-Kiljunen, S., Alenius, H., Reunala, T., & Palosuo, T. (1996). *In vivo* and *in vitro* evaluation of allergenicity of natural rubber latex (NRL) gloves used in health care: A nationwide study. *Journal of Allergy and Clinical Immunology, 97,* 325 (Abstract No. 570).

Researchers measured latex allergen content of 20 brands of surgical and examination gloves representing over 90 percent of glove brands marketed in Finland. Coded glove extracts were blindly skin prick tested in 20 latex-allergic patients and assayed by a RAST inhibition test. Allergenicity varied over 1,000-fold. Allergen content was high (> 100 AU/ml) in 7 brands, moderate (100-10 AU/ml) in 2 brands, and low (> 10 AU/ml) in 9 brands. Researchers informed glove marketing companies and glove purchasing personnel in hospitals.

Wrangsjo, K., & Lundberg, M. (1996). Prevention of latex allergy. *Allergy, 5,* 60–65.

Researchers in Sweden measured the latex allergen content and randomly sampled medical and surgical gloves used in 1994 and 1995 at two university hospitals. Latex allergens were measured by the EAI IgE antibody inhibition method using sera from latex-allergic patients. Latex antigens (immunologically reactive latex proteins) were measured by the Gutherie LEAP assay using rabbit anti-latex antisera. Latex allergen levels varied (< 0.1 to 86 units/ml), and were higher in powdered examination and surgical gloves than in powder-free gloves. Results of the EAI and LEAP assays did not correlate, and researchers preferred the EAI. Researchers concluded that glove buyers can measure latex allergen content by immunologic methods, and ask for documentation of how manufacturers handled the problem of latex allergens in their products.

Yunginger, J. W., Jones, R. T., Fransway, A. F., Kelso, J. M., Warner, M. A., & Hunt, L. W. (1994). Extractable latex allergens and proteins in disposable medical gloves and other rubber products. *Journal of Allergy and Clinical Immunology, 93,* 836–842.

Researchers at Mayo Medical Center, Rochester, MN, measured extractable latex allergens in 71 lots of examination gloves, surgical gloves, and chemotherapy gloves from 22 different manufacturers in routine use at their center and the U.S. Navy Hospital in San Diego, CA in late 1991 and 1992. Allergens were measured by anti-latex IgE inhibition immunoassay with a rubber glove extract as the solid phase allergen and pooled sera from 5 latex-sensitized healthcare workers as the IgE antibody source. A raw latex preparation provided by the FDA was used as the standard and assigned an arbitrary potency of 100,000 allergy units (AU).

Allergen levels in 15 lots of powdered examination gloves from 10 different manufacturers varied by more than 3,000-fold (< 5–16,300 AU/ml), and were generally higher than in 10 lots of powder-free examination gloves or chemotherapy gloves. Allergen levels in 46 lots of surgical gloves varied 3,000-fold (< 5 to 16,000 AU/ml) and were appreciably higher in 37 lots of powdered gloves than in 9 lots of powder-free gloves.

Additionally, a high allergen level in a toy balloon (4,700 AU/ml) was comparable to levels in powdered gloves. Allergen was measurable in a latex condom and anesthesia rebreathing bag (50 AU/ml), but no extractable allergen could be measured in IV tubing, an IV T-connector, or 3 types of baby bottle nipples and a pacifier by these assay techniques.

Part VI

Characteristics of Women

Chapter 6

Sexual Harassment

Judith A. Roos

Since the Thomas-Hill and Navy Tailhook incidents, the public's awareness of and sensitivity to the topic of sexual harassment has increased. Similarly, research studies and descriptive and anecdotal articles have increased rapidly. Writings in journals and anthologies or research papers by psychologists, sociologists, and academicians account for most of these articles. The abstracts in this review are by no means exhaustive but are a representative sample of classic and thought-provoking theoretical, analytical, and research writings from different disciplines. Definitions, theoretical perspectives, research findings, and directions, consequences, and policy implications are addressed.

Although sexual harassment was not publicized to any extent until the mid-1970s, it is not a new problem for women. In their accounts of historical conditions of sexual harassment, Bularzik (1978) and Segrave (1994) cite records of the sexual exploitation of working women dating as far back as colonial times. However, it was the resurgence of feminism during the 1960s and the increased participation of women in the labor force that brought greater attention and visibility to sex discrimination and sexual harassment; both became targets of feminist inquiry and political organization. The Civil Rights Act was amended in 1964 to include a ban on sex discrimination. It authorized the Equal Employment Opportunity Commission (EEOC) to review complaints and recommend cases for federal litigation (Rhode, 1989). In 1972, Congress enacted Title IX of the Education

Amendments prohibiting sex discrimination in education institutions (Dowell, 1992).

DEFINITIONS

The most well-known legal definitions of sexual harassment are MacKinnon's and the EEOC's. In her influential book, MacKinnon (1979) argued that sexual harassment was a form of sex discrimination. She divided women's experiences of sexual harassment into: (a) *"quid pro quo in which sexual compliance is exchanged, or proposed to be exchanged, for an employment opportunity,"* and (b) "a persistent *condition of work*" (p. 32). Although Title VII of the Civil Rights Act prohibited employment discrimination against any individual with respect to sex, most early legal complaints met with little success in establishing sexual harassment as sex discrimination: courts largely considered the matter trivial and private. It was not until a decade later that the federal courts heard the first case in which sexual harassment was the primary complaint (*Barnes v. Train*, 1974).

In 1980, the EEOC established its now well-known guidelines. Consistent with MacKinnon's position, it identified two types of sexual harassment: *quid pro quo* and *hostile environment*. Although the guidelines do not have the force of law, courts generally rely on them. Most of the early cases were of the nature of exchange conditions; however, they soon gave way to the hostile environment cases that are more widespread and difficult to prove. In 1986, the landmark *Meritor Savings Bank v. Vinson* case set the precedent for deferring to the EEOC guidelines when the Supreme Court concurred with the D.C. court of appeals' decision that sexual harassment which creates a hostile environment is just as discriminatory as quid pro quo harassment (Dowell, 1992; Fitzgerald, Swan, & Magley, in press). Since the *Meritor* decision, it is generally accepted that actionable behavior extends to "gender harassment" (Franklin, Moglen, Zatlin-Boring, & Angress, 1981) which refers to negative and belittling behaviors and remarks directed at women because they are women.

Empirical definitions are usually derived from research participants' descriptions or ratings of their experiences or judgments of sexual harassment. Gruber (1992) used content analysis or research studies and court cases to identify three categories of sexual harassment: verbal requests, verbal remarks, and nonverbal displays. Based on a series of survey studies of diverse samples and settings and on a series of confirmatory factor analyses, Fitzgerald and her colleagues (1997) have suggested three broader categories that not only encompass Gruber's classifications but also include perceived offensive behaviors and illegal behaviors. The three categories are: gender harassment, unwanted sexual attention, and sexual coercion.

THEORETICAL EXPLANATIONS

A number of theoretical explanations of sexual harassment have been suggested. Male power and privilege have long been considered important explanatory concepts of sexual harassment (Farley, 1978; MacKinnon, 1979; Tangri, Burt, & Johnson, 1982). It is often said of sexual harassment that it is "more about power than about sex." Power appears to play a role in sexual harassment interactions, especially those of the quid pro quo class. In such cases, the usual perpetrator is a male boss or professor who holds coercive or reward power over women as a result of his position and authority.

Research findings do not support power as the *sole* determinant of sexual harassment. Fiske (1993) and Fiske and Glick (1995) argue that sex role socialization and gender stereotyping of women and jobs also promote sexual harassment. They encourage research and further testing of their theory. Organizational climate and structure are also potential contributors to sexual harassment. Organizational factors that have some research support include norms of tolerance of harassing behaviors (Hulin, Fitzgerald, & Drasgow, 1996; Pryor, 1987; Pryor, Giedd, & Williams, 1995), lack of effective policies and procedures (Hulin et al., 1996; Riger, 1991), hierarchical structures (Gruber & Bjorn, 1986; Tangri et al., 1982) and skewed occupation sex ratios (Gruber & Bjorn, 1986; Gutek & Cohen, 1987; Gutek & Morasch, 1982).

WOMEN AT RISK

Among rigorous large scale surveys, estimates of prevalence of sexual harassment range from 17 percent of females when considering only supervisor harassment to the more typical 40 to 50 percent when including coworker or peer harassment (Brooks & Perot, 1991; Gutek, 1985; Fitzgerald et al., 1988). Single women are significantly more frequently harassed than other groups (Fain & Anderson, 1987; Gutek, 1985) suggesting that sexual pursuit of unmarried women is likely considered more acceptable and provides a context in which sexual harassment may be rationalized as normal courtship behavior. Sexual harassment vulnerability also increases with a history of previous sexual victimization (Fitzgerald et al., 1997). Women in nontraditional jobs seem to be at increased risk (Gruber & Bjorn, 1986; Gutek, 1985). Although a number of studies report that younger women are the most vulnerable, Fitzgerald, Hulin, and Drasgow (1995) suggest that age may correlate with type of harassment: there appears to be weaker correlation with age for gender harassment than for unwanted sexual attention and sexual coercion. Data regarding race, ethnicity, and sexual orientation are inconclusive, primarily because so few researchers explicitly examine or report these categories in their samples.

PERPETRATORS

Most perpetrators of sexual harassment are males whether in academic or work settings. While quid pro quo harassment is usually inflicted by a superior toward a subordinate, it is infrequent. More often gender harassment and unwanted sexual attention occur. In these cases, the typical offender tends to be a male coworker or peer who is likely to have harassed other women (Gutek, 1985; Shoop & Hayhow, 1994). Beyond this findings vary. For example, some studies report that the coworker is likely to be married and older than the victim (Gutek, 1985); however, in a survey of male academics, Fitzgerald and her colleagues (1988) found no significant difference between harassers on age, marital status, rank, or academic discipline.

In summary, sexual harassment is not merely an event but a process that is simultaneously a legal, social, and organizational issue for female workers and students. As time elapses, theoretical perspectives and models are emerging to help explain the multiple dimensions of sexual harassment. It is much more complex and multifaceted than once thought: sex role norms and socialization, stereotypes, power dynamics, individual dynamics, and organizational climate and structure converge to explain and predict type and severity of harassment.

IMPLICATIONS

Unravelling the complexities of sexual harassment is not easy. Given its multidimensional nature, a systemic approach is needed to reduce or eradicate it.

Legal parameters are important. Laws and regulations have defined unacceptable and illegal behavior and have been especially successful in sanctioning quid pro quo harassment. They have punished offenders and helped to establish the moral standards that are necessary if sexual harassment is to be combatted. However, incremental legal reforms and policies have not dismantled sex discrimination and sexual harassment. Hostile environment and gender harassment continue to be extensive problems.

Frequency of harassment is influenced by the weakness or absence of local harassment policies, procedures, and remedies. Some argue that, even if organizations where sexual harassment is discouraged and formal policies and procedures are in place and reviewed, few women will use them because such formal models of conflict resolution better fit a male orientation to problem solving (Charney & Russell, 1994; Riger, 1991). They suggest that women are more likely to take informal actions to resolve the harassment. Formal models tend to be more adversarial in nature and tend to cast judgment on both the harasser and the harassed; informal models tend to simply put an end to the problem. Desire for informal resolution may also be due to women's subordinate status and their socialization to put the needs of others first. Formal reporting or complaint filing may threaten a woman's "relatedness" and sense of herself as caring and empathic. Formal procedures also imply that both parties involved have equal power in the process. Such an assumption is false. Women are more often in subordinate and lower paying positions in organizations. Use of formal grievance and litigation can be risky business for women since it can result in retaliation, being ostracized by coworkers and significant others, and being treated as a whistleblower (Fitzgerald & Shullman, 1993; Gutek & Koss, 1993).

In addition to the need to change organizational climate and establish woman sensitive policies and procedures, education of both men and women is important in combatting sexual harassment. Educational sessions need to provide employees and students with the knowledge and skills to decrease sexual harassment. Awareness of sexual harassment, its process, causes, and consequences for both harassers and those who are harassed should be discussed. Learning how to resolve conflict without resorting to stereotypical gender retorts and behavior is necessary (Barak, 1992; Shoop & Hayhow, 1994). Barak (1992) advocates training workshops that teach women workers and students to overcome those traits and attributes that have been empirically observed as typical to women that facilitate sexual advances toward them and make it difficult to rebuff unwanted ones. Based on research findings, Beauvais (1986) stressed the need to hold workshops that emphasize practical skills for coping with sexual harassment, informal and formal response options, and how to make use of applicable laws and complaint processes. Parents, educators, and administrators need to be educated to develop appropriate policies and procedures in educational and work settings and to supportively respond to those who report sexual harassment incidents.

Counsellors also need to be knowledgeable so that they can recognize manifestations and treat harassed women. Studies documenting incidence and severity of sexual harassment show that harassment often results in harmful effects, especially if the harassment is frequent, intense, and of long duration (Fitzgerald et al., 1997; Gutek & Koss, 1993; Loy & Stewart, 1984). Effects include physical symptoms, for example, headaches, loss of appetite, inability to sleep, and weight loss, and impaired mental health. Victims appear to progress through stages of feelings—confusion/self-blame, fear/anxiety, depression/anger, and disillusionment. Women also report detrimental effects on academic and career achievements and job performance as well as increased stress and "second injury" when they choose to engage in a formal complaint process (Gutek & Koss, 1993; Frazier & Cohen, 1992; Salisbury, Ginorio, Remick, & Stringer, 1986). However, counsellors and other health professionals need to recognize that women seldom seek help in early stages of harassment. When first encountering harassing incidents, most women believe it will stop or level off or that they are responsible. It is often not until they suffer from depression and are exhibiting symptoms of post-traumatic stress disorder that they seek help (Gutek & Koss, 1993; Salisbury et al., 1986).

There is little doubt that sexual harassment of women is a serious and widespread problem. Use of multiple research methods over time has helped to identify sexual harassment as a complex construct. However, other methodological problems remain and several areas have been insufficiently researched.

The multidimensional nature of sexual harassment, especially the issue of severity, has not been sufficiently researched. Although many researchers have equated severity with type, Fitzgerald et al. (1997) argue that severity relates to parameters that have yet to be revealed. Although many institutions have or are developing policies and procedures to deal with sexual harassment and some are regularly educating all levels of employees, there has been little research attention to the effectiveness and outcomes of such policies, grievance procedures, and training programs. Harassed women's coping skills also need to be uncovered. The women's stories in Sumrell and Taylor (1992) indicate that women survive and develop humorous and creative ways of coping.

Definitions of sexual harassment and range of behaviors considered harassing vary widely in research studies. Lack of a shared definition and a broad classification system as well as use of convenience samples and low response rates have resulted in conflicting prevalence estimates. A standardized classification of sexual harassment, such as that developed and validated by Fitzgerald and colleagues (1997), offers a promising beginning and needs to be used regularly in developing content valid instruments for measuring sexual harassment parameters.

Another problem in research is the lack of inclusion as research participants of women in blue collar and nontraditional areas of work as well as women of color, ethnic women, and lesbians (DeFour, 1990; Fitzgerald & Shullman, 1993; Fitzgerald et al., 1997). Because federal funding for research is minimal, the majority of studies have examined local or convenience samples in which these women are typically underrepresented.

Fitzgerald (1993) suggests a need for a research initiative concerned with prevalence data. Because the study of sexual harassment is relatively new and is a civil rights violation rather than a crime, it is not included in large database reports or in national victimization surveys. Statistics are compiled by the EEOC for the number of complaints filed annually with the federal government, however, figures represent only a fraction of the true incidence of sexual harassment in the population since evidence suggests that very few victims ever report their experiences or file formal complaints (Fitzgerald et al., 1988; Gutek & Koss, 1993).

In summary, greater precision and agreement in defining and measuring sexual harassment, its parameters and solutions, and inclusion of diverse random samples of women are needed to accurately and meaningfully inform and shape policy and effectively resolve harassment problems.

REFERENCES

Barak, A. (1992). Combatting sexual harassment. *American Psychologist, 47*(6), 818–819.

Barnes v. Train, 13 FEP Cases 123, 124 (D.D.C. 1974).

Beauvais, K. (1986). Workshops to combat sexual harassment: A case study of changing attitudes. *Signs: Journal of Women in Culture and Society, 12*(1), 130–144.

Brooks, L., & Perot, A. (1991). Reporting sexual harassment: Exploring a predictive model. *Psychology of Women Quarterly, 15*(1), 31–47.

DeFour, D. (1990). The interface of racism and sexism on campuses. In M. A. Paludi (Ed.), *Ivory power: Sexual harassment on campus* (pp. 45–52). Albany: State University of New York Press.

Equal Employment Opportunity Commission. (1980). Guidelines on discrimination because of sex. *Federal Register, 45,* 74.676–74.677.

Fain, T., & Anderton, D. (1987). Sexual harassment: Organizational context and diffuse master status. *Sex Roles, 17,* 291–311.

Farley, L. (1978). *Sexual shakedown: The sexual harassment of women on the job.* New York: McGraw-Hill.

Fiske, S. (1993). Controlling other people: The impact of power on stereotyping. *American Psychologist, 48,* 621–628.

Fiske, S., & Glick, P. (1995). Ambivalence and stereotypes cause sexual harassment: A theory with implications for organizational change. *Journal of Social Issues, 51,* 97–115.

Fitzgerald, L., Hulin, C., & Drasgow, F. (1995). The antecedents and consequences of sexual harassment in organizations: An integrated model. In G. Keita & J. J. Huvvell, Jr. (Eds.), *Job stress in a changing workforce: Investigating gender* (pp. 55–73). Washington, DC: American Psychological Association.

Fitzgerald, L. F., & Shullman, S. L. (1993). Sexual harassment: A research analysis and agenda for the 1990s. *Journal of Vocational Behavior, 42,* 5–27.

Fitzgerald, L., Shullman, S., Bailey, N., Richards, M., Swecker, J., Gold, Y., Ormerod, M., & Weitzman, L. (1988). The incidence and dimensions of sexual harassment in academia and the workplace. *Journal of Vocational Behavior, 32,* 152–175.

Fitzgerald, L., Swan, S., & Magley, V. (1997). But was it really sexual harassment: Legal, behavioral, and psychological definitions of the workplace victimization of women. In O'Donohue (Ed.), *Sexual harassment: Theory, research, and treatment* (pp. 5–28). Needham Heights, MA: Allyn & Bacon.

Franklin, P., Moglen, H., Zatlin-Boring, P., & Angress, R. (1981). *Sexual and gender harassment in the academy.* New York: Modern Language Association of America.

Frazier, P., & Cohen, B. (1992). Research on the sexual victimization of women: Implications for counselor training. *The Counseling Psychologist, 20,* 141–158.

Gruber, J. (1992). A typology of personal and environmental sexual harassment: Research and policy implications for the 1990s. *Sex Roles, 26,* 447–464.

Gutek, B. (1985). *Sex and the workplace.* San Francisco: Jossey-Bass.

Hulin, C., Fitzgerald, L., & Drasgow, F. (1996). Organizational influences on sexual harassment. In M. S. Stockdale (Ed.), *Sexual harassment in the workplace* (pp. 127–150). Thousand Oaks, CA: Sage.

Loy, P., & Stewart, L. (1984). The extent and effects of the sexual harassment of working women. *Sociological Focus, 17,* 31–43.

Meritor Savings Bank v. Vinson, 477 U.S. 57, 40 FEP Cases 1822 (1986).

Pryor, J., Giedd, J., & Williams, K. (1995). A social psychological model for predicting sexual harassment. *Journal of Social Issues, 51,* 69–84.

Riger, S. (1991). Gender dilemmas in sexual harassment policies and procedures. *American Psychologist, 46,* 497–505.

Salisbury, J., Ginorio, A., Remick, H., & Stringer, D. (1986). Counseling victims of sexual harassment. *Psychotherapy, 23,* 316–324.

Segrave K. (1994). *The sexual harassment of women in the workplace, 1600 to 1993.* Jefferson, NC: McFarland.

Shoop, R. J., & Hayhow, J. W. (1994). *Sexual harassment in our schools: What parents and teachers need to know to spot it and stop it.* Boston: Allyn & Bacon.

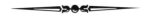

BOOKS AND ARTICLES

Borgida, E., & Fiske, S. T. (Eds.). (1995). Gender stereotyping, sexual harassment, and the law. *Journal of Social Issues, 51,* 1–207.

The entire issue of this journal is devoted to the topic of sexual harassment. Researchers, theoreticians, and legal experts who have contributed to the study of sexual harassment discuss issues related to the definition and measurement of sexual harassment, the interpersonal and intrapersonal forces contributing to harassment, individual and organizational responses to sexual harassment, and use of research in gender stereotyping and sexual harassment by the courts.

Bularzik, M. (1978). *Sexual harassment at the workplace: Historical notes.* Somerville, MA: New England Free Press.

This paper originally appeared in *Radical America* (July–August, 1978) and frames sexual harassment as a form of violence and social and economic control in a patriarchal society that oppresses women. It reviews the historical condition of sexual harassment and uses anecdotes and reports from publications as far back as the 1700s. Its primary focus is on white, single working class urban women in Northern U.S. cities. Perceptions of sexual exploitation of working women, individual and group reactions of women, women's responses, and effects on women are identified. Type of sexual harassment is related to social class and occupational differences. The roles of unions and coworkers are also examined.

Chan, A. A. (1994). *Women and sexual harassment: A practical guide to the legal protections of Title VII and the hostile environment claim.* New York: Harrington Park Press.

This is a comprehensive easy-to-use resource on the hostile environment claim. The background and history of the hostile environment claim is detailed and related law summarized. A guide to locating resources relevant to hostile environment harassment and related issues is provided, including online service, paper indices, and special libraries and organizations. Primary and secondary sources on the topic are also listed. This is an invaluable guide for all types of researchers including victims considering filing a claim, feminist scholars, students, attorneys, and employers.

Charney, D. A., & Russell, R. C. (1994). An overview of sexual harassment. *American Journal of Psychiatry, 151,* 10–17.

Computerized literature searches of psychology and psychiatry journals were used to locate and review research and papers on sexual harassment with particular attention to demographic information, psychological consequences, interventions, and related psychological issues. The highly publicized cases of Dr. Frances Conley and the Hill-Thomas Supreme Court hearings are mentioned and current legislation is briefly reviewed. Incidence figures for occupational settings, educational settings, and medical training are given. Other topics or findings discussed include low rates of formal complaints; psychological and physical symptoms; perceptions of sexual harassment; the "reasonable woman" standard; the problems of formal complaint structures as a male model; "second injury"; and therapeutic interventions of empathy, validation, and empowerment.

Dowell, M. (1992). Sexual harassment in academia: Legal and administrative challenges. *Journal of Nursing Education, 31,* 5–9.

Dowell reviews the historical development of federal laws and guidelines dealing with sexual harassment: Title VII of the Civil Rights Act (1964), Title IX of the Educational Amendments (1972), EEOC Guidelines (1980), and the Civil Rights Restoration Act (1987), and the effects of the legislation on litigation and policy making in education settings. Examples of actual court cases are used to demonstrate the nebulous definition and narrow interpretation of sexual harassment, particularly cases alleging hostile environment harassment. Much of the educational litigation does not focus on the issue of sexual harassment per se, but on the charge or challenge of denial of procedural due process to the accused perpetrator. Lack of research studies on the impact of harassment on nursing students in the classroom and practice area as well as a need for proactive and clear policies are discussed.

Dzeich, B. W., & Weiner, L. (1990). *The lecherous professor: Sexual harassment on campus* (2nd ed.). Urbana: University of Illinois Press.

This edition continues the in-depth discussion and updates the finding of sexual harassment of women college students by male professors that was initially revealed in the stories and surveys of women students, faculty, administrators, and alumni published in the first edition in 1984. Stories and comments are supported by cases and statistics. The book also addresses issues such as defining sexual harassment, the "chilly climate" for women on campus, the dilemma of teacher-student dating, and faculty concerns about administrative directives on sexual harassment. Included in the appendices are the 1980 Title VII federal guidelines on sexual harassment, the *Student's Guide to Legal Remedies for Sexual Harassment*, and examples of university statements and policies on sexual harassment.

Fitzgerald, L. F. (1993). Sexual harassment. Violence against women in the workplace. *American Psychologist, 48,* 1070–1076.

A brief review of historical incidents and current sexual harassment related legislation is given. Following this, the author summarizes major publicized legal cases; significant survey research studies on prevalence in the workplace and in educational settings; psychological research generated on topics such as structure, definition, measurement, perceptions, coping, and characteristics of harassers; costs and consequences to institutions and victims; similarities between sexual harassment and other forms of violence; and social policy implications, including research initiatives, legislation, and primary prevention.

Fitzgerald, L. F., & Hesson-McInnis, M. (1989). The dimensions of sexual harassment:

A structural analysis. *Journal of Vocational Behavior, 35,* 309–326.

The main purpose of this research study was to examine the concept of sexual harassment and to determine the factors influencing individuals' perceptions. It tests directly the multidimensional structure of sexual harassment as represented by Till's five levels of severity typology and operationalized by Fitzgerald's Sexual Experiences Questionnaire ($N = 28$; 11 male and 17 female higher education students). Data analysis included nonmetric multidimensional scaling analysis and multiple regression. Results support the multidimensionality hypothesis of sexual harassment. Although the analysis covered Till's five levels, gender harassment appeared to be distinct from the other aspects of the general construct of sexual harassment. It appeared that required sexual exchange (quid pro quo) accounted for most of the variance in perceptions of sexual harassment. An unexpected finding was that sex role ideology did not differentiate among subjects in the study.

Fitzgerald, L. F., & Shullman, S. L. (1993). Sexual harassment: A research analysis and agenda for the 1990s. *Journal of Vocational Behavior, 42,* 5–27.

This paper presents an overview of sexual harassment research with a focus on methodological problems and gaps. Research on incidence, prevalence, perceptions, and attributions is reviewed. Also examined are two emerging areas of interest: victim responses and coping behavior and organizational factors and variables. Critical omissions from research are analyzed, including evaluation of outcomes of training interventions; examination of organizational responses and contextual issues (potential for "whistleblower effect" is mentioned); and lack of conceptual clarity and specificity. The authors conclude with an overview of explanatory models and then propose an integrative model.

Fitzgerald, L. F., Shullman, S. L., Bailey, N., Richards, M., Swecker, J., Gold, Y., Ormerod, M., & Weitzman, L. (1988). The incidence and dimensions of sexual harassment in academia and the workplace. *Journal of Vocational Behavior, 32,* 152–175.

These authors note that sexual harassment has proven difficult to study due to the lack of a commonly accepted definition and standardized instrumentation. The research of this paper describes the results of the Sexual Experiences Questionnaire (SEQ). Study 1 details the instrument's development, results of psychometric analyses and results of the use of the instrument in a survey of graduate and undergraduate students at two large public universities ($N = 2599$ women and men). The item pool of the instrument was based on Till's five levels of sexual harassment. Study 2 describes the development of a second form of the SEQ for working women and reports the results for a population of academic, professional, clerical and blue-collar women ($N = 642$). Factor analysis resulted in a three-factor solution (rather than Till's five): bribery and threat collapsed into one factor, seduction and sexual imposition collapsed into a second factor, and gender harassment was a separate third factor. Discussion of conclusions from the data relate to type and extent of harassment experienced, perceptions and labeling of harassment, and gender differences in incidence of sexual harassment.

Goodner, E. D., & Kolenich, D. B. (1993). Sexual harassment: Perspectives from the past, present practice, policy, and prevention. *The Journal of Continuing Education in Nursing, 24,* 57–60.

The article discusses the need for proactive policies and prevention programs in controlling and eradicating sexual harassment, particularly in hospital settings. According to these authors, necessary components of an effective policy include a statement of purpose, a legal definition, a list of intolerable behaviors, delineation of what constitutes a harassment complaint, a complaint process, an investigation process, mechanisms to ensure confidentiality and due process, an appeals process, and potential disciplinary measures. Education of all levels of staff is emphasized. Sexual harassment is discussed as a form of treating the other as a sexual object and as a form of expressing power and social control. Other topics reviewed are key pieces of legislation; Florence Nightingale's writings on sexual harassment; nursing and medicine as sex-typed occupations; effects of sexual harassment on the victims; the reasons for and effect of not reporting sexual harassment; and consequences for the organization.

Gruber, J. E. (1990). Methodological problems and policy implication in sexual harassment research. *Population Research and Policy Review, 9,* 235–254.

Gruber claims that the ability of research on sexual harassment to influence the courts and policy decisions has been hampered by methodological flaws in many major studies. He discusses the difficulties associated with (a) determining incidence, for example, low response rates to surveys, and small sample sizes; (b) instrument construction; and (c) failure to include severity of harassment as a variable. Solutions to these problems are presented and include determining estimates of subtypes of sexual harassment, developing a mutually exclusive yet exhaustive set of harassment categories, and outlining factors that could be used to assess sexual harassment severity.

Gruber, J. E., & Bjorn, L. (1986). Women's responses to sexual harassment: An analysis of sociocultural, organizational, and personal resource models. *Social Science Quarterly, 67,* 814–826.

This research paper addresses the assumption that more powerful women will respond more assertively to sexual harassment than less powerful women. The sociocultural and organizational models that have received support when predicting targets of sexual harassment are reviewed and used as the basis for predicting response differences to sexual harassment. The authors also propose and test a personal resource model; similarities of this model to social exchange theory, Goffman's concepts of role playing, and Rosenberg's self-esteem theory are identified. Women ($N = 150$) in blue-collar jobs in an assembly auto plant were interviewed. Content analysis yielded 11 ways of responding that were categorized as passive, deflective, or assertive. Sociocultural power was not found to be important in determining response but it was important in predicting targets of harassment (black, young, unmarried women). Organizational power had some bearing on response: low skill, low status positions, and work area sex compositions predicted targets and determined response. Personal resources also had some bearing on response: low self-esteem and low life satisfaction predicted a passive response. The significant variables from these three models were included in a multiple regression to determine which factors would be most predictive of women's responses to sexual harassment. The two strongest responses were from the organizational model: job skills and work area sex composition. Life satisfaction and self-esteem were significant but weaker factors.

Gutek, B. A. (1993). Responses to sexual harassment. In S. Oskamp & M. Costanzo (Eds.), *Gender issues in contemporary society* (pp. 197–216). Newbury Park, CA: Sage.

Gutek focuses on the pervasiveness of the problem as well as the extent to which strategies have been sufficient in eliminating sexual harassment in the workplace. A brief history of the discovery and documentation of sexual harassment is provided. Based on research findings, the frequency of harassment and nonharassing sexual behavior at work is assessed. Research studies on consequences of sexual harassment and reactions of victims are also examined. An actual court case is used to illustrate some of the problems confronting the person who decides to seek legal redress for being sexually harassed.

Gutek, B. A., & Cohen, A. G. (1987). Sex ratios, sex role spillover, and sex at work: A comparison of men's and women's experiences. *Human Relations, 40,* 97–115.

Using the sex-role spillover model, this paper reviews and extends the work of Gutek and Morasch in regard to women's experiences of sexual behavior at work, examines the same issues from the perspective of working men, and compares the experiences of women and men. The reasons sex-role spillover exists are that (a) sex is the most salient social characteristic and noticed immediately, (b) gender roles learned early in life remain powerful influences in nearly all domains of life, and (c) both men and women are usually comfortable interacting with the opposite sex in ways that are congruent with these gender roles even when this conflicts with optimal work-role behavior. As a result, people frequently interact according to gender role at work and sex-role spillover occurs. Descriptive statistics are presented based on data from a representative sample survey about sexual harassment from the research program begun at UCLA (See Gutek & Morasch). Two levels of dependent measures were considered: the experience of behaviors directed personally toward the respondent and the generalized sexualization of the work environment. The fallout of sex-role spillover was more visibly negative for women than for men. Women in traditional jobs who worked a great deal with men faced being seen as sex-objects. Women in nontraditional jobs were seen as role deviants and experienced more of almost all kinds of social-sexual overtures and more frequently reported sexual harassment as a problem. Very few men worked in integrated or female-dominated jobs.

Gutek, B. A., & Koss, M. P. (1993). Changed women and changed organizations: Consequences of and coping with sexual harassment. *Journal of Vocational Behavior, 42,* 28–48.

This article focuses on some consequences of the sexual harassment of women. It reviews research on the work-related, psychological, and somatic effects on women. Of particular note is the discussion on retraumatization and the "catch-22" quality inherent in such research: showing sexual harassment is harmful requires demonstration that it has caused physical/emotional distress; however, evidence of breakdown undermines the woman's credibility and competence. The scant research on the effects on the organization is also reviewed as is the response of organizations to charges of sexual harassment. The whistleblower effect on the worker alleging sexual harassment is mentioned. The last portion of the article deals with victims' direct and indirect coping responses to sexual harassment and discusses the effectiveness and stages of responses. The authors identify shortcomings and gaps in the available research on responses and outcomes.

Gutek, B. A., & Morasch, B. (1982). Sex-ratios, sex-role spillover, and sexual harassment of women at work. *Journal of Social Issues, 38,* 55–74.

This article discusses factors that facilitate the occurrence and perpetuate the existence of sexual harassment of working women. The strong points and possible shortcomings of the prevalent power differential hypothesis are considered. A second perspective is then proposed and elaborated; it considers the effects of the sex-ratio at work on sex-role spillover. Some supporting data is provided from a survey conducted as part of a program of research on interaction between the sexes at work begun at UCLA and continued at the Claremont Graduate School.

Hoffmann, F. L. (1986). Sexual harassment in academia: Feminist theory and institutional practice. *Harvard Educational Review, 56,* 105–121.

This paper explores the issue of elimination of sexually harassing behavior by elimination of gender inequality. It critically assesses the relationship between sexual harassment theories and institutional remedies with a particular focus on student-professor "amorous relationships" statements in policies of educational institutions as perpetuation of patriarchy. Hoffmann provides a feminist critique of the problem of sexual harassment, its underlying structural conditions, and institutional responses. Guidelines are offered for formulating policies and procedures that clarify the connection between sexual harassment and sociocultural conditions and empower women in order to avoid backlash from procedures established in the name of women's emancipation.

MacKinnon, C. (1979). *Sexual harassment of working women: A case of sex discrimination.* New Haven, CT: Yale University Press.

MacKinnon, a feminist legal scholar, analyzes sexual harassment of working women. She contends that sexual harassment is primarily a problem for women. Sexual harassment law in its early stages is critiqued. She argues that sexual harassment is a form of sex discrimination and its victims deserve the same legal protection available to victims of sex discrimination under the Civil Rights Act of 1964. Many of the issues raised and examined in this book have yet to be resolved.

Morrison, T. (Ed.). (1992). *Race-ing justice, engendering power: Essays on Anita Hill, Clarence Thomas, and the construction of social reality.* New York: Pantheon.

This book is a collection of 18 essays by prominent and distinguished academicians—black and white, female and male—in response to the Hill-Thomas Supreme Court hearings. Contributors evaluate and analyze various aspects of the controversial and profound social issues raised during the hearings. They raise insights from a range of views and aspects: racial, sexual, historical, political, cultural, legal, psychological, and linguistic. Morrison claims that the time of undiscriminating gender and racial unity has passed and calls for new conversations. The contributors begin this new conversation with thoughtful, incisive and far-reaching dialogue on the issues coming from the Hill-Thomas hearings.

Paludi, M. (Ed.). (1990). *Ivory power: Sexual harassment on campus.* Albany: University of New York Press.

Contributors to this book include professors, deans, students, and counsellors. They discuss research and theory on sexual harassment on college campuses. Issues covered are defining and measuring sexual harassment, the interrelationships between rape and sexual harassment, the impact of sexual harassment on physical and emotional health, legal issues, incidence and dimensions of sexual and gender harassment of women of color, a developmental model for helping women cope and label their harassment experiences, and characteristics of male harassers. Clinical interventions, suggestions for handling sexual harassment complaints, and strategies for prevention and change are identified. In addition, a student contributor describes her personal experiences with sexual harassment. Helpful appendices include a bibliography of articles and books on sexual harassment on campus, a listing of audiovisual materials, a listing of organizations concerned with sexual harassment, and materials for training faculty about sexual harassment.

Pryor, J. B. (1987). Sexual harassment proclivities in men. *Sex Roles, 17,* 269–289.

This paper describes three studies conducted to develop and validate a method of studying individual differences in the tendency to sexually harass. It focuses exclusively on proclivities in males as they pertain to women

victims. Based on a review of previous studies of sexual harassment, a gap in the knowledge of the characteristics of sexual harassers is identified. Pryor discusses Malamuth's studies on rape proclivities and the bearing it has on his development of the Likelihood to Sexually Harass (LSH) measurement tool. Study 1 ($N = 117$ male undergraduate students) examined the reliability and convergent validity of the LSH scale. It found that high LSH men are likely to hold adversarial sexual beliefs, find it difficult to assume other's perspectives, and have higher rape proclivities. Study 2 ($N = 185$ male undergraduate students) examined reliability and discriminant validity. It found that high LSH men are more likely to be high in authoritarianism, low in Machiavellianism, and have negative feelings about sexuality. Study 3 ($N = 130$ male undergraduate students) explored the behavioral validity of the LSH scale. It found that high LSH men are more likely to describe themselves in socially undesirable masculine terms or masculine terms that strongly differentiate them from stereotypical femininity and have a tendency to behave in sexually exploitive ways when their motives can be disguised by situational excuses.

Pryor, J. B., LaVite, C. M., & Stoller, L. M. (1993). A social psychological analysis of sexual harassment: The person/situation interaction. *Journal of Vocational Behavior, 42,* 68–83.

The authors develop a social psychological framework for the study of sexual harassment. The framework conceptualizes sexual harassment of women as a behavior that some men perform some of the time. It implies that both situational and individual factors contribute to sexual harassment. Evidence for this framework is reviewed. Norms set by local management contribute to the occurrence of sexual harassment. The multivariate analysis of this study confirmed that men high in LSH tend to behave in a sexually harassing way when local norms suggest that they can get away with it. Studies of individual factors demonstrate that measurable individual differences exist in the men who possess a proclivity to harass and that the difference lies in a link between social dominance and sexuality. Finally, research is reviewed that demonstrates that sexual harassment behavior can be studied in laboratory conditions where individual and situational factors are systematically combined.

Rhode, D. L. (1989). *Justice and gender: Sex discrimination and the law.* Cambridge, MA: Harvard University Press.

In the chapter on "Sex and Violence" (pp. 230–237), Rhode discusses the legal definition of sexual harassment; historical findings on the adverse effects of sexual harassment on victims, employers, and society; differences in gender perceptions; and popular myths about sexual harassment. Inadequacies of legal responses and the power and limitations of legal rights as a strategy for ending sexual harassment are examined. Less attention to difference and more attention to disadvantage is advocated.

Riger, S. (1991). Gender dilemmas in sexual harassment policies and procedures. *American Psychologist, 46,* 497–505.

This article proposes that the reason for the lack of use of formal grievance lies not with the women who are harassed but with the gender bias in the definitions (reasonable person rather than reasonable woman) and the grievance procedures themselves. Attribution theory is discussed as an explanation for sex differences in what behaviors are labeled as harassment. Other obstacles to reporting complaints include belief that sexual harassment of women is normative, negative outcomes for victims who report, and worry about being believed and about retaliation. Feminist approaches to prevention of sexual harassment are discussed including educating individuals, creating organizational cultures and practices that promote equal opportunities for women, and attacking structural roots of gender inequalities in educational and workplace organizations such as the

chilly classroom and laboratory climate for women students, inferior athletic programs for women, sex-segregation of occupations, and hierarchical sex stratification.

Sex and power in the office. (1991, October 18). *The Wall Street Journal,* pp. B1–B4.

The entire Marketplace section addresses various topics and public concerns about sexual harassment. Some of the topics deal with polarization of men and women at work, interoffice romance, the gap between women's consciousness and political power, variation in women's views, men's sexual harassment experiences, consequences of filing formal complaints and pursuing litigation, and greater frequency of occurrence of sexual harassment in small rather than large businesses.

Shoop, R. J., & Hayhow, J. W. (1994). *Sexual harassment in our schools: What parents and teachers need to know to spot it and stop it.* Boston: Allyn & Bacon.

The premises of this book are that (a) the costs and consequences of sexual harassment in elementary through high schools are extreme and (b) resolving the conflict or "contentious relations" between the sexes at a young age will reduce sexual harassment. Based on research and legal expertise, the authors probe the causes and consequences of sexual harassment and suggest actions parents and educators can take to gain public support and initiate change at the policy level. Appendices include: (a) sample state and school district policies, a sample posting notice, a sample letter to an harasser, and sample complaint forms; (b) summary of the Equal Employment Opportunity Commission (EEOC) guidelines and list of EEOC offices; (c) gender equity resources; and (d) the Kids' Bill of Rights.

Shrier, D. (1990). Sexual harassment and discrimination: Impact on physical and mental health. *New Jersey Medicine, 87,* 105–107.

This paper focuses on women's experience of sexual harassment. Sexual harassment and sex discrimination are defined. Its prevalence and impact, including retaliation, adverse job effects, common physical and emotional effects, and alcohol and drug use are discussed. Options for handling incidents of sexual harassment and their hazards (whistleblowing effect and revictimization) are reported.

Stockdale, M. S. (Ed.). (1996). *Sexual harassment in the workplace: Perspectives, frontiers and response strategies.* Thousand Oaks, CA: Sage.

This volume integrates sexual harassment research and theory from a variety of disciplines and provides a comprehensive look at what is known. Stockdale provides two models for organizing concepts and theories on past research in order to provide direction for future research. One framework organizes current knowledge and theory on antecedents and causes of sexual harassment. A second framework focuses on processes that connect sexual harassment experiences with outcomes. Well-known contributors to the field of sexual harassment theory and research discuss or analyze the dynamics of sexual harassment of women professors, the impact of race and ethnicity on sexual harassment experiences and responses, emerging theory on hostile environment harassment, and an ethical decision-making model. Research frontiers focus on organizational influences on sexual harassment occurrences, implications of type and severity of sexual harassment on policy, individual and organizational outcomes, and a model estimating costs. Strategies for change and integration of dispute resolution systems are suggested. The concluding chapter applies the principles, findings, and concepts discussed in the book to one organization's actual experience with an allegation of sexual harassment.

Stockdale, M. S. (1993). The role of sexual misperceptions of women's friendliness in an emerging theory of sexual harassment. *Journal of Vocational Behavior, 42,* 84–101.

This paper examines the role of sexual interpretations of women's friendly behavior as part of an explanation or theory of some forms of sexual harassment but not the only explanation; Stockdale also argues that sexual harassment is a complex construct. First, the relationship between men's tendency to misperceive and beliefs supporting sexually aggressive behavior are examined. Reference is made to rape study findings and to Pryor's Likelihood to Sexually Harass scale. Second, factors affecting misperceptions are outlined and the role of misperception in theories of acquaintance rape is discussed. Third, the dimensions of sexual harassment and the role of misperceptions in different forms of harassment are examined. Fourth, misperception theory is integrated with other theories of sexual harassment: the natural/biological model, the organizational model, and the sex-role spillover model. Finally, an alternative perspective and unasked questions regarding the role of women's misperceptions and their potential implications are suggested.

Sumrall, A. C., & Taylor, D. (Eds.). (1992). *Sexual harassment: Women speak out.* Freedom, CA: Crossing Press.

This anthology of women's stories of sexual harassment is one way the editors and publisher responded to the testimony of Anita Hill and their outrage over the outcome. Women's long repressed memories are given voice. Women write not only of their experiences, responses, and consequences of sexual harassment but also of humorous and creative ways of dealing with their experiences. Stories are interspersed with quotes and cartoons. Included at the end of the book is a list of resources women can contact for information or assistance in dealing with sexual harassment.

Tangri, S. S., Burt, M. R., & Johnson, L. B. (1982). Sexual harassment at work: Three explanatory models. *Journal of Social Issues,* *38*, 33–54.

This article explores three models of sexual harassment derived from previous research, court cases, and legal defenses: the natural/biological model, the organizational model, and the sociocultural model. Assumptions and predictions of each model are reviewed. Data from a large random sample survey of federal workers (*N* = 20,083) is analyzed in relation to these models. Survey results are presented in relation to the models' predictions. Although the organizational and sociocultural models received more support than the natural/biological model, no clear cut support for any of the models emerged. Sexual harassment was not a unitary phenomenon, especially across the sexes. Male and female victims had different experiences and different views about sexual behavior at work. The picture painted by this data appeared to be more complex and varied than previous studies suggested. Results are discussed in view of the difficulties of using large-scale survey techniques to investigate complex cultural phenomena. Suggestions are made for future research approaches that could complement survey techniques.

Terpstra, D. (1986). Organizational costs of sexual harassment. *Journal of Employment Counselling, 23,* 112–119.

This article discusses the organizational costs of sexual harassment, such as turnover and litigation, ways to prevent costs, and implications for employment counsellors. University employed women (*N* = 71) were surveyed regarding their initial reactions to several different forms of sexual harassment. Incidents were developed from cases and examples found in the *Fair Employment Practices Guidelines* published by the Bureau of Business Practices. Categories of reactions included: quit, report externally, report internally, resolve personally, and uncodable. Fourteen percent said they would quit; a substantial number said they would externally

report although the range varied from 3 percent for gender harassment to 18 percent for sexual coercion to 83 percent for sexual assault or rape; a majority said they would report internally. Turnover cost factors are delineated.

Vaux, A. (1993). Paradigmatic assumptions in sexual harassment research: Being guided without being misled. *Journal of Vocational Behavior, 42,* 116–135.

The aim of this paper is to examine how the generalizations—men are violent toward women, most women are potential victims, and most men are potential perpetrators—have misled as well as guided research. While placing sexual harassment in the context of other forms of gender-related violence serves a function of synthesis, Vaux claims that it has also discouraged addressing problems with the concept of sexual harassment, impaired recognition of limitations in relevant research, and contributed to unresolved conceptual and theoretical problems and conflicting estimates. An alternate view is proposed in which sexual harassment can be viewed as a form of moral exclusion reflecting cultural views on the proper use of power and the extent of our moral community. Vaux claims this view suggests the antidote to sexual harassment is redefinition of civil conduct.

Webb, S. L. (1991). *Step forward: Sexual harassment in the workplace.* New York: Master Media.

This is an easy-to-follow, practical and very readable book that begins with an historical and a legal overview followed by a discussion of behavioral and legal definitions. The author identifies factors for assessing a sexual harassment incident, how to investigate complaints, and a six-step program on how to stop sexual harassment that both employers and employees will find useful. Also included are practical tips for action for employees experiencing sexual harassment.

Part VII

Reproductive Health

Chapter 7

Controversies Over Perinatal HIV/AIDS Testing Policies: A Critical Issue in Women's Health

Kathleen Fordham Norr

M. Ryan Gantes

Agatha Lowe

When an infant is infected with human immunodeficiency virus (HIV) from its mother perinatally, it places heavy burdens on the infant, the mother, her family, and society as a whole. Autoimmune deficiency syndrome (AIDS) prevention during the perinatal period (pregnancy, birth, and early infancy) is a women's health issue because mothers and their infants are the ones most directly affected by this burden. The discovery in 1994 that antiretroviral therapy could substantially reduce the rate of vertical transmission of HIV offered the first major drug treatment success story in the AIDS pandemic. This news was greeted with enormous enthusiasm by healthcare providers, AIDS researchers and the general public. However, controversy erupted almost immediately about how to take advantage of this major new weapon in the fight against perinatal HIV/AIDS. The scientific community as a whole proposed a dissemination model built around voluntary testing and informed consent. Others, including politicians and pubic policy spokespersons, have campaigned aggressively for mandatory testing either prenatally or after birth.

This policy debate raises serious ethical issues for women. All of those potentially subject to mandatory testing would be women, and the majority of them would be low-income women of color. It is highly unlikely that the same ethical standards and violation of individual rights would be suggested for a group of men only. It is unclear whether these policies are feasible or cost-effective. Moreover, this debate obscures public policies and healthcare delivery alternatives that potentially have far greater impact on perinatal transmission.

In this chapter, we review the issue of voluntary versus mandatory perinatal testing from three perspectives: ethical issues, the likelihood that the policy can be implemented effectively, and cost-effectiveness. To facilitate comprehension of the issues, we first provide a brief overview of the relative importance of perinatal HIV/AIDS as a public health issue in the United States and internationally, the rate and factors affecting perinatal transmission, and the current evidence regarding the perinatal HIV/AIDS prevention strategies. Finally, we propose a policy regarding perinatal HIV/AIDS prevention that is ethically sound, consonant with principles of primary healthcare and women's health, and potentially more efficacious and cost-effective.

PERINATAL HIV/AIDS AS A PUBLIC HEALTH ISSUE

In framing public debate around perinatal HIV/AIDS, it is important to recognize that perinatal HIV/AIDS prevention can have only a modest impact on the continued spread of the AIDS pandemic. As of July 1996, the World Health Organization (WHO) estimated that the cumulative number of persons infected with HIV was 25.5 million, 2.4 million of whom are children (8.6 percent) (Shelton, 1996). Nearly all of the children were infected by perinatal transmission. Two-thirds of all HIV infected infants born in 1995 were in sub-Saharan Africa and 30 percent were in Asia ("Status and Trends," 1996). By the year 2000, a cumulative total of 30 to 40 million persons, including 5 million children (12.5 percent to 17 percent), will be infected with HIV (WHO, 1996). Thus, pediatric AIDS is growing as a proportion of total infections. Any efforts to reduce perinatal transmission will help to slow the epidemic. However, what is fueling the growth of AIDS cases among children is the explosive growth of HIV infection among women in their childbearing years, estimated by WHO to include 3,000 new infections each day. Children who get AIDS do not currently live long enough to engage in risky sexual or drug use behaviors that can spread AIDS.

As of 1993, there has been an estimated cumulative total of 1.0 to 1.5 million HIV infections in the United States (Karon et al., 1996), including 14,920 children or 1.5 percent of the total infections (Davis et al., 1995). Perinatal HIV/AIDS is a much smaller proportion of total infections in the United States than it is worldwide because the epidemic here and in other industrialized countries first spread mainly among homosexual men and then to injecting drug users (IDUs). Today heterosexual infection is the fastest growing mode of transmission in the United States, increasing by 15 percent to 20 percent per year and affecting more and more young women (Shelton, 1996). Currently half of all women with AIDS in the United States contracted their infection through injected drug use, and another quarter through sexual contact with a drug-using partner (Michaels, 1992). Minority women have substantially higher rates of HIV infection, recently estimated at 5.3 to 6.9 per 1000 for African-American women and 2.2 to 3.3 for Latino women, compared to only 0.3 to 0.4 for Caucasians (Karon et al., 1996).

Perinatal HIV/AIDS has grown as an increasing number of women in their childbearing years have become infected, but since 1989 has stabilized at approximately 6,500 to 7,000 births to HIV positive women and 600 to 760 HIV infected infants per year (Davis et al., 1995). This represents the exposure to HIV of approximately 24,000 fetuses and newborns in the United States. The current prevalence rate for all pregnant women is about 1.5 per 1,000, but many cities have much higher prevalence, around 4 to 6 per 1,000, and 11 states account for 80 percent of perinatal HIV transmission (National Minority AIDS Council, 1995). These substantial differences in the prevalence rates suggests that different perinatal prevention approaches might be needed in different regions of the United States.

When viewed from the perspective of infant and child mortality reduction, perinatal HIV/AIDS looms as a more important public health issue. In the United States, AIDS is now the third leading cause of death for children (Chu, Buehler, Oxtoby, & Kilbourne, 1991). Since African-American women have a higher fertility rate and a higher incidence of HIV infection than Caucasians [U.S. Department of Health and Human Services (USDHHS), 1986, p. 36], the majority of HIV infected infants are African-American, exacerbating their already disproportionately high mortality rates. Rates are also disproportionately high for Latinos. Thus, the stress of caring for these infants continues to fall heavily on disadvantaged minority groups. In developing countries, the absolute number of infant and child deaths to pediatric AIDS is large, but higher overall infant and child mortality rates means pediatric AIDS is just one of many important causes of premature death. Although the majority of perinatal AIDS cases occur in developing countries, the greater proportion of child mortality due to perinatal AIDS in the United States helps to explain why perinatal AIDS prevention has become a major political as well as health issue here.

Perinatal HIV/AIDS also needs to be considered from the perspective of the human suffering it causes. The outlook for the HIV infected infant is not as hopeful as it is for those infected as adults. A cohort study of children with AIDS found 8.9 percent died by one year and half had died by age nine (Tovo et al., 1992). About 10 percent to 20 percent of the infants who are born HIV positive show signs of immunodeficiency early in life, most of whom die within the first two years of life (David et al., 1995; Mayaux et al., 1996). Even with new prophylactic treatment for pneumocystic carinii pneumonia (PCP) and other opportunistic infections, the prognosis for these infants remains poor. Many researchers believe that these infants are the ones infected early in pregnancy. The majority of HIV positive infants develop AIDS only in later childhood, with a mean age at diagnosis of AIDS at 6 years, and many live to adolescence (Mayaux et al., 1996). Internationally the life span of HIV positive infants is far shorter. A recent study in the Congo found over half of a group of HIV positive infants had died by 18 months from AIDS-related causes (Lallemant et al., 1994).

In addition to the suffering infants experience, all HIV positive mothers and their families suffer emotional, social, and financial stress. Wissow, Hutton, and McGraw (1996) provide an excellent overview of these issues. While only children born after the mother is infected are at risk of HIV infection, all of her children, whether infected or not, are likely to be orphaned at a young age. In the United States alone, 125,000 to 150,000 children of HIV infected women alive in 1992 will be affected by their mothers' illness and death (Michaels, 1992). The number affected internationally is staggering. Living long enough to care for an infected child and providing for a secure future for all their children are major concerns for HIV positive mothers.

FACTORS AFFECTING THE PERINATAL HIV TRANSMISSION PROCESS

Perinatal transmission of HIV infection can occur during pregnancy, during the birth process, and postnatally through breastfeeding. A review of 13 prospective cohort studies found a transmission rate (TR) of 14 percent to 25 percent in industrialized countries and 21 percent to 43 percent in developing countries, with most studies in developing countries between 25 percent to 30 percent (Working Group on Mother-to-Child Transmission of HIV, 1995). Studies in the United States report a TR between 20 percent to 25 percent despite many differences by study site in mothers' demographic, health and obstetric characteristics (Matheson et al., 1996). Possible explanatory factors for a higher TR in developing countries include higher rates of breastfeeding thus increasing post-delivery transmission, poorer overall physical health including malnutrition and sexually transmitted diseases, and identification of women as HIV positive at later stages of infection. Since all infants of HIV positive mothers have passively acquired HIV antibodies in their blood for up to a year, it has been difficult to establish the timing of transmission. A recent study using advanced test methods found detectable virus in about 25 percent of infants by 48 hours after birth, suggesting they were infected during pregnancy (Kalish et al., 1996).

Maternal Factors and Transmission

Various indicators of the mother's stage of HIV/AIDS and her viral load have been the most consistent and most important factors associated with transmission identified thus far. All studies where laboratory indicators were available, whether in industrialized or developing countries, found that women with more compromised immune systems (usually measured by CD4), higher viral load and/or more HIV antibodies, or AIDS-related symptoms during pregnancy or at delivery were considerably more likely to transmit the infection to the infant (Bredberg-Raden et al., 1995; Burns et al., 1994; Burns et al., 1996; Coll et al., 1996; Kovacs, Thurston, Rother, Rasheed, & Chan, 1996; Lallemant et al., 1994; Nesheim et al., 1994, 1996; Povolotsky, Baron, Polsky, & the Ariel Project Cohort Investigators, 1996; Rodriguez et al., 1996; Rubini et al., 1996; Shaffer et al., 1996). These studies also found that mothers with premature labor and/or low birthweight infants were more likely to transmit the infection, but the causal linkage is unclear. Thus far, none of these markers of transmission has been accurate enough to use clinically to evaluate the likelihood that a particular mother will transmit the virus.

Maternal drug use is the second factor consistently related to fetal transmission. While only a few studies have examined maternal drug use during pregnancy, they have all found significant effects (Nesheim et al., 1994; Rodriguez et al., 1996). Women who continue using intravenous drugs or cocaine during pregnancy have higher HIV transmission rates. Cocaine users also have poorer pregnancy outcomes, perhaps attributable to the negative impact of cocaine on placental function, premature labor, and poor fetal growth. Another study found that smoking, which also affected placental functioning and fetal growth, related to higher rates of transmission (Burns et al., 1994). These placental problems may mean a greater likelihood of HIV transmission across the placenta and of greater exposure to maternal blood for the fetus. Placental membrane inflammation was related to transmission in a Ugandan study (Wabwire-Mangen et al., 1996), but physical breaks in the placental surface in a U.S. study were not (Burton et al., 1996).

Since the hepatitis C virus (HCV) can be transmitted by shared needles, co-infection with HCV is relatively common among HIV positive women infected from injecting drug use by themselves or their partners. Three recent studies all found high rates of perinatal HCV transmission but only one found an increase in HIV transmission (Bossi et al., 1996; Sanchez, Fortuny, Ercilla, Sorni, & Jimenez, 1996; Villano et al., 1996).

Maternal nutritional status, specifically Vitamin A deficiency, has also been related to a higher risk of transmission. A study of 330 HIV positive pregnant women in Malawi found that 60 percent had Vitamin A deficiency during pregnancy and that the TR increased steadily with decreasing levels of Vitamin A: 7.2 percent for the high adequate group, 16 percent for the adequate group, and 26 percent and 32 percent for the deficient and very deficient groups (Semba et al., 1994). While vitamin A deficiency is not highly common in industrialized countries, a recent study in the United States also found that mothers who transmitted the infection were more likely to have Vitamin A deficiency than nontransmitters (16 percent versus 5 percent) (Greenberg et al., 1996). It is not known whether Vitamin A plays a causal role in transmission or is merely a marker of HIV progression in the mother. However, the known role of Vitamin A in maintaining skin integrity lends support to the idea that it may be a contributing factor. This is especially important because Vitamin A deficiency is likely to be widespread in many developing countries.

In contrast to the important effects of the maternal health-related factors of immune status, drug use and nutritional status, most studies have found few or no independent relationships with maternal demographic characteristics or previous obstetric factors. This is noteworthy because all studies have included these factors. Even having had a previous birth of an infant with HIV does not change the TR for the subsequent birth.

Intrapartum Factors

Evidence from numerous studies suggest that a substantial portion of HIV transmission from mother to infant occurs during labor and birth. A meta-analysis of 11 studies found that vaginal birth carried a relatively small but consistent and significantly higher TR than delivery by cesarian section (CS) (Dunn et al., 1994). One large study has documented higher TR in births where the membranes are ruptured more than four hours prior to birth (Rodriguez et al., 1996). The most compelling evidence of intrapartum transmission comes from twin studies, which have consistently demonstrated a substantially higher rate of transmission for the firstborn twin who is directly exposed to maternal vaginal secretions and blood (Duliege et al., 1995). For the firstborn twin, CS reduced the TR from 35 percent to 16 percent; for the second-born, CS reduced the TR from 15 percent to 8 percent. All these findings, taken together, suggest that the critical factor is the length of time the infant is exposed to vaginal fluids, so that elective cesarean section (ECS) where the procedure is performed before the infant enters the birth canal might have a great effect on transmission.

However, a study of diagnostic procedures such as fetal internal monitoring and fetal scalp samples that potentially expose the fetus more directly to maternal blood and secretions had only a minimal effect on transmission (Viscarello, Copperman, & DeGennaro, 1994).

Postpartum Factors

There is growing evidence that breastfeeding, the only mechanism for transmission from mother to infant after birth, is a major factor in transmission. HIV is present in 70 percent of milk samples at days 0 to 4 and 50 percent of samples collected 6 to 12 months postpartum (Ruff et al., 1994). A meta-analysis of published prospective studies in 1992 estimated the additional risk of perinatal transmission from breastfeeding at 14 percent, and as high as 29 percent if the mother became infected after the infant's birth (Dunn, Newell, Ades, & Peckham, 1992). Mothers in early stages of infection may have a higher viral load and therefore be more likely to transmit the infection. Three recent studies comparing the TR for breastfed versus bottle fed babies also found large differences: 49.3 percent for breastfed babies versus 18.8 for bottle fed babies in Brazil (Rubini et al., 1996) and 46 percent versus 18 percent in one South African study (McIntyre, Gray, & Lyons, 1996) and 49 percent versus 23 percent in another South African study (Lyons et al., 1996). The nearly universal and extended breastfeeding in developing countries may be one factor contributing to a higher TR.

STRATEGIES TO REDUCE PERINATAL TRANSMISSION

Development of sound public policy regarding perinatal HIV/AIDS requires an understanding that perinatal HIV/AIDS is a women's health issue affected by biological, psychological, social and environmental factors (McElmurry & Huddleston, 1991). The birth of an infant infected with HIV is the endpoint of a complex process that may stretch over many years: a woman must become sexually active, contract HIV, become pregnant and carry the pregnancy to term. Although we do not fully understand which infants will be infected, transmission is affected by the way the pregnancy, birth, and postpartum period is managed. Underlying gender inequality is an important factor affecting women's opportunities and available choices, the relationships between women and men, physical and psychological health, and healthcare policies and services affecting women. An important element of the debate about AIDS prevention is the degree to which prevention efforts need to address long-term changes in these underlying sociocultural factors to achieve significant reduction in HIV infection for women and their infants. The two major approaches to intervention focus on (1) factors that contribute to pregnancy in an HIV positive woman, thus exposing an infant to infection, and (2) perinatal factors that affect which infants exposed to HIV will be infected.

PREVENTING UNPLANNED PREGNANCIES OF HIV POSITIVE WOMEN

The most effective way to prevent perinatal transmission is to reduce the number of HIV positive women who become pregnant unintentionally. Preventing HIV infection among women is clearly an important way to both reduce perinatal transmission and help halt the overall AIDS pandemic. In the United States and most other industrialized countries, as well as parts of Latin America, both IV drug use and heterosexual contact are important mechanisms of infection for women, while in sub-Saharan Africa and most of the developing world heterosexual infection is the major cause of infection ("Status and Trends," 1996).

A related approach would focus on the reduction of unintended pregnancies. In the United States, unintended pregnancy is a frequent occurrence among impoverished women of color, and it is even more true for HIV positive women. Most pregnant HIV positive women either did not know that they were pregnant or conceived unintentionally because of inconsistent or ineffective contraceptive use (Chu, Hanson, Jones & the Adult/Adolescent HIV Spectrum of Disease Project group, 1996; Kline, Strickleer & Kemp, 1995). However, relatively few HIV positive women elect to terminate their pregnancy because of strong moral values against abortion. This contrasts with other industrialized countries; a recent European study found that only 26 percent of HIV positive women who become pregnant carry the pregnancy to term (De Vincenzi, 1996). Limited data from developing countries suggest that reducing unintended pregnancy might be less successful there, where many HIV positive women express a desire for pregnancy despite the risk of perinatal transmission (Batter et al., 1991).

It is beyond the scope of this article to review all of the factors that make women vulnerable to drug use, unprotected sex with infected partners, and unintended pregnancy. However, recent studies have documented the many ways underlying gender inequalities contribute to the risk of HIV transmission for women in the United States (Amaro, 1995; Levine & Dubler, 1990) and internationally (Gupta & Weiss, 1993). Women are biologically more vulnerable to sexual transmission than men. Psychological factors of low self-esteem, feelings of powerlessness and lack of control, depression, and a need to defer to male partners all make women vulnerable to drug use and sexual risk taking. Social contributing factors include lack of knowledge about sexuality and AIDS transmission, lack of ability to negotiate with partners, and social pressures to keep a partner happy as well as systemic factors of gender discrimination in education and employment, poverty, the profitability of drug trafficking and commercial sex, and lack of attention to women's needs in the development of health and social policies. Factors that contribute to unintended pregnancies for women in both industrialized and developing countries include psychological factors of low self esteem, depression, lack of control and lack of negotiation skills and social factors including lack of sex education, lack of accessible, affordable and acceptable family planning services, and economic dependency on male partners—many of the same underlying factors that make women vulnerable to sexual risk taking and drug use.

Possible short-term interventions to reduce HIV infection among women include targeted AIDS prevention interventions with proven effectiveness such as peer education to build self-esteem and negotiating skills to avoid unsafe sex, drug treatment programs for women, needle exchanges, and increased access to treatment of sexually transmitted diseases (Adjorlolo, 1996; Des Jarlais, Hagen, Paone & Friedman, 1996; Strand et al., 1996). Strengthening family planning services and reducing barriers to their use and providing more effective sex education have already proven their effectiveness in the United States and internationally (Barnett, 1994; Blaney, 1993; Finger, 1991). Many women become HIV positive and/or unintentionally pregnant in their teens, and prevention should especially target the pre-adolescent to build social skills and self-esteem to avoid early sexual activity and drug use. Community level interventions that focus on changing community norms that foster early sexuality and childbearing, restricting drug trafficking, and providing more adult supervision to young people are important in beginning structural change (Parker, 1996; Sikkema et al., 1996). More long-term efforts might include efforts to reduce school drop-out and homeless youth, gender inequalities, violence within and outside the home, poverty, drug trafficking, and the commercial sex industry. While these efforts are costly, the same empowerment process would simultaneously help women reduce drug use, unprotected sex and unintended pregnancies.

REDUCING TRANSMISSION DURING THE PERINATAL PERIOD

While much remains to be learned about the process of transmission, many authorities believe that most infants acquire HIV infection late in pregnancy and during birth. The Sienna Consensus Workshop II (1995) and Saba (1995) provide an excellent overview of current approaches to perinatal HIV/AIDS. They include drug treatment, prenatal vitamins, vaccines, intrapartum labor management approaches, and bottle feeding.

Drug Treatments

In 1994, results from a double-blind study conducted in Paris, Puerto Rico, and multiple sites in the United States, demonstrated that when Ziduvodine (ZDV, formerly known as AZT) was given to HIV positive women orally during pregnancy, intravenously during labor, and to their infants for six weeks after birth, only 8 percent (13 of 180) of their babies were infected with HIV, in contrast to 25 percent (40 of 183) of the babies in the other group. (Connor et al., 1994). Several later studies have now confirmed the effectiveness of ZDV (Fiscus et al., 1996; Landsberger, McGuinness, & Biggers, 1996; Lapointe et al., 1996; Wiznia et al., 1996). The large multi-site Perinatal AIDS Transmission Study (PACTS) found a decline in TR associated with ZDV and shorter duration of ruptured membranes for infants born after 1994 compared to those born in prior years (Simonds et al., 1996). However, among infants born in 1994–95, whether they received full, partial, or no ZDV therapy did not relate to the rate of transmission (Steketee et al., 1996). A small study in Canada found a TR of only 7.1 percent for women receiving the full treatment, but those receiving incomplete treatment (mostly intrapartum and postpartum only) had a transmission rate of 18.2 percent, not very different from the 21.4 percent rate for untreated mothers (Forbes, Burdge, & Money, 1996). The CDC has reported a 48 percent decline in observed versus expected perinatal HIV/AIDS cases in 1994. This decline is only partly due to increased perinatal ZDV treatment, because fewer children were born to HIV positive women and the average time from the birth of an HIV positive infants to a diagnosis of AIDS has gotten longer due to improved prophylactic treatment (Lindegren et al., 1996).

Alternative treatments now being tested for industrialized countries include mixed-drug and alternative drug protocols using therapies that have shown promising results in treatment of adults (Siena Consensus Workshop II, 1995; Saba, 1995). Internationally, the ZDV protocol and alternative drug treatments are so costly and so intensive in personnel and organizational costs that they are not feasible (Saba, 1995). Many developing countries cannot afford large testing programs (Dabis, Mandelbrot, Msellati, & van de Perres, 1995). However, more limited treatments may offer important public health benefits even if not as efficacious as the full-course treatment, and at least some short-course treatment protocols might be affordable in many of the better-off developing countries (Lallemant, Le Coeur, Shepard, & Marlink, 1996; Mansergh et al., 1996). Several major clinical trials of these alternative drug and short-course treatment protocols are already in progress and will provide important results soon (Siena Consensus Workshop II, 1995; Mansergh et al., 1996).

Non-Drug Preventive Strategies

During pregnancy, vitamin A supplementation is a promising strategy. Preparations are underway for a clinical trial of vitamin A supplementation in Tanzania now (Fawzi et al., 1996). Prenatal treatment with vitamin A could be highly beneficial in countries where HIV positive women are likely to be nutritionally compromised. This treatment poses almost no risks, can be offered to all mothers without testing, is low cost and can be readily incorporated into existing prenatal care services.

There are a variety of passive and active immunizations in various stages of development and testing. A trial of HIV immunoglobulin containing concentrated antibodies against the HIV virus is planned for the United States and Uganda (Sienna Consensus Workshop II, 1995). Two trials are also underway of a vaccine to provide active immunity to infants and children, and results should be available soon. The complexity, rapid mutation, and geographic variation of the HIV virus has made development of vaccines a very difficult process. It is not likely that immunization interventions, which have the potential to be highly effective, will be available in the near future.

During the intrapartum period, there are several promising strategies for intervention. In the United States and other industrialized countries, birth by elective cesarian section (ECS) is one possible strategy. A study in Switzerland was able to examine the relative impacts of both drug treatment and ECS because ECS was used at some of the sites where they conducted a trial of ZDV. They found no cases of transmission among the nine women receiving both ZDV and ECS, 8.6 percent for ECS only, 14.3 percent for drug treatment only and 20.8 percent for those receiving neither treatment (Kind, 1996). These results present a strong argument for ECS, which may be as efficacious as drug treatment, but the data are too limited to generalize with confidence at present.

Vaginal washing during labor has been proposed for developing countries because it is simple to do, low cost, and can be done without a system of prenatal testing. However, a trial of vaginal washing with chlorhexidine during labor in Malawi had disappointing results in that transmission was not reduced overall (Biggar et al., 1996). Vaginal washing did reduce the TR from 39 percent to 25 percent for mothers with ruptured membranes more than four hours before delivery, and the overall rates of maternal and neonatal sepsis were lower. Washing with a more concentrated solution or a different viricide might prove more effect. Alternatively, the lack of impact may mean that the intrapartum period is less important or that early breastfeeding plays a larger role than anticipated. In many developing countries, the use of gloves for all deliveries is also important to implement immediately. Where such safeguards are not in place, the delivery attendant is at high personal risk of contracting HIV and there is also a risk of infection transfer from attendant to mother or infant. Where many births take place with traditional birth attendants, educating these women and supplying protective equipment is very important.

Reducing breastfeeding is another preventive strategy that needs to be re-examined in the light of growing evidence of its importance in perinatal transmission. In industrialized countries, HIV positive mothers are routinely advised not to breastfeed. However, the documented health benefits of breastfeeding for infant survival in developing countries coupled with the high cost and relative unavailability of infant formula and safe water has made health officials reluctant to recommend bottle feeding in developing countries. Two randomized trials are now underway in Africa, with adequate amounts of safe formula supplied to participants. Extrapolating from these will be difficult unless similar subsidization of bottle feeding is possible on a wider scale (Siena Consensus Workshop II, 1995).

This review of the range of potential interventions to reduce perinatal transmission highlights several important considerations. There are many potentially effective strategies, and it is important to continue to explore a wide range of interventions. Most of the recent advances in both perinatal prevention and preventive therapies for children and adults are simply not affordable in developing countries. Less costly and simpler interventions may offer important public health benefits even if these interventions prove to be less efficacious than the full course ZDV treatment. In both the United States and developing countries, primary prevention to reduce unwanted pregnancies and HIV infection is especially important but often overlooked. Primary prevention not only reduces perinatal transmission but also reduces the spread of AIDS and promotes community health and development. The development and provision of interventions in the countries where the majority of mothers and infants affected by perinatal HIV/AIDS live must be an international priority if the AIDS pandemic is to be controlled.

EVALUATING PRENATAL TESTING: A WOMAN'S HEALTH PERSPECTIVE

A policy has importance on two different levels: it sends an important message about the values of the society, government and healthcare systems that produced the policy and it should lead to desired changes in healthcare delivery and health outcomes. Three alternative policies have been proposed in the USA for HIV testing and drug treatment for pregnant women and newborns. Immediately following the release of the evidence that ZDV could reduce perinatal transmission, the members of congress debated the issue of requiring *mandatory testing of all pregnant women*. Pressure for mandatory prenatal testing continues, as in the 1995 passage of the Ryan

White bill funding AIDS services with a rider directing mandatory testing if states cannot demonstrate knowledge of the HIV status of at least 95 percent of newborn infants within two years. In June, 1996, the American Medical Association (AMA) narrowly approved a resolution making it the only professional organization to support mandatory testing (AMA, 1996). The second policy alternative is *mandatory testing of newborns*. With the postponement of mandatory prenatal testing, mandatory newborn testing was proposed in several state legislatures. Thus far this policy has also been averted by strong public pressure, but a vocal group of supporters continues to work for it. The third policy is for *voluntary prenatal testing and treatment*, but in a changed context where prenatal testing is destigmatized and made a normal and routine procedure for all pregnant women. This policy has been recommended by the Center for Disease Control (CDC) (1994, 1995) and by a joint statement of the American Academy of Pediatrics (AAP) and the American College of Obstetricians and Gynecologists (ACOG) in 1995 that specifically rejects mandatory testing approaches (AAP & ACOG, 1995).

Ethical Issues

Perinatal testing policy does not emerge in a vacuum but reflects the more general issue of reproduction for HIV positive women. Ethical issues around reproductive decision-making are always complex. A delicate balance must be achieved between the rights of the mother, the best interests of the fetus, and the legitimate interests of society. Women are justifiably concerned by policies affecting their right to bodily autonomy. Historically, such policies have given primacy to the interests of the infant and society rather than the rights of the woman, and enforcement has been directed almost entirely against poor women, women of color, and women with disabilities, especially the mentally incompetent (Banks, 1996). The area of AIDS research and treatment generally has not been responsive to the needs of women, reflecting systemic biases of gender inequality that perpetuate insensitivity to women's different needs (Faden, Kass, & McGraw, 1996). The experiences of drug-using women with mandatory testing further documents that women have much to fear from policies that violate their autonomy and bodily integrity. Despite numerous rulings of unconstitutionality and an inadequate number of drug treatment programs, pregnant women have been jailed as well as threatened with prosecution or loss of custody to compel them to enter drug treatment programs (Acuff, 1996). Although drug use is prevalent across class lines, poor women of color have been the ones prosecuted (Acuff, 1996).

   Official health policy recommendations from both the CDC in 1985 and ACOG in 1987 have been that HIV positive women should not bear children

(Banks, 1996). However, a growing number of bioethicists, HIV positive women, clinicians and researchers argue that reproductive decisions should be evaluated from the ethical perspective of caring rather than justice (Levine & Dubler, 1990; Locher, 1996; McFadden, 1996; Pinch, 1994). While not exclusive to women, Gilligan (1988) identifies the caring perspective as more prevalent among women and more congruent with women's views of self-in-relations and higher valuing of relationships. Both ethicists and researchers put forth the view that the costs of having a child for an HIV positive woman, while high, are not higher than many other situations where only nondirective counseling has been regarded as ethical (Arras, 1990; Powers, 1996). Others argue that it is not ethical to ask HIV positive women to forgo the fulfillment of motherhood that many of them value so highly for the overall benefit of a society that has provided so little for them (Levine & Dubler, 1990; McFadden, 1996). The balance of costs and benefits varies greatly from one situation to the next, so that ethical decision-making must be contextualized (Arras, 1990; McFadden, 1996). Counselors must also be sensitive to the potential coercion inherent in the nature of counseling in a framework of unequal power (Bloche, 1996). Faden et al. (1996) recommend that counselors help HIV positive women make a more informed ethical decision that is congruent with her individual life context and personal moral values. It is highly relevant that this is also the perspective of the HIV positive women and their caregivers identified by Allen (1996) and Kass and Faden (1996a, 1996b). Both groups felt strongly that the role of counselors and friends should be to help HIV positive women struggling with reproductive decisions and even to offer their personal opinions, but to respect women's rights to make their own decisions. They also acknowledged the extraordinary difficulty of such decisions and that women could make ethically responsible decisions that differed from their personal values and feelings.

Individual Costs and Benefits of Testing

Although there is controversy about the weight that should be given to each factor, there is general agreement on what the risks and benefits of prenatal testing are for women, children, and society (Britton, 1995; Crawford, 1995; Dumois, 1995; Minckoff & Willoughby, 1995). For infants and the mothers who will nurture them, the most important benefit of prenatal HIV testing is the opportunity to use ZDV and other interventions to substantially reduce the risk of transmitting HIV infection to the infant. Testing in early pregnancy also allows HIV positive women time to consider their situation and the possibility of elective abortion. Women may also benefit personally, since knowing their HIV status allows them to avoid infecting others and to receive earlier and closer monitoring of their health and preventive treatment (Agency for Health Care Policy and Research, 1994). These benefits are especially important to women who are less likely to present with the classical symptoms of HIV infection. Mandatory post-natal testing of infants does not offer this benefit, but only confirms infant exposure to HIV infection to allow monitoring and preventive treatment. Even postnatal ZDV treatment or restricting breastfeeding is unlikely to be feasible since obtaining test results and locating families is likely to take several weeks. While proponents have argued that testing is important, especially for infants in foster care (Crawford, 1995), this problem could be addressed by improving the timeliness and effectiveness of process already in place for providing healthcare, including diagnostic tests, for wards of the state.

Balanced against these individual benefits are unknown but not improbably long-term negative health consequences of administering large doses of a powerful drug over an extended period of time (Britton, 1995). For the mother, there is also the threat that taking ZDV at this time may cause her to develop resistant strains of HIV and limit the usefulness of this drug later when she may need it (Minckoff & Willoughby, 1995). The rapid development of alternative antiretroviral drugs and combination therapies has somewhat reduced this threat, but it cannot be discounted entirely. To date, no adverse health impacts on HIV positive women from pregnancy itself have been identified.

The most immediate cost to most women is the testing itself. Finding out that she has a long-term infection that will probably lead to her early death and which she may pass on to her fetus is burdensome and may have serious psychological effects such as depression. Social and economic stigmas mean that being identified as HIV positive threatens a woman's healthcare insurance, job promotions, credit, housing, and social relationships. Her partner may become abusive or desert her even when the woman is carrying his child and may have contracted the infection from him (Rothenberg, Paskey, Reuland, Zimmerman, & North, 1995). If a woman is HIV positive and chooses the extended ZDV treatment, she is not likely to retain control over when and to whom her condition is disclosed.

Although many policy makers view post-test ZDV treatment as the only logical option for pregnant HIV positive women, there are sufficient uncertainties so that a woman's decision to decline prenatal testing and/or ZDV treatment can be ethically justified. Some HIV positive women, considering their personal moral values and the burdens for themselves and their infants, may choose pregnancy termination. Others may decide to refuse treatment. A substantial majority of infants will not be infected even without treatment. For every 100 pregnancies, treatment will prevent transmission for approximately 17 infants. Some women may decide that this benefit does not outweigh the unknown long-term risks of treatment (Minckoff & Willoughby, 1995). If a mother intends to refuse treatment, then she might reasonably decide not to test or to have an anonymous test.

Societal Costs and Benefits

Clearly society as a whole will benefit from any reduction in the number of HIV positive infants born. A substantial portion of the costs of caring for an HIV infected infant and for children orphaned by AIDS fall to the general public, especially when the mother and her family are poor. Another social benefit of all three proposed testing policies over current practice is greater social justice than prior practice, where prenatal HIV testing occurred mainly in high prevalence areas, in public more than private facilities, and for women of color and women who were identified as engaging in high risk behaviors. This approach was both discriminatory and ineffective. It is well documented that neither caregiver assessment nor self-assessment of risks adequately identify HIV positive women, providing a strong rationale for mandating the offering of testing to all pregnant women (Lindsay et al., 1989; Walter et al., 1995). Mandated testing, especially when funding to support both testing and treatment is provided, also ensures that all mothers and infants benefit equally from the recently discovered treatment, regardless of their ability to pay.

Mandatory counseling and voluntary testing for all pregnant women provide all women with the information they need to make informed decisions about HIV testing and perinatal treatment. This policy also sends important messages: that all sexually active women are potentially at risk; that all women should be treated equally regardless of ethnic or racial origin, income, drug use history, or other factors; that the health of women and their infants is important; and that women can be trusted to make decisions in the best interests of themselves and their infants when given adequate information. This policy message may have a social benefit of increasing women's trust in the healthcare system. Thus, voluntary prenatal testing is ethically acceptable from a woman's health perspective.

Mandatory prenatal testing is not ethically acceptable because it undermines the rights of bodily autonomy and reproductive freedom and perpetuates gender inequality. Mandatory testing implies that the rights of infants and society are far more important than the rights of women to retain autonomy over their bodies, that there is only one "correct" choice regarding prenatal testing, and that women cannot be trusted to make the correct choice even if well informed. The policy stops short of mandating treatment, but it is couched in a framework that strongly suggests all pregnant women should accept treatment. In mandating a single course of action, public policy may be going beyond the scientific evidence and inappropriately limiting a woman's freedom of choice. This is especially problematic when it is the mother who assumes most of the risks. The government may be legally liable for any long-term adverse effects on mothers and infants from this policy. Social costs may include exacerbating the mistrust of both government and healthcare felt by many women, poor people, persons living with HIV, and people of color.

The policy of *mandatory postnatal testing* is also unethical because it violates women's rights and does not promote social justice. It sends the same negative messages to women that mandatory prenatal testing does. However, the major benefit of prenatal testing, the opportunity to prevent perinatal HIV transmission, is absent when testing occurs after birth. This means that the potential risks of harmful long-term effects are also not present. Since what the test really identifies is whether the mother is HIV positive, all the burdens of testing and disclosure for the mother remain the same. The only benefit of postnatal testing is the identification that a particular infant may be HIV positive, enabling the care provider to institute more careful monitoring and prophylactic treatment. Arguments for this policy are built on the assumption that prenatal counseling and testing will fail (Crawford, 1995).

All three of the proposed policies have potentially very high opportunity costs for society as a whole. All three policies will be expensive and will require extensive organizational skills and professional expertise. This major effort will draw resources away from other alternatives for perinatal HIV/AIDS prevention, especially in today's climate of dwindling resources for public health and social services generally. Primary prevention efforts toward preventing HIV infection and unintended pregnancy among women offer the best long-term strategy for reducing perinatal HIV/AIDS. Early prevention also offers many additional public health and development benefits in both the United States and internationally. If we consider just interventions during the perinatal period, the other alternatives reviewed above are also promising but have garnered little attention compared to prenatal testing and drug treatment. When we take a global perspective, it is especially important to test and implement affordable prevention strategies that can reach the developing countries where perinatal HIV/AIDS prevention is most needed.

Feasibility and Probable Efficacy

Once a public policy is determined to be ethical, the policy's feasibility of implementation and whether it will have the desired public health impacts must be assessed. As in any expansion of a protocol from a clinical trial, the less controlled conditions usually lead to less favorable outcomes than in the clinical trial. To date, the reports of ZDV use outside the original trial already reviewed are reassuring that the full course of ZDV is effective in a wider range of conditions, but that partial treatment may have less benefit. Developing and sustaining a high-quality testing and follow-up program will be the major challenge in implementing all three of these policies and the factor most critical for success. The most practical way to implement prenatal testing programs is within existing prenatal care networks. Most public prenatal clinics in urban areas already have some sort of voluntary testing program in place, but the quality and success are highly variable. Many rural prenatal services and private practices have less extensive programs currently in place and also serve populations with lower prevalence rates. Implementing an effective prenatal testing program for all pregnant women in these healthcare facilities may first require convincing providers that it is important.

Barriers to prenatal care, including financial cost, inaccessible clinic hours, long waiting times, culturally unacceptable patterns of care, transportation, and child care, mean that 15 percent of all women in the United States receive no prenatal care (Turner, Markson, Hauck, Cocroft, & Fanning, 1995). This is even more true of HIV positive women. A recent study found that 20 percent of HIV positive women in New York state received no prenatal care, and 65 percent received inadequate care (Turner et al., 1995). Thus, even a mandatory prenatal testing program that does not draw women into care could not achieve more than 80 percent coverage. If programs were adequately funded to address barriers to prenatal care, this would offer major public health benefits for all women and infants.

Many critics fear that mandatory testing is likely to have the unintended consequence of driving those it seeks to help further away from care. The women who are already the most alienated from care, especially those using drugs, are the most likely to be affected (Britton, 1995). HIV positive drug users are already heavily stigmatized by the general public, healthcare professionals, and even other HIV positive women. About half of all HIV positive women are current or former injecting drug users, and others use crack or cocaine, so this is a substantial part of the target population. These women are already heavily stigmatized by caregivers as well as the general public. Both their current drug use and their fears of negative experiences already make them suspicious of the healthcare system and less likely to get prenatal care or comply with instructions (McCaul, Lillie-Blanton, & Svikis, 1996). Adding a new reason for suspicion is not likely to build the caregiver trust that would bring these women into prenatal care or drug treatment.

Postnatal testing might seem to have a distinct advantage in terms of achieving universal coverage, since nearly all women in the United States do deliver their babies in the hospital. However, one study of voluntary post-birth testing was able to reach only 75 percent of mothers before discharge, and most of those who agreed to be tested after birth had already been tested (Walter et al., 1995).

Voluntary testing programs need to achieve a high rate of acceptance of testing among the women they reach. Three U.S. studies found that the rate of acceptance of testing varied from 50 percent to more than 94 percent, even in the same city perinatal network (Lindsay et al., 1989; Mason et al., 1991; Walter et al., 1995), while a study in Sweden had a testing acceptance rate of 93 percent (Mason et al., 1991). There is strong evidence that the acceptance rate can be substantially improved by strengthening the quality of the counseling program; one study increased testing acceptance from 50 percent to 80 percent after initiating a group educational program. Moreover, all of these studies were conducted before ZDV was shown to reduce perinatal HIV transmission; women now have a much stronger reason to accept testing than they did at the time of these studies.

Once tests are performed, there is a need to follow and treat those identified as HIV positive. This is especially problematic for the postnatal testing of infants, since there is no prior link with the mother and women will have left the hospital long before test results are known. Many HIV positive mothers are living in poverty and unstably housed, making them hard to locate. Potential alienation due to the mandatory nature of the tests may increase the difficulty and may mean that women will avoid the healthcare system and thus preventive care for their infants. Locating pediatric care providers is an alternative approach, but establishing these links would also be difficult, especially for large public clinics, and this approach fails to reach those who avoid the healthcare system.

The major advantage of prenatal testing is that once women are in the prenatal care system, they are uniquely accessible to healthcare providers for long-term follow-up. In an ideal program, HIV positive women would receive sensitive counseling regarding treatment options, and most would decide to accept treatment. A well-coordinated program would then ensure that the prenatal, intrapartum and postpartum drug treatment was delivered in a timely fashion. However, the many women who enter prenatal care late in pregnancy would seldom receive the full prenatal course of ZDV and it is not clear how effective partial treatment will be. Providing IV drug therapy during labor is even more problematic, and seems to be especially difficult for drug-using mothers. One study in New York City found that 75 percent of the 49 HIV-positive women identified prenatally agreed to ZDV treatment, but one-third did not receive the full course of treatment. Twelve of the women, half of whom tested positive for cocaine, arrived at the hospital too close to delivery to initiate intrapartum ZDV treatment (Wiznia et al., 1996).

Two studies, both conducted after the ZDV trials, highlight both the possibilities and the difficulties in implementing universal voluntary prenatal testing. In North Carolina, statewide directives to provide testing and treatment to all pregnant women were issued in April, 1994. The proportion of HIV-exposed infants identified and tested increased from 60 percent to 82 percent for all of 1994 and more than 90 percent in the last quarter of 1994. Three-quarters of the mothers received drug therapy, with a transmission rate of only 5.7 percent, compared to 18.9 percent for infants of untreated women. The state transmission rate declined from 21 percent to 8.4 percent between 1993 and 1994 (Fiscus et al., 1996). The authors attribute this success to a statewide coordinated counseling and testing program in public health clinics where most of the HIV-positive women received their care. However, in a large hospital in the Bronx, only 49 of the 125 HIV positive women who delivered at the hospital were identified prenatally (Wiznia et al., 1996). It is unclear what proportion of these women did not receive prenatal care, did not receive counseling, or refused to be tested.

A primary healthcare system that serves mothers and babies in an integrated system would be ideal to maximize treatment. This is especially important since both mother and infant should receive continued intensive monitoring. In areas of high prevalence, a primary healthcare system for HIV positive families integrating health and social services in Chicago would be ideal. One such example is the Women and Children's HIV Program of the HIV Primary Care Center at Cook County Hospital in Chicago. Their MCH/HIV Integration Project has developed standards for education, counseling, and testing of women and established linkages between Chicago's perinatal system. Another example is the Ryan White funded agencies that provides for continuity of care for HIV positive women and their families during and after pregnancy. [MCH/HIV Integration Project, & Midwest AIDS Training & Education Center (MATEC), 1996]. Holistic models integrating woman-centered drug treatment with prenatal care have shown improved outcomes for mother and infant (McCaul, Lillie-Blanton, & Svikis, 1996). The actual cost and difficulty of a prenatal counseling and testing program may vary considerably depending on how it is implemented. Before moving to a national mandate, it would probably be a wise investment to pilot a variety of models and to consider whether different areas with different rates of seroprevalence for women should have somewhat different programs. One possible model is that of "informed refusal" where clients receive a brief explanation that blood is routinely tested for HIV unless the client specifically declines. Costly individual counseling is then reserved for HIV positive women and those with questions (Gunderson, Mayo, & Rhame, 1996; Minckoff & Willoughby, 1995). While the benefits of HIV negative women of a counseling opportunity would be lost, the cost reduction would be considerable. This might be particularly appropriate in areas of relatively low seroprevalence. Another relatively low cost model is that used in some Chicago public health clinics where a group information session is followed by an individual counseling with a nurse and a signed consent if testing is elected. This model also reduces costs while retaining the benefits of education and counseling for all pregnant women. Other possible strategies to reduce costs and increase effectiveness might include using peer educators to do community outreach and more intensive education and counseling.

Cost Effectiveness

There have been no studies of cost-effectiveness for mandatory testing of newborns. Clearly the program would be costly, and the potential infant health benefits are far fewer than with prenatal testing.

Since preventing perinatal HIV infection through drug treatment has been documented for only two years, cost-effectiveness is not well established. To some degree, analysis at present is speculative, given that the actual effectiveness of treatment outside a clinical trial is not yet well established. One study used formal modeling and found that treatment improved infants' average quality of life under a wide variety of assumptions, but did not look at costs (Rouse, Owen, Goldenberg, & Vermud, 1995). Two recent studies using current estimated costs found that drug treatment of pregnant women known to be HIV positive is clearly cost effective in the United States (Farnham, Holtgrave, Rogers, & Guinan, 1996; Mauskopf, Paul, Witchman, White, & Tilson, 1996), with an estimated net savings of over $1.5 million per 100 HIV positive women treated according to Mauskopf et al. For both studies, even when the authors assumed that treatment would be much less effective than in the original trial, it remained cost-effective. However, Mauskopf et al. (1996) estimated that universal screening of all pregnant women would only be cost-effective when the prevalence of HIV infection among those screened is 4.5 per 1,000 or greater, even assuming that all women who are reached agree to testing and treatment. This reflects both the high cost of establishing universal screening and the few HIV positive women identified per 100 women screened. While many cities in the United States meet or exceed this level, the estimated prevalence rate nationally is only 1.1 per 1,000 for pregnant women. Thus, it is not clear that universal screening of all pregnant women would be cost effective, whether voluntary or mandatory. This analysis included only the narrow healthcare costs and savings of screening programs, so it might well be cost-effective if more social costs and economic costs to the infant's family or the benefits of education and testing for the large number of HIV negative women were also included. Cost-effectiveness also would be greatly enhanced if screening costs were reduced.

The lack of established cost-effectiveness of prenatal screening programs can be viewed two ways. If the societal benefits of the program are important despite their high cost, then the mandating of such programs, together with funding to support them, is a way to ensure that these benefits are not denied to anyone because of costs. From another perspective, the question might be raised as to whether these programs maximize the social good obtained from the expenditure required.

Practical implementation will not be easy for any of the three proposed policies. All three policies require the development of sophisticated and well coordinated systems for counseling, testing, and follow-up. The current state of maternal-child health in the United States suggests that development and coordination of these systems will not happen overnight and that an extraordinary effort will be required to implement the best of what we already know about counseling and testing nationwide. Differences in success rates will probably vary far more due to quality than due to whether testing is mandatory, especially since mandatory testing may drive some women out of the healthcare system entirely. The politicians who have made these policy statements seem very poorly informed about the magnitude of what they have proposed in terms of financial, personnel and organizational costs.

TOWARD A PRIMARY HEALTHCARE PERINATAL PREVENTION POLICY

Public health policy regarding perinatal HIV/AIDS in the United States stands at a critical crossroad today. One path, mandatory prenatal or infant testing, sends a message of continued disregard for women as persons, their rights to autonomy and reproductive freedom, and their capacity to make reasoned and ethical decisions for themselves and their infants. This policy does not promote social justice because it restricts only women and disproportionately affects low income women of color. Ironically, this approach is likely to drive women away from care and thus achieve testing for fewer women than a policy of voluntary testing. Postnatal infant tests also fail to achieve substantial health benefits, making it clearly inappropriate as national health policy. Mandatory testing offers no compelling social benefits that cannot be achieved through voluntary testing and it is ethically unacceptable.

The second policy of universal counseling for all pregnant women with voluntary testing and treatment is ethically acceptable and potentially efficacious in helping to reduce the number of HIV positive infants born. Universal counseling achieves social justice, while voluntary testing preserves women's rights. An effective prenatal counseling and testing program provides the foundation for implementation of both current and future interventions to reduce transmission. The policy should encourage counseling from an ethical perspective of caring that helps each woman make decisions that are well informed and consistent with her moral values. Because establishing effective counseling and testing programs is likely to be cost-effective only in areas of relatively high prevalence of HIV infection among women, establishing voluntary testing as public policy is one way to ensure that the effort is made.

A third possible path would support voluntary prenatal testing and treatment as one component of a holistic approach to the interlocking health promotion goals of women's health, AIDS prevention, and infant health. The WHO Primary Health Care (PHC) model emphasizes provision of acceptable, accessible, affordable healthcare for all through the collaboration of healthcare providers and the community (WHO, 1978). A policy based on a PHC model would allocate resources so that primary prevention to reduce unwanted pregnancy and HIV infection in women would receive equal attention. To preserve human and financial resources for primary prevention, prenatal counseling and testing would need to be implemented in a cost-saving manner that also is responsive to the different needs of diverse communities and regions. This approach would integrate perinatal HIV/AIDS prevention into a context of improved overall healthcare for women and children, including HIV prevention, IV drug use prevention and rehabilitation, family planning and prenatal services. A cornerstone of these efforts would be long-term efforts to enhance self-esteem and partner negotiation and decision-making skills for all women and an emphasis on reproductive responsibility for men as well as women.

Holistic public policy should also recognize the need for social justice that goes beyond national borders. It is in the developing world, especially sub-Saharan Africa and Asia, where the majority of infants born with HIV infection live. These countries have neither the money nor the human resources to implement prenatal testing and ZDV treatment. They need far more help than the United States and other industrialized countries currently provide. The United States should support both primary prevention and continued development and implementation of more affordable and feasible perinatal interventions. Greater commitment to international perinatal HIV/AIDS prevention would emphasize the need for international solutions to an international epidemic and the importance of worldwide gender inequality as an underlying factor that fuels the AIDS pandemic affecting us all, men, women and children.

CITED LITERATURE

Acuff, K. (1996). Perinatal drug use: State interventions and the implications for HIV-infected women. In R. R. Faden & N. E. Kass (Eds.), *HIV, AIDS & childbearing. Public policy, private lives* (pp. 214–257). New York: Oxford University Press.

Adjorlolo, G. (1996). *Positive developments in interventions* (Abstract Th.16). In XI International Conference on AIDS Abstract Book (Vol. 2, p. 208). Vancouver, Canada.

Agency for Health Care Policy and Research. (1994). *Evaluation and management of early HIV infection* (AHCPR Publication No. 94-00572). Rockville, MD: Author.

Allen, A. (1996). Moral multiculturalism, childbearing, and AIDS. In R. R. Faden & N. E. Kass (Eds.), *HIV, AIDS & childbearing. Public policy, private lives* (pp. 367–410). New York: Oxford University Press.

Amaro, H. (1995). Love, sex, and power: Considering women's realities in HIV prevention. *American Psychologist, 50*(6), 437–447.

American Academy of Pediatrics & American College of Obstetricians and Gynecologists. (1995). *Joint statement on human immunodeficiency virus screening.* Glenview, IL: Authors.

American Medical Association. (1996). *House of Delegates Resolution 425, A-96: Counseling and testing of pregnant women for HIV.* (Available from the American Medical Association) Chicago, IL.

Arras, J. D. (1990). AIDS and reproductive decisions: Having children in fear and trembling. *The Milbank Quarterly, 68*(3), 353–382.

Banks, T. L. (1996). Legal challenges: State intervention, reproduction, and HIV-infected women. In R. R. Faden & N. E. Kass (Eds.), *HIV, AIDS & childbearing. Public policy, private lives* (pp. 143–177). New York: Oxford University Press.

Barnett, B. (1994). Family planning reduces mortality. *Network: Family Health International 14*(3), 4–7.

Batter, V., Malulu, M., Mbuyi, K., Mbu, L., Kamenga, M., & St. Louis, M. (1991). *HIV seronotification and counselling of childbearing women in Kinshasa, Zaire* (Abstract M.D.4013). In VII International Conference on AIDS Abstract Book (Vol. 1, p. 86). Florence, Italy.

Biggar, R. J., Miotti, P. G., Taha, T. E., Mtimavalye, L., Broadhead, R., Justesen, A., Yellin, F., Liomba, G., Miley, W., Waters, D., Chiphangwi, J. D., & Goedert, J. J. (1996, June 15). Perinatal intervention trial in Africa: Effects of a birth canal cleansing intervention to prevent HIV transmission. *Lancet, 347,* 1647–1650.

Blaney, C. L. (1993). Sex education leads to safer sex. *Network: Family Health International 14*(2), 7–11.

Bloche, M. G. (1996). Clinical counseling and the problem of autonomy-negating influence. In R. R. Faden & N. E. Kass (Eds.), *HIV, AIDS & childbearing. Public policy, private lives* (pp. 257–319). New York: Oxford University Press.

Bossi, G., Maccabruni, A., Caselli, D., Arlandi, L., Silini, E., & Mondelli, M. U. (1996). *Mother-to-child HIV transmission: Role of maternal HIV infection* (Abstract Th.B.4326). In XI International Conference on AIDS Abstract Book (Vol. 1, p. 306). Vancouver, Canada.

Bredberg-Raden, U., Urassa, W., Laymuya, E., Msemo, G., Kawo, G., Kazimoto, T., Massawe, A., Grankvist, O., Mbena, E., Karlsson, K., Mhalu, F., & Biberfeld, G. (1995). Predictive markers for mother-to-child transmission of HIV-1 in Dar es Salaam, Tanzania. *Journal of Acquired Immune Deficiency Syndromes and Human Retrovirology, 8*(2) 182–187.

Britton, C. B. (1995). An argument for universal HIV counseling and voluntary testing of women. *Journal of the American Medical Women's Association, 50*(3-4), 85–86.

Burns, D. N., Landesman, S., Muenz, L. R., Nugent, R. P., Goedert, J. J., Minkoff, H., Walsh, J. H., Mendez, H., Rubinstein, A., & Willoughby, A. (1994). Cigarette smoking, premature rupture of membranes, and vertical transmission of HIV-1 among women with low CD4$^+$ levels. *Journal of Acquired Immune Deficiency Syndromes, 7*(7), 718–726.

Burns, D. N., Landesman, S., Rubinstein, A., Waters, D., Willoughby, A., & Goedert, J. J. (1996). *HIV-RNA levels during pregnancy and vertical transmission of HIV-1* (Abstract Tu.C.345). In XI International Conference on AIDS Abstract Book (Vol. 1, p. 247). Vancouver, Canada.

Burton, G. J., O'Shea, S., Rostron, T., Mullen, J. E., Aiyer, S., Smith, R., & Banatvala, J. E. (1996). *Physical breaks in the placental trophoblastic surface: Significance in vertical transmission of HIV* (Abstract Tu.C.2587). In XI International Conference on AIDS Abstract Book (Vol. 1, p. 366). Vancouver, Canada.

Centers for Disease Control. (1995). U.S. Public Health Service recommendations for human immunodeficiency virus counseling and voluntary testing for pregnant women. *Morbidity and Mortality Weekly Report, 44*(RR.7).

Chu, S. Y., Buehler, J. W., Oxtoby, M. J., & Kilbourne, B. W. (1991). Impact of the human immunodeficiency virus epidemic on mortality in children, United States. *Pediatrics, 87,* 806–810.

Chu, S. Y., Hanson, D. L., Jones, J. L., & Adult/Adolescent HIV Spectrum of Disease Project Group. (1996). Pregnancy rates among women infected with human immunodeficiency virus. *Obstetrics & Gynecology, 87*(2), 195–198.

Coll, O., Hernandez, M., Boucher, C., Fortuny, C., Canet Espanol, T., & Martinez-Tejada, B. (1996). *Vertical transmission of HIV is correlated with high maternal viral load at delivery* (Abstract Tu.C.2580). In XI International Conference on AIDS Abstract Book (Vol. 1, p. 365). Vancouver, Canada.

Connor, E. M., Sperling, R. S., Gelber, R., Kiselev, P., Scott, G., O'Sullivan, M. J., VanDyke, R., Bey, M., Shearer, W., Jacobson, R. L., Jimenez, E., O'Neill, E., Bazin, B., Delfraissy, J. F., Culnane, M., Coombs, R., Elkins, M., Moye, J., Stratton, P., & Balsley, J. (for the Pediatric AIDS Clinical Trials Group Protocol 076 Study Group). (1994). Reduction of maternal-infant transmission of human immunodeficiency virus type 1 with Zidovudine treatment. *New England Journal of Medicine, 331*(18), 1173–1180.

Crawford, C. (1995). Protecting the weakest link: A proposal for universal, unblinded pediatric HIV testing, counseling and treatment. *Journal of Community Health, 20*(2), 125–141.

Dabis, F., Mandelbrot, L., Msellati, P., & van de Perres, P. (1995). Zidovudine to decrease mother-to-child transmission of HIV-1: Is it good for developing countries? [Correspondence] *AIDS, 9*(2), 204–206.

Davis, S. F., Byers, R. H., Jr., Lindegren, M. L., Caldwell, B., Karon, J. M., & Gwinn, M. (1995, September 27). Prevalence and incidence of vertically acquired HIV infection in the United States. *Journal of the American Medical Association, 274*(12), 952–955.

Des Jarlais, D., Hagen, H., Paone, D., & Friedman, S. (1996). *HIV incidence among syringe exchange participants: The International data* (Abstract Tu.C.322). In XI International Conference on AIDS Abstract Book (Vol. 1, p. 244). Vancouver, Canada.

De Vincenzi, I. (1996). *Incidence of pregnancy in a European cohort of HIV-infected women* (Abstract Mo.B.542). In XI International Conference on AIDS Abstract Book (Vol. 1, p. 29). Vancouver, Canada.

Duliege, A. M., Amos, C. I., Felton, S., Biggar, R. J., & Goedert, J. J. (1995). International Registry of HIV-Exposed Twins: Birth order, delivery route, and concordance in the transmission of human immunodeficiency virus type 1 from mothers to twins. *Journal of Pediatrics, 126*, 625–632.

Dumois, O. A. (1995). The case against mandatory newborn screening for HIV antibodies. *Journal of Community Health, 20*(2), 143–159.

Dunn, D. T., Newell, M. L., Ades, A. E., & Peckham, C. S. (1992). Risk of human immunodeficiency virus type 1 transmission through breast-feeding. *Lancet, 340*, 585.

Dunn, D. T., Newell, M. L., Mayaux, M. J., Kind, C., Hutto, C., Goedert, J. J., Andiman, W., & Perinatal AIDS Collaborative Transmission Studies. (1994). Mode of delivery and vertical transmission of HIV-1: A review of prospective studies. *Journal of Acquired Immune Deficiency Syndromes, 7*(10), 1064–1066.

Faden, R., Kass, N., Acuff, K., Allen, A., Anderson, J., Banks, T., Bloche, M. G., Chaisson, R., Cohn, S., Hutton, N., King, P., Lillie-Blanton, M., McCaul, M., Powers, M., Rothenberg, A., Saah, A., Solomon, L., & Wissow, L. (1996). HIV infection and childbearing: A proposal for public policy and clinical practice. In R. R. Faden & N. E. Kass (Eds.), *HIV,*

AIDS & childbearing. Public policy, private lives (pp. 426–446). New York: Oxford University Press.

Faden, R., Kass, N., & McGraw, D. (1996). Women as vessels and vectors: Lessons from the HIV epidemic. In S. M. Wolf (Ed.), *Feminism and bioethics, beyond reproduction* (pp. 252–281). New York: Oxford University Press.

Farnham, P. G., Holtgrave, D. R., Rogers, M. F., & Guinan, M. E. (1996). *Preventing perinatal HIV infection: Costs and effects of a recommended intervention in the U.S.* (Abstract Th.C.4817). In XI International Conference on AIDS Abstract Book (Vol. 2, p. 379). Vancouver, Canada.

Fawzi, W., Hunter, D. J., Spiegelman, D. L., Msamanga, G. I., Mwakagile, D. S., McGrath, N., & Kagoma, C. (1996). *Design and demographic, immunologic, and clinical profile in the trial of vitamins in HIV infection, Tanzania* (Abstract Tu.C.2598). In XI International Conference on AIDS Abstract Book (Vol. 1, p. 368). Vancouver, Canada.

Finger, W. (1991). Worldwide surveys show sharp decline in fertility rates. *Network: Family Health International 12*(3), 19–22.

Fiscus, S. A., Adimora, A. A., Schoenbach, V. J., Lim, W., McKinney, R., Rupar, D., Kenny, J., Woods, C., & Wilfert, C. (1996, May 15). Perinatal HIV infection and the effects of Zidovudine therapy on transmission in rural and urban counties. *Journal of the American Medical Association, 275*(19), 1483–1488.

Forbes, J., Burdge, D., & Money, D. (1996). *Outcome of infants born to HIV seropositive mothers in British Columbia, Canada* (Abstract Tu.C.2574). In XI International Conference on AIDS Abstract Book (Vol. 2, p. 364). Vancouver, Canada.

Gibb, D., MacDonagh, S. E., Masters, J., Helps, B., Gupta, R., Tuck, P., Tookey, P. A., Peckham, C., & Ades, A. E. (1996). *Evaluating antenatal HIV testing in London, UK* (Abstract Th.C.4615). In XI International Conference on AIDS Abstract Book (Vol. 2, p. 349). Vancouver, Canada.

Gilligan, C. (1988). Remapping the moral domain: New images of self in relationship. In C. Gilligan, J. V. Ward, J. M. Taylor, & B. Bardige (Eds.), *Mapping the moral domain* (pp. i–xxxix). Cambridge, MA: Harvard University Press.

Greenberg, B. L., Semba, R. D., Vink Peter, E., Schoenbaum, E. E., Weedon, J., & Perinatal AIDS Collaborative Transmission Study (PACTS). (1996). *Serum vitamin A and perinatal transmission of HIV among a cohort of HIV-infected women in the United States* (WITS) (Abstract Tu.C.2592). In XI International Conference on AIDS Abstract Book (Vol. 1, p. 367). Vancouver, Canada.

Gunderson, M., Mayo, D., & Rhame, F. (1996). Routine HIV testing of hospital patients and pregnant women: Informed consent in the real world. *Kennedy Institute of Ethics Journal, 6*(2), 161–182.

Gupta, G. R., & Weiss, E. (1993). Women's lives and sex: Implications for AIDS prevention. *Culture, Medicine and Psychiatry, 17,* 399–412.

Joao Esau, C., Menezes, J., Resende, O., Aleixo, P., Souza, J., Lourenco, N., D'Ippolito, M., Anderson, J., & Lambert, J. (1996). *HIV testing for pregnant women in a public maternity hospital located in inner city Rio de Janeiro* (Abstract Tu.C.2571). In XI International Conference on AIDS Abstract Book (Vol. 1, p. 363). Vancouver, Canada.

Kalish, L. A., Pitt, J., Hershow, R., Hollinger, B., Landesman, S., Lew, J., Pagano, M., & Moye, J. [for the Women and Infants Transmission Study (WITS)]. (1996). *Age at first positive HIV-1 culture in prenatally infected infants: Implications for determining the roles of intrauterine and intrapartum transmission* (Abstract Tu.C.2596). In XI International Conference on AIDS Abstract Book (Vol. 1, p. 370). Vancouver, Canada.

Karon, J. M., Rosenberg, P. S., McQuillan, G., Khare, M., Gwinn, M., & Peterson, L. R. (1996, July 10). Prevalence of HIV infection in the United States, 1984 to 1992. *Journal of the American Medical Association, 276*(2), 126–131.

Kass, N., & Faden, R. (1996a). In women's words: The values and lived experiences of HIV-infected women. In R. R. Faden & N. E. Kass (Eds.), *HIV, AIDS & childbearing. Public policy, private lives* (pp. 426–446). New York: Oxford University Press.

Kass, N., & Faden, R. (1996b). Practices and opinions of health-care providers serving HIV-infected women. In R. R. Faden & N. E. Kass (Eds.), *HIV, AIDS & childbearing. Public policy, private lives* (pp. 411–425). New York: Oxford University Press.

Kelly, J., Murphy, D., Washington, C., Wilson, T., Koob, J., Davis D., Ledezma, G., & Davantes, B. (1994). The effects of HIV/AIDS intervention groups for high-risk women in urban clinics. *American Journal of Public Health, 84*(12), 1918–1922.

Kind, C. (for the Swiss Neonatal HIV Study Group). (1996). *Effects of Zidovudine prophylaxis and elective cesarean section on vertical HIV transmission* (Abstract Tu.C.442). In XI International Conference on AIDS Abstract Book (Vol. 1, p. 249). Vancouver, Canada.

Kline, A., Strickleer, J., & Kemp, J. (1995). Factors associated with pregnancy and pregnancy resolution in HIV seropositive. *Social Science & Medicine, 40*(11), 1539–1547.

Kovacs, A., Thurston, L., Rother, C., Rasheed, S., & Chan, L. (1996). *Effects of maternal viral load on prenatal transmission* (Abstract Tu.C.2597). In

XI International Conference on AIDS Abstract Book (Vol. 1, p. 368). Vancouver, Canada.

Lallemant, M., Le Coeur, S., Samba, L., Cheynier, D., M'Pele, P., Nzingoula, S., Essex, M., & Congolese Research Group on Mother-to-Child Transmission of HIV. (1994). Mother-to-child transmission of HIV-1 in Congo, Central Africa. *AIDS, 8*(10), 1451–1456.

Lallemant, M., Le Coeur, S., Shepard, D., & Marlink, R. (1996). *Preventing mother-to-child HIV transmission in developing countries: A cost effectiveness perspective* (Abstract Th.C.4822). In XI International Conference on AIDS Abstract Book (Vol. 2, p. 380). Vancouver, Canada.

Landsberger, E. I., McGuinness, K., & Biggers, S. D. (1996). *The impact of Zidovudine on the reduction of prenatal transmission in NYC Parturients* (Abstract Tu.C.2595). In XI International Conference on AIDS Abstract Book (Vol. 1, p. 368). Vancouver, Canada.

Lapointe, N., Samson, J., Ag Bazet, A., Boucher, M., Fauvel, M., Tran, T., & Hankins, C. (1996). *Mother-to-child HIV transmission associated with duration of the second stage of labor* (Abstract Tu.C.340). In XI International Conference on AIDS Abstract Book (Vol. 1, p. 246). Vancouver, Canada.

Larsson, G., Spanfberg, L., Lindgren, S., & Bohlin, A. B. (1990). Screening for HIV in pregnant women: A study of maternal opinion. *AIDS Care, 2*(3), 223–228.

Levine, C., & Dubler, N. N. (1990). HIV and childbearing. Uncertain risks and bitter realities: The reproductive choices of HIV-infected women. *The Milbank Quarterly, 68*(3), 321–349.

Lindegren, M. L., Byers, B., Fleming, P., Thomas, P., Davis, S., Simonds, R. J., Valappil, T., & Ward, J. W. (1996). *A decline in the incidence of perinatally acquired (PA) AIDS in the United States* (Abstract Tu.C.2593). In XI International Conference on AIDS Abstract Book (Vol. 1, p. 367). Vancouver, Canada.

Lindsay, M. K., Peterson, H. B., Feng, T. I., Slade, B. A., Willis, S. W., & Klein, L. (1989). Routine antepartum human immunodeficiency virus infection screening in an inner-city population. *Obstetric & Gynecology, 74*(1), 289–294.

Locher, A. W. (1996). Ethics, women with HIV, and protection: Implications for nursing practice. *Journal of Obstetric, Gynecologic & Neonatal Nursing, 25*, 465–469.

Lyons, S., Bredell, W. J., McGillivray, G. M., Whistler, T., Gray, G., & McIntyre, J. A. (1996). *Mother-to-infant transmission of HIV-1 in South Africa* (Abstract Tu.C.2579). In XI International Conference on AIDS Abstract Book (Vol. 1, p. 365). Vancouver, Canada.

Maldonado, M. (1995) National Minority AIDS Council. Update 10/95. http://www.the body.com/nma/careact:htm/.

Mansergh, G., Haddix, A. C., Steketee, R. W., Nieburg, P. I., Hu, D. J., Simonds, R. J., & Rogers, M. (1996). Cost-effectiveness of short-course Zidovudine to prevent perinatal HIV type 1 infection in a Sub-Saharan African developing country setting. *Journal of the American Medical Association, 276*(2), 139–145.

Mason, J., Preisinger, J., Sperling, R., Walther, V., Berrier, J., & Evans, V. (1991). Incorporating HIV education and counseling into routine prenatal care: A program model. *AIDS Education and Prevention, 3*(2), 118–123.

Matheson, P. B., Farley, J., Greenberg, B., Nesheim, S., Simonds, R. J., & Perinatal AIDS Collaborative Transmission Studies (PACTS). (1996). *Perinatal HIV-1 transmission rates (TR), USA* (Abstract Tu.C.2599). In XI International Conference on AIDS Abstract Book (Vol. 2, p. 369). Vancouver, Canada.

Mauskopf, J. A., Paul, J. E., Witchman, D. S., White, A. D., & Tilson, H. H. (1996). Economic impact of treatment of HIV-positive pregnant women and their newborns with Zidovudine. Implications for HIV screening. *Journal of the American Medical Association, 276*(2), 132–138.

Mayaux, M. J., Blanche, S., Rouzioux, C., Chenadec, J. L., Chambrin, V., Firtion, G., Allemon, M. C., Vilmer, E., Vigneron, N. C., Tricoire, J., Guillot, F., Courpotin, C., & French Pediatric HIV Infection Study Group. (1995). Maternal factors associated with perinatal HIV-1 transmission: The French cohort study: 7 years of follow-up observation. *Journal of Acquired Immune Deficiency Syndromes and Human Retrovirology, 8*(2), 188–194.

Mayaux, M. J., Burgard, M., Teglas, J. P., Cottalorda, J., Krivine, A., Simon, F., Puel, J., Tamalet, C., Dormont, D., Masquelier, B., Doussin, A., Rouzioux, C., & Blanche, S. (for the French Pediatric HIV Infection Study Group). (1996, February 28). Neonatal characteristics in rapidly progressive perinatally acquired HIV-1 disease. *Journal of the American Medical Association, 275*(8), 606–610.

McCaul, M. E., Lillie-Blanton, M., & Svikis, D. S. (1996). Drug use, HIV status, and reproduction. In R. R. Faden & N. E. Kass (Eds.), *HIV, AIDS & childbearing. Public policy, private lives* (pp. 110–142). New York: Oxford University Press.

McElmurry, B. J., & Huddleston, D. S. (1991). Self-care and menopause: Critical review of research. *Health Care for Women International, 12*, 15–16.

McFadden, M. A. (1996). Moral development and reproductive health decisions. *Journal of Obstetric, Gynecologic & Neonatal Nursing, 25*, 507–512.

MCH/HIV Integration Project & Midwest AIDS Training & Education Center. (1996). *Universal HIV counseling and voluntary testing for women: A resource manual.* (Available from Cook County Hospital, CCSN Suite 1200, 1838 W. Harrison, Chicago, IL 60612)

McIntyre, J. A., Gray, G. E., & Lyons, S. F. (1996). *Maternal and obstetrical factors in mother-to-child transmission of HIV in Soweto, South Africa* (Abstract Tu.C.342). In XI International Conference on AIDS Abstract Book (Vol. 1, p. 246). Vancouver, Canada.

Michaels, D. (1992). Estimates of the number of motherless youth orphaned by AIDS in the United States. *Journal of the American Medical Association, 268*, 3456–3461.

Minckoff, H., & Willoughby, A. (1995). Predicting HIV diseases, Zidovudine in pregnancy, and unblinding heelstick surveys. Reframing the debate on prenatal HIV testing. [Commentary]. *Journal of the American Medical Association, 274*(14), 1165–1168.

Nesheim, S. R., Lindsay, M., Sawyer, M. K., Mancao, M., Lee, F. K., Shaffer, N., Jones, D., Slade, B. A., Ou, C. Y., & Nahmias, A. (1994). A prospective population-based study of HIV perinatal transmission. *AIDS, 8*(9), 1293–1298.

Nesheim, S. R., Sawyer, M. K., Meadows, L., Grimes, V., Nahmias, A., & Lindsay, M. (1996). *Perinatal HIV transmission among women with primary infection during pregnancy* (Abstract Tu.C.2600). In XI International Conference on AIDS Abstract Book (Vol. 1, p. 368). Vancouver, Canada.

Parker, R. (1996). *Empowerment, community mobilization and social change in the face of AIDS* (Abstract Tu.D.06). In XI International Conference on AIDS Abstract Book (Vol. 1, p. 214). Vancouver, Canada.

Pinch, W. (1994). Vertical transmission in HIV infection/AIDS: A feminist perspective. *Journal of Advanced Nursing, 19*, 36–44.

Povolotsky, J., Baron, P., Polsky, B., & Ariel Project Cohort Investigators. (1996). *Anti-HIV-1 p24 antibody reactivity as a predictor of maternal-infant HIV-1 transmission* (Abstract Tu.C.2591). In XI International Conference on AIDS Abstract Book (Vol. 1, p. 367). Vancouver, Canada.

Powers, M. (1996). The moral right to have children. In R. R. Faden & N. E. Kass (Eds.), *HIV, AIDS & childbearing. Public policy, private lives* (pp. 320–366). New York: Oxford University Press.

Rodriguez, E. M., Mofenson, L. M., Chang, B. H., Rich, K. C., Fowler, M. G., Smeriglio, V., Landesman, S., Fox, H. E., Diaz, C., Green, K., & Hanson, I. C. (for the Women and Infants Transmission Study). (1996). Association of maternal drug use during pregnancy with maternal HIV culture positively and perinatal HIV transmission. *AIDS, 10*(3), 273–282.

Rothenberg, K. H., Paskey, S. J., Reuland, M. M., Zimmerman, S. I., & North, R. L. (1995). Domestic violence and partner notification: Implications for treatment and counseling of women with HIV. *Journal of the American Medical Women's Association, 50*(3-4), 87–93.

Rouse, D. J., Owen, J., Goldenberg, R. L., & Vermud, S. H. (1995). Zidovudine for the prevention of vertical HIV transmission: A decision analytic approach. *Journal of Acquired Immune Deficiency Syndromes and Human Retrovirology, 9*(4), 401–407.

Rubini, N. P., Arabe, J., Cordovil, A. V., Sion, F. S., Morais-de-sa, C. A., Lima, A. J., Linares, J. C., Rocco, R., & Borges, M. R. (1996). *HIV vertical transmission in Rio de Janeiro: Rates and risk factors* (Abstract Tu.C.2570). In XI International Conference on AIDS Abstract Book (Vol. 2, p. 369). Vancouver, Canada.

Ruff, A. J., Coberly, J., Halsey, N. A., Boulos, R., Desormeaux, J., Burnley, A., Joseph, D. J., McBrien, M., Quinn, T., Losikoff, P., O'Brien, K. L., Louis, M. A., & Farzadegan, H. (1994). Prevalence of HIV-1 DNA and p24 antigen in breast milk and correlation with maternal factors. *Journal of Acquired Immune Deficiency Syndromes, 7*(1), 68–73.

Saba, J. (1995, July). Prevention of mother-to-child transmission of HIV. *International AIDS Society, 2,* 6–7.

Sanchez, E., Fortuny, C., Ercilla, M. G., Sorni, A., & Jimenez, R. (1996). *Children born to HIV-1 and HCV coinfected mothers* (Abstract Tu.C.2581). In XI International Conference on AIDS Abstract Book (Vol. 1, p. 365). Vancouver, Canada.

Semba, R. D., Miotti, P. G., Chiphangwi, J. D., Saah, A. J., Canner, J. K., Dallabetta, G. A., & Hooveer, D. R. (1994, June 25). Maternal vitamin A deficiency and mother-to-child transmission of HIV-1. *Lancet, 343,* 1593–1597.

Shaffer, N., Bhiraleus, P., Chinayon, P., Kalish, M., Roongpisuthipong, A., Siriwasin, W., Chearskul, S., Chotpitayasunondh, T., Sangkarat, S., Young, N., Brown, T., Batter, V., & Mastro, T. D. (1996). *High viral load predicts perinatal HIV-1 subtype transmission, Bangkok, Thailand* (Abstract Tu.C.343). In XI International Conference on AIDS Abstract Book (Vol. 1, p. 247). Vancouver, Canada.

Shelton, D. (1996, July 22). HIV prevention helping, but not enough. *American Medical News, 39*(27), 1, 52.

Siena Consensus Workshop II. (1995). Strategies for prevention of perinatal transmission of HIV infection. Report of a Consensus Workshop, Siena, Italy, June 3–6, 1993. *Journal of Acquired Immune Deficiency Syndromes and Human Retrovirology, 8*(2), 161–175.

Sikkema, K., Kely, J., Heckman, T., Roffman, R., Solomon, L., Cargill, V., & Winett, R. (1996). *Effects of community-level behavioral change intervention for women in low income housing developments* (Abstract Tu.C.453). In XI International Conference on AIDS Abstract Book (Vol. 1, p. 250). Vancouver, Canada.

Simonds, R. I., Nesheim, S., Matheson, P., Abrams, E., Vink, P., Palumbo, P., & Steketee, R. (for the Perinatal AIDS Collaborative Transmission Study (PACTS). (1996). *Declining mother-to-child HIV transmission following prenatal Zidovudine recommendations, United States* (Abstract Tu.C.441). In XI International Conference on AIDS Abstract Book (Vol. 1, p. 248). Vancouver, Canada.

Simonds, R. J., & Rogers, M. (1996). Preventing perinatal HIV infection. How far have we come? [Editorial]. *Journal of the American Medical Association, 275*(19), 1514–1515.

The status and trends of the global HIV/AIDS pandemic. Final Report (pp. 1–32). (1996, July). Symposium conducted at the meeting of the Eleventh International Conference on AIDS, Vancouver, Canada.

Stekettee, R. W., Simonds, R. J., Abrams, E., Nesheim, S., Vink, P., & Palumbo, P. (for the AIDS Collaborative Transmission Study (PACTS). (1996). *Perinatal HIV transmission risk and the effect of pregnancy or infant Zidovudine use in a multiethnic study, 1994–1995* (Abstract Tu.C.441). In XI International Conference on AIDS Abstract Book (Vol. 1, p. 249). Vancouver, Canada.

Strand, J., Rosenbaum, J., Middlestadt, S., Baume, C., Schechter, C., & Jimerson, A. (1996). *"Fill in the blanks"—A practical theory-based model for designing HIV prevention programs to promote behavioral change* (Abstract We.C.580). In XI International Conference on AIDS Abstract Book (Vol. 2, p. 42). Vancouver, Canada.

Tovo, P. A., DeMartino, M., Gabiano, C., (1992). Prognostic factors and survival in children with perinatal HIV-1 infection. *Lancet, 339*(63), 1249–1253.

Turner, B. J., Markson, L., Hauck, W., Cocroft, J., & Fanning, T. (1995). Prenatal care of HIV-infected women: Analysis of a large New York State cohort. *Journal of Acquired Immune Deficiency Syndromes and Human Retrovirology, 9*(4), 371–378.

U.S. Department of Health and Human Services, Health Resources and Services Administration. (1986). *Health Status of the Disadvantaged*

Chartbook 1986 (HRS-P-DV86-2). Washington, DC: U.S. Government Printing Office.

Villano, S. A., Thomas, D., Chang, B., Hershow, R., Mofenson, L., Lew, J., Davenny, K., Cotton, D., Hanson, C., Tang, B., Hillyer, G., Landesman, S., & Quinn, T. (1996). *Hepatitis infection and concurrent drug use is associated with increased vertical transmission of HIV* (Abstract Tu.C.2589). In XI International Conference on AIDS Abstract Book (Vol. 1, p. 367). Vancouver, Canada.

Viscarello, R. R., Copperman, A. B., & DeGennaro, N. J. (1994). Is the risk of perinatal transmission of human immunodeficiency virus increased by the intrapartum use of spiral electrodes or fetal scalp pH sampling? *American Journal of Obstetrics and Gynecology, 170*(3), 740–743.

Wabwire-Mangen, F., Gray, R. H., Mmiro, F. A., Wabinga, H., Abramowsky, C., Ndugwa, C., & Saaah, A. J. (1996). *Placental risk factors for the vertical transmission of HIV-1 in Uganda* (Abstract Tu.C.341). In XI International Conference on AIDS Abstract Book (Vol. 1, p. 246). Vancouver, Canada.

Walter, E. B., Elliott, A. J., Regan, A. N., Drucker, R., Clements, D. A., & Wilfert, C. M. (1995). Maternal acceptance of voluntary human immunodeficiency virus antibody testing during the newborn period with the Guthrie card. *Pediatric Infectious Disease Journal, 14*(5), 376–381.

Wissow, L., Hutton, N., & McGraw, D. C. (1996). Psychological issues for children born to HIV-infected mothers. In R. R. Faden & N. E. Kass (Eds.), *HIV, AIDS & childbearing. Public policy, private lives* (pp. 78–95). New York: Oxford University Press.

Wiznia, A., Crane, M., Lambert, G., Sansary, J., Harris, A., & Solomon, L. (1996, May 15). Zidovudine use to reduce perinatal HIV type 1 transmission in an urban medical center. *Journal of the American Medical Association, 275*(19), 1504–1506.

Working Group on Mother-To-Child Transmission of HIV. (1995). Rates of mother-to-child transmission of HIV-1 in Africa, America, and Europe: Results from 13 perinatal studies. *Journal of Acquired Immune Deficiency Syndromes and Human Retrovirology, 8*(5), 506–510.

World Health Organization. (1978). *Primary Health Care.* Geneva, Switzerland: Author.

World Health Organization. (1996). AIDS Update, Internet.

CURRENT INFORMATION SOURCES ON PERINATAL HIV/AIDS PREVENTION

There is an explosion of research, clinical studies and policy debates in the area of perinatal transmission. We have chosen to focus on providing the best sources for the most recent information on various topics. Summaries of most articles would quickly become out of date. We have included a few key articles that are reviews of multiple studies or especially thoughtful discussions of these complex issues.

HIV/AID STATISTICS

International data are best obtained via the World Health Organization (WHO) which publishes the current global situation of the HIV/AIDS pandemic from its base in Geneva, Switzerland. WHO publications can be obtained free of charge from the WHO headquarters but this is a slow process. WHO AIDS data is now obtainable on the Internet through the WHO home page.

National data can be found in *The Morbidity and Mortality Weekly Report* series *(MMWR)* prepared by the Centers for Disease Control and Prevention (CDC) for publication by the US Department of Health and Human Services/Public Health Service. It is published weekly, and regularly reports summary data on AIDS and HIV infection, and regularly offers integrative and interpretive discussions of recent statistics. It is the best source of statistics on AIDS/HIV occurring in the United States. The CDC has recently put AIDS statistics on the Internet.

Local and State HIV/AIDS statistics are generally compiled by State Departments of Public Health. In Illinois, both the state and the city of Chicago regularly publish data which can be obtained free on request. Because the prevalence of HIV infection and the types of persons most affected vary greatly by local area, local statistics are critical in developing local programs or policies.

PERINATAL TRANSMISSION AND PREVENTION RESEARCH

At present, many advances in basic research on the process of transmission and clinical trials of a wide range of drug therapies and other interventions are ongoing. The initial report of major breakthroughs are usually published in the traditionally most prestigious medical journals, including *Journal of the American Medical Association, New England Journal of Medicine,* and *Lancet.* Because there is often a long gap between acceptance and publication, the Internet is useful to search for preliminary reports as well as new published studies. New developments in perinatal prevention and in monitoring and treatment of HIV positive infants strongly affect the benefits and costs of prenatal testing. It is likely that as prevention improves prenatal testing will become increasingly beneficial to women and infants.

Dabis, F., Mandelbrot, L., Msellati, P., & van de Perres, P. (1995). Zidovudine to decrease mother-to-child transmission of HIV-1: Is it good for developing countries? [Correspondence] *AIDS, 9*(2), 204–206.

Saba, J. (1995, July). Prevention of mother-to-child transmission of HIV. *International AIDS Society, 2,* 6–7.

Siena Consensus Workshop II. (1995). Strategies for prevention of perinatal transmission of HIV infection. Report of a Consensus Workshop, Siena, Italy, June 3–6, 1993. *Journal of Acquired Immune Deficiency Syndromes and Human Retrovirology, 8*(2), 161–175.

These three articles provide excellent overviews of the approaches to perinatal HIV/AIDS transmission and how soon each is likely to be feasible for widespread use. The Siena Workshop provides the most comprehensive review, while Saba is more recent, written after the ZDV trial results were available. Dabis et al. provide an especially thoughtful discussion of the inequity between developing countries and industrialized nations which make drug therapy almost irrelevant internationally.

Key Studies Today

Biggar, R. J., Miotti, P. G., Taha, T. E., Mtimavalye, L., Broadhead, R., Justesen, A., Yellin, F., Liomba, G., Miley, W., Waters, D., Chiphangwi, J. D., & Goedert, J. J. (1996, June 15). Perinatal intervention trial in Africa: Effects of a birth canal cleansing intervention to prevent HIV transmission. *Lancet, 347,* 1647–1650.

The first trial of birth canal cleansing during labor with a viricidal solution was disappointing in that no overall reduction in transmission was achieved, although the transmission rate was improved for women whose membranes were ruptured at least four hours prior to delivery.

Connor, E. M., Sperling, R. S., Gelber, R., Kiselev, P., Scott, G., O'Sullivan, M. J., VanDyke, R., Bey, M., Shearer, W., Jacobson, R. L., Jimenez, E., O'Neill, E., Bazin, B., Delfraissy, J. F., Culnane, M., Coombs, R., Elkins, M., Moye, J., Stratton, P., & Balsley, J. (for the Pediatric AIDS Clinical Trials Group Protocol 076 Study Group). (1994). Reduction of maternal-infant transmission of human immunodeficiency virus type 1 with Zidovudine treatment. *New England Journal of Medicine, 331*(18), 1173–1180.

This is the classic study that first documented the effectiveness of perinatal transmission. The study was conducted with great care, and the evidence is very clear that ZDV given during the prenatal, intrapartum and postpartum period substantially reduces HIV transmission from mother to child.

Duliege, A. M., Amos, C. I., Felton, S., Biggar, R. J., International Registry of HIV-Exposed Twins, & Goedert, J. J. (1995). Birth order, delivery route, and concordance in the transmis-

sion of human immunodeficiency virus type 1 from mothers to twins. *Journal of Pediatrics, 126,* 625–632.

This study documented the importance of vaginal contact through a careful examination of the relationship between birth order and whether vaginal or cesarian delivery for a large series of twin births.

Kind, C. (for the Swiss Neonatal HIV Study Group). (1996). *Effects of Zidovudine prophylaxis and elective cesarean section on vertical HIV transmission* (Abstract Tu.C.442). In XI International Conference on AIDS Abstract Book (Vol. 1, p. 249). Vancouver, Canada.

This small but exciting study indicates that both ZDV and elective cesarean section reduce transmission and for the small group of infants receiving both there were no HIV positive infants. A more detailed study is likely to be published soon.

For ongoing updates, see:
Harvard AIDS Institute [HAI] on the Internet. The HAI Home Page provides information on four areas of research, Basic Science, Clinical Science & Care, Epidemiology/Public Health and Prevention, and Social Science & Policy, as well as Useful Tools for the Researcher, which provides information on how to access relevant bibliographic services and government agencies.

ETHICAL ISSUES IN PERINATAL TESTING

Prenatal Testing

Britton, C. B. (1995). An argument for universal HIV counseling and voluntary testing of women. *Journal of the American Medical Women's Association, 50*(3-4), 85–86.

Minckoff, H., & Willoughby, A. (1995). Predicting HIV diseases, Zidovudine in pregnancy, and unblinding heelstick surveys. Reframing the debate on prenatal HIV testing. [Commentary]. *Journal of the American Medical Association, 274*(14), 1165–1168.

Simonds, R. J., & Rogers, M. (1996). Preventing perinatal HIV infection. How far have we come? [Editorial]. *Journal of the American Medical Association, 275*(19), 1514–1515.

These three articles all present strong justifications for a policy of universal testing and voluntary testing, integrating ethical issues with feasibility, cost and effectiveness issues. While the articles overlap a good deal each offers a somewhat different perspective. Britton points out that counseling and voluntary testing begin the development of a trusting collaboration between HIV positive mothers and their caregivers, and emphasizes the role of informed consent in documenting at least minimal adherence to ethical standards of disclosure and non-coercion. Minckoff and Willoughby argue for integration of HIV testing into prenatal care with a model of routine testing and right of refusal, while Simonds and Rogers focus on the organizational and financial challenges of implementing universal counseling nationwide.

Postnatal Infant Testing

Crawford, C. (1995). Protecting the weakest link: A proposal for universal, unblinded pediatric HIV testing, counseling and treatment. *Journal of Community Health, 20*(2), 125–141.

Dumois, O. A. (1995). The case against mandatory newborn screening for HIV antibodies. *Journal of Community Health, 20*(2), 143–159.

These companion articles offer arguments for and against mandatory infant HIV testing in the context of proposed legislation pending in New York State. Crawford (1995) argues that mandatory testing is necessary to enable infants born to HIV positive mothers to receive appropriate care and recounts bureaucratic difficulties in getting tests authorized for children who are wards of the state. He charges that voluntary testing has been a failure. Dumois points out that voluntary testing has already succeeded in many programs, and that a strong rationale for testing has only

emerged since ZDV treatment has been shown to be effective. She also points out that mandatory newborn testing is both ineffective and high-cost, and will draw resources away from excellent statewide programs of counseling and testing both prenatally and in family planning and STD clinics where women are not pregnant.

Background Materials on HIV/AIDS and Women's Reproductive Rights

Faden, R. R., & Kass, N. E., (Eds.). (1996). *HIV, AIDS & childbearing. Public policy, private lives.* New York: Oxford University Press.

This reader provides an excellent background on a variety of issues related to reproduction for HIV positive women, including a history of reproductive rights, women's legal issues, and the health considerations for women and infants. Especially noteworthy is the inclusion of three chapters presenting the ethical perspectives of women living with HIV/AIDS and their caregivers. The authors recommend counseling from a caring perspective that helps HIV positive women make better informed ethical decisions that are in accord with their personal moral perspectives (not necessarily that of their caregivers.

McFadden, M. A. (1996). Moral development and reproductive health decisions. *Journal of Obstetric, Gynecologic and Neonatal Nursing, 25,* 507–512.

This article provides an excellent overview of the caring ethical perspective compared to the justice perspective. McFadden also discusses the reasons why this perspective may be appropriate for counseling HIV positive women regarding ethical decisions.

Clinicians Perspectives

Lindberg, C. (1995). Perinatal transmission of HIV: How to counsel women. *Maternal Child Nursing, 20,* 207–212.

This very straightforward article reviews the factors affecting perinatal transmission, the interventions currently available, and the need to adapt counseling to fit the diverse situations of HIV positive women in their childbearing years.

Consumers Perspectives

There are now many consumer-oriented publications on the Internet. They all provide recent and highly readable information for women. However, consumers need to be cautious in using these materials because the quality of contents varies and often material is older than it seems at first glance.

Two services with health professional affiliation that offer a degree of peer review to ensure accuracy and balanced presentations are the AIDS Information Newsletter (www.cmpharm.ucsf.edu) published by the San Francisco VA Medical Center and Perinatal HIV/AIDS published by the March of Dimes (www.noah.cuny/edu/pregnancy/march_of _dimes/stds/periaids.html).

The Women's Wire (www.women.com) home page offers access to many interesting newsletters, many by women for women, including SisterLove (www.hidwater.com /sisterlove/slhome.html).

Women Alive is an online journal targeted to women living with HIV/AIDS (WomenAlive, BngAlive@aol.com). This journal offers lively discussion of issues from a woman's perspective. The views expressed are very sensitive to the political context of AIDS research, but the views expressed regarding the ZDV trials contained a few inaccuracies or misinterpretations.

Part VIII

Physical Diseases and Health Problems

Chapter 8

Autoimmunity and Gender Effects: Lupus Erythematosus

Ayhan Aytekin Lash

Partly due to the recognition of the importance that the immune system plays in the development of cancer and acquired immune deficiency syndrome, the last decade witnessed an exponential growth in the understanding of the mechanisms involved in the immune response. The availability of increased funds for more animal research to combat these diseases combined with advances in biotechnology transformed our understanding of how the immune system works in relation to health and disease.

It is widely accepted that the immune system interacts with most, if not all, body systems responsible for the maintenance of homeostasis (Ahmed & Talal, 1993; Da Silva, 1995; Grossman, 1984; Lahita, 1992). For example, the hormones of the endocrine system influence the immune system through several feedback mechanisms that also involve the central nervous system. The evidence linking both the immune with the endocrine, and the immune with the nervous system is so substantial that a new field called psychoneuroimmunology undertakes the study of the nature of interactions between the immune, endocrine, and the nervous systems. This three-way interaction has implications for women's health in terms of resisting infection and tumor formation, on the one hand, but also increased susceptibility to autoimmune disorders on the other.

The interaction of the immune system with other biological systems is accomplished by the widespread presence of immune cells, (T and B cells or lymphocytes), immune molecules, and immune organs throughout the body for defense against infection. To accomplish this defense, the cells and the molecules of the immune system, "talk" with one other to continuously identify the unknown antigens (pathogens) and to alert the nervous and endocrine system of the impending confrontation. The accuracy of this communication is the key to the delivery of specific immune responses against foreign antigens. The immune response against the antigen is complex and sophisticated. It includes the following actions: recognition of the antigen's foreignness and its breakage into peptides by B cells and macrophages; the specific identification of the antigen peptide in relation to self-tissue markers, the major histocompatibility complex, by T cells with assistance from chemical mediators called cytokines; the creation and storage of a memory for antigen's instant re-identification in case it re-enters the body by B and T cells; the manufacturing of powerful antibodies to render the antigen harmless by B cells; further destruction of the antigen by T cells and cytokines; cessation of antibody production by B cells with guidance from suppressor T cells; and finally, ousting the antigen from the body by the phagocytic cells.

This process of normal immune reactivity, however, requires that the immune system distinguishes the friend (self-tissues) from foe (pathogens). This process of differentiating self- from nonself-tissues is so consequential that some immunologists even define immunology as the science of self-nonself discrimination (Klein, 1982). This discrimination, which has important implications for women's health, is made possible by an intricate specific-recognition system involving immune cells, cytokines, body proteins associated with the complement, kinin and fibrolytic systems (Goodman, 1994), as well as the endocrine and the nervous systems (Talal, 1987).

In addition, the human body is equipped with numerous safeguards to prevent immune cells from attacking self-tissues. For example, immature (incompetent) lymphocytes have the potential to respond to self-tissues. There is, however, a mechanism called apoptosis, or programmed cell death, that drives these autoreactive cells to self-destruct. Moreover, if these cells survive to maturity and react to self-tissues, they are usually killed or become deactivated by other immune cells (Mountz, Wu, Cheng, & Zhou, 1994; Steinburg, 1994).

Despite numerous safeguards, however, at times, the immune cells fail to recognize the body cells they are programmed to tolerate. When this recognition fails, an attack on the body cells ensues causing a disease condition called autoimmunity. Central to the concept of autoimmunity is the concept of defect in self-tolerance and incessant injury of self-tissues (Beeson, 1994).

Autoimmunity affects 5 percent of the U.S. and European populations, and even more if the suspected link between autoimmunity and atherosclerosis becomes confirmed (Steinman, 1993). Among the genetically susceptible individuals, the triggering factors include infections (viruses), certain drugs (for example, hydralazine, procainamide, and oral contraceptives are associated with onset of lupus-like syndromes), change in hormonal environment, and physical and/or psychological trauma. Once formed, autoantibodies may attack any organ, such as the white matter of the brain and the spinal cord as in multiple sclerosis; the lining of the joints as in rheumatoid arthritis (RA); the insulin secreting cells as in juvenile diabetes mellitus; destruction of the connection between muscles and nerves as in myasthenia gravis; excessive thyroid hormone production as in Grave's disease; red blood cells as in immune hemolytic anemia (Atkinson, 1995), and the heart, the kidneys, lungs, and the brain as in systemic lupus erythematosus (SLE).

Autoimmunity is a chronic, destructive disease condition that is either organ specific or systemic that occurs mostly in women. Table 8.1 shows some of the most common autoimmune diseases and their rate of prevalence in women. Research in this area during the last four decades identified gender differences in immune reactivity, and also that the female immune system was more potent than male (Ahmed, Penhale, & Talal, 1985; Grossman, 1984; Grossman, Roselle, & Mendenhall, 1991; Lahita, 1990). Studies with laboratory animals, mostly with New Zealand White (NZW) and New Zealand Black (NZB) mice, for example, revealed that females responded better to immunization than males, generating a stronger antibody-mediated immunity (Eidinger & Garret, 1972).

During the 1980s and 1990s, research on the role of sex hormones revealed that the immune system was partially regulated by sex steroids and that this regulation was steroid-hormone dependent (Ahmed & Talal, 1990; Grossman, 1984; Grossman, Roselle, & Mendenhall, 1991; Lahita, 1990; McCruden & Stimsom, 1991). Research with both humans and laboratory animals, particularly with NZW and NZB mice, allowed researchers to identify how estrogens, progesterone, and androgens influenced the rate and amplitude of immune reactivity. Lahita (1990), for example, found that high levels of serum estrogen were associated with high immune reactivity and that high levels of androgens attenuated the immune response.

Writing about the importance of sex hormones during the mid-1990s, Ahmed and Talal (1993)—prominent researchers of immunity, autoimmunity, and sex hormones—stated that sex hormones were immunomodulators capable of affecting oncopathological and allergic processes. Additional evidence showed females to have higher levels of immunoglobulins (Igs or antibodies) than age-matched males (Ahmed & Talal, 1993). This immune reactivity of the female was also evident in the rapid reactivity of females to allograft (Ahmed & Talal, 1993).

Moreover, Lahita (1990) reported that sex hormones produce immunologically active cytokines that regulate the initiation, amplitude, and duration of the immune response. More significantly for women's health, cytoxines play a significant role in tumor surveillance, thereby, giving

Table 8.1
Selected Autoimmune Diseases with 50 Percent or
More Prevalence in Women

Autoimmune Diseases	% Females (All Ages)
Sjogren's syndrome	95
Systemic lupus erythematosus	90
Primary biliary cirrhosis	90
Erythema nodosum	90
Hashimoto's thyroiditis	85
Takayasu's arteritis	85
Thyrotoxicosis	85
Scleroderma	80
Addison's disease	75
Myasthenia gravis	75
Thrombocytopenic purpura	75
Dermatomyositis	70
Giant cell arteritis/polymyalgia	65
Chronic active hepatitis	65
Rheumatoid arthritis	65
Sydenham's chorea	65
Multiple sclerosis	65
Pernicious anemia	60
Sarcoidosis	60
Polymyositis/dermatomyositis	55
Bullous pemphigoid	55
Pemphigus vulgaris	50
Polychondritis	50
Ulcerative colitis	50
Wegener's granulomatosis	50
Polyglandular syndromes	50
Rheumatic fever	50

Source: Modified from Beeson (1994).

females greater protection against certain tumors. Lahita (1990) and Petri, Howard, and Repke (1991), for example, reported that estradiol, the most potent and plentiful of the three estrogens, influenced the lymphocyte count as the number of B and T cell counts escalated during the normal menstrual cycle and in pregnancy. By contrast, men treated with estrogen for prostate cancer showed compromised T cell mediated immunity later playing a major role in regulating (initiating and terminating) the antibody response. These observations suggested that females have greater resistance to infections than males due to their highly reactive immune system.

In reviewing the immunomodulation by sex steroids, Ahmed and Talal (1985, 1993) stated that the female immune system may have given them a selective advantage for protection against infection and tumor formation so as to ensure fetal survival. These investigators also asserted that the endocrine, the immune, and the central nervous system were all under the influence of higher centers in the brain, so were affected by stress, mood, and emotions. Talal (1987) believed that these connections were part of the evolutionary process and were designed to ensure species survival. Talal (1987) stated that the immunological strength of women, however, could become a double-edged sword as it predisposed women to excessive immune reactivity and, therefore, put women at risk to acquire autoimmune diseases such as SLE.

SLE: AN OVERVIEW

As Table 8.1 showed, women are more susceptible to autoimmune diseases such as the Sjogren's syndrome, SLE, RA, primary biliary cirrhosis, thyroiditis, scleroderma, myasthenia gravis, multiple sclerosis, and ulcerative colitis. This susceptibility has far-reaching implications for women's health, in terms of body image, role performance at home and work, professional career, social and sexual life, and reproductive health. Very few autoimmune diseases, however, exemplify the autoimmune reactivity in women better than SLE in terms of its physical and psychosocial ramifications. According to an informal survey by the Lupus Foundation of America (LFA, 1994), there are over 1.5 million SLE patients in the United States; 90 percent of these patients are women. A recent epidemiological survey by McCarthy et al. (1995), for example, showed that the relative frequency of SLE for white females was 3.2 while it was 0.4 for white males per 100,000 population.

SLE is three times more common among African-American and Hispanic women. In the aforementioned survey, McCarthy et al. (1995) found SLE rates for African-American females to be 9.2/100,000 showing the persistence of earlier estimates for this group. Moreover, SLE is age dependent; the prevalence of the disease peaks during reproductive years and tapers off after menopause. It has also been reported that oral contraceptives affect the course of SLE (Ahmed & Talal, 1993). In addition, there is a high correlation between SLE onset and lupus flares during menses, pregnancy, and the postpartum period (Legun, 1990; Petri, Howard, & Repke, 1991; Repke & Petri, 1991), all of which give credence to research linking female hormones to autoimmunity.

SLE is a prototypical autoimmune disorder that is characterized by the production of antibodies against host tissues that results in a generalized inflammatory response (hot, swollen, and painful tissues) in the organs attacked. Space limitations prevent extensive review of the etiology, pathophysiology, and the wide variance seen in clinical manifestations of the disease (SLE is known as "the great imitator"). In general, since autoantibodies circulate throughout the body, no organ is exempt from the attack. The most commonly affected organs are the mucocutaneous, pulmonary, cardiovascular, hematologic, and renal systems (Stevens, 1991). Among the most typical manifestations are the butterfly rash over the bridge of the nose and the cheeks, erythematous patches around fingers, palms, and periungual areas, extreme fatigue, painful joints, and hair loss. Kidney involvement is seen in 50 percent of the SLE patients occasionally progressing to kidney failure requiring kidney transplant. Cardiac involvement (lupus carditis) occurs in up to 48 percent of SLE patients, an ominous sign of an advanced stage, and contributes significantly to mortality and morbidity (Stevens, 1991).

Hematological alterations are among the most common features of SLE due to the formation of autoantibodies against blood cells such as erythrocytes (red blood cells), leukocytes (infection-fighting white blood cells), thrombocytes (or platelets, those blood cells that form clots to prevent blood loss), and other coagulation factors. Among SLE patients, the presence of antibodies against blood cells cause anemia in 98 percent, mild leukopenia in up to 80 percent, and thrombocytopenia (low platelet count) in about 30 percent of SLE patients (Mudge-Groud, 1992; Stevens, 1991; Ziminski, 1991).

One of the most puzzling aspects of hematological involvement of SLE is the presence of both bleeding and clotting tendencies that have implications for birth control, child bearing, and reproductive health. Because of its significance for women's health, SLE and reproductive health will be briefly reviewed later. More significantly, and relevant to the diagnosing of the disease, is the presence of antinuclear antibodies (ANA) in 90 percent of SLE patients' blood serum. The positive ANA blood test indicates that antibodies attack the nucleus of the body cells as foreign. When the pivotal role of the cell nucleus in overall functioning of all living organisms is considered, the contribution of antinuclear antibodies to overall poor health becomes obvious.

Although still without a cure, the survival of SLE patients has improved significantly over the last four decades. For example, while in the 1950s the 5-year survival rate was about 50 percent, in the 1990s the 10-year survival exceeded 90 percent both nationally and internationally (Gripenberg & Helve, 1991; Pistiner, Wallace, Nessim, Metzger, & Klineberg, 1991). Because of the wide spectrum of clinical manifestations, treatment is individualized. Among the pharmacological interventions are the use of nonsteroidal anti-inflammatory (aspirin, ibuprofen), immunosuppressive (prednisone), antimalarial (plaquenil), and anticancer (cytoxan) drugs that are individualized according to the severity of the illness.

The nursing care of patients with SLE must aim to manage symptoms, prevent organ damage, and provide supportive care both to the individual and the family. Nonpharmacological interventions in the form of fatigue management, pain control, and daily, mild-to-moderate weight-bearing exercises, such as walking and low-impact dancing, have been shown to minimize joint problems. Sunlight is one of the most common triggering factors—about 30 percent of patients show sun sensitivity. Therefore, sunlight must be avoided with the use of sunblocking agents. Moreover, stress, which is identified as one of the most insidious factors triggering SLE onset or lupus flares, must be controlled. The LFA and its local chapters are among the important resources for patients and families. Many countries such as Australia, England, Egypt, and South Africa have active lupus organizations that provide patients with information and support services.

SLE and Reproductive Health

Because of the link between sex hormones and immune reactivity, issues related to menses, pregnancy, and the use of birth control pills are important for SLE patients. As would be expected, there is increased SLE activity (lupus flares) among those taking oral contraceptives (Bucala, Lahita, Fishman, & Cerami, 1987). However, some women with SLE have been able to use birth control pills without flares, suggesting that the decision should be made individually. Also, the use of intrauterine devices are contraindicated due to the susceptibility of SLE patients to infections. The use of barrier methods, however, such as condoms, foams, and diaphragms, is without additional risk.

Available data suggest that pregnancy puts SLE women at great risk. Between 25 percent to 50 percent of SLE patients experienced lupus flares during pregnancy (Petri, Howard, & Repke, 1991; Repke & Petri, 1991). Among serious complications are miscarriages due to the placental thrombosis that is associated with the formation of antibodies against clotting factors. In addition, hypertension, pre-eclampsia, and kidney damage can develop during, and most frequently immediately after, the delivery. Moreover, a few infants can develop congenital heart block and neonatal lupus from mothers with SLE. These complications, however, may be prevented or minimized if women become pregnant during remission and receive close supervision from both rheumatologist and obstetrician throughout pregnancy. Therefore, women with SLE planning pregnancy must consult a rheumatologist for guidance on timing and management of pregnancy. Without close supervision from healthcare professionals, pregnant women with SLE and their fetuses would be at risk.

SLE is a chronic illness that requires the active involvement of the patient and the family. Therefore, the skills necessary for competent self-care are essential to extend survival and improve the quality of life.

IMPLICATIONS FOR EDUCATION, PRACTICE, RESEARCH AND HEALTH POLICY

The research related to autoimmunity has been robust. The prevalence of auto-immune disorders among women is now a well-established pathophysiological phenomena. However, studies related to auto-immune disorders from the perspective of women have been limited. For example, currently we know very little about individual and family coping, psychosocial adjustment, changes in the body image, and QOL in SLE. Similarly, fatigue, one of the most debilitating symptoms of SLE remains understudied in terms of its link to disease activity, disease severity, and QOL. Moreover, auto-immunity as a pathophysiological phenomena that puts women at risk has yet to be recognized as an area of research by nurse investigators. Autoimmunity, particularly SLE, however, can put women at risk not only for heart and kidney diseases, but also for stroke, osteoporosis, psychosis, and premature death. In addition, there is an urgent need to curtail the time it takes to diagnose SLE. The traditional underrating of women's health problems by healthcare professionals coupled with the deceptive nature of the disease continue to delay its definitive diagnosis that currently takes up to ten years after its onset.

Nursing research can identify, and propose ways to eliminate, those factors delaying diagnosis. Moreover, prevention of organ damage through symptom management and self-care management among the newly diagnosed patients is an area that needs the attention of all healthcare professionals and researchers. Although no cure has yet to be found, successful control of SLE has been possible with the use of pharmacological and non-pharmacological means. The fit between these interventions and the individual, however, can be improved with the investigation of psychosocial factors that contribute to prolonged survival with the disease.

Moreover, several investigators have reported that SLE is more aggressive among African-Americans, contributing to higher morbidity and mortality. The identification of culturally sensitive interventions that would improve the management of the disease would make an invaluable contribution to the healthcare of women in this population. Most importantly, government funding for SLE remains limited. Studies that would investigate the link between the biomedical and behavioral aspect of SLE would be most beneficial in preventing and curtailing the physical, biological, and emotional cost of SLE.

REFERENCES

Ahmed, A. S., Penhale, W. J., & Talal, N. (1985). Sex hormones, immune and autoimmune responses, and mechanisms of sex hormone action. *American Journal of Pathology, 121*, 531–551.

Ahmed, A. S., & Talal, N. (1985). The survival value of nonclassical sites for sex hormone action in the immune and central nervous systems. *Clinical Immunology Newsletter, 6*, 97.

Ahmed, A. S., & Talal, N. (1990). Sex hormones and immune system: Part 2. Animal data. *Bailliere's Clinical Rheumatology, 4*, 13–81.

Ahmed, A. S., & Talal, N. (1993). Importance of sex hormones in systemic lupus erythematosus. In D. J. Wallace & B. H. Hahn (Eds.), *Dubois' lupus erythematosus* (pp. 148–156). Philadelphia: Lea & Febinger.

Atkinson, J. P. (1995). Some thoughts on autoimmunity. *Arthritis & Rheumatism, 38*(3), 301–305.

Beeson, P. B. (1994). Age and sex associations of 40 autoimmune diseases. *The American Journal of Medicine, 96*, 457–462.

Bucala, R., Lahita, R. G., Fishman, J., & Cerami, A. (1987). Anti-estrogen antibodies in users of oral contraceptives and in patients with systemic lupus erythematosus. *Clinical and Experimental Immunology, 67*, 167–175.

Da Silva, J. A. P. (1995). Sex hormones, glucocorticoids and autoimmunity: Facts and hypotheses. *Annals of Rheumatic Diseases, 54*, 435–455.

Eidinger, D., & Garret, T. J. (1972). Studies of the regulatory effects of the sex hormones on the antibody formation and stem cell differentiation. *Journal of Experimental Medicine, 136*, 1098–2116.

Goodman, J. W. (1994). The immune response. In D. P. Stites, A. I. Terr, & T. G. Parslow (Eds.), *Basic and clinical immunology* (pp. 40–49). Norwalk, CT: Appleton & Lange.

Gripenberg, M., & Helve, T. (1991). Outcome of systemic lupus erythematosus: A study of 66 patients over 7 years with special reference to the predictive value of anti-DNA antibody determination. *Scandinavian Journal of Rheumatology, 20*, 104–109.

Grossman, C. J. (1984). Regulation of the immune system by sex steroids. *Endocrine Review, 5*(3), 435–455.

Grossman, J. C., Roselle, G. A., & Mendenhall, C. L. (1991). Sex steroid regulation of autoimmunity. *Journal of Steroid Biochemical Molecular Biology, 40,* 649–659.

Klein, J. (1982). *Immunology: The science of self-nonself discrimination.* New York: John Wiley & Sons.

Lahita, R. G. (1990). Sex hormones and the immune system—Part 1. *Baillieres Clinical Rheumatology, 4,* 1–12.

Lahita, R. G. (1992). Sex, age and systemic lupus erythematosus. In R. G. Lahita (Ed.), *Systemic lupus erythematosus* (pp. 527–542). New York: Churchill Livingstone.

Legun, L. A. (1990). Systemic lupus erythematosus during pregnancy. *Journal of Obstetric, Gynecologic & Neonatal Nursing, 19,* 304–310.

LFA study shows between 1,400,000 and 2,000,000 people diagnosed with lupus. (1994). *Lupus News, 14*(3), 12.

Liang, M. H., Roger, M., Larson, M., Eaton, H. M., Murawski, B. J., Taylor, J. E., Swafford, J., & Shur, P. (1984). The psychological impact of lupus erythematosus and rheumatoid arthritis. *Arthritis & Rheumatism, 27*(1), 13–19.

McCarthy, D., Manzi, S., Medsger, T. A., Jr., Ramsey-Goldman, R., LaPorte, R. E., & Kwoh, K. C. (1995). Incidence of systemic lupus erythematosus. *Arthritis & Rheumatism, 38*(9), 1260–1270.

McCruden, A. B., & Stimson, W. H. (1991). Sex hormones and immune function. In R. Ader, D. L. Felton, & N. Cohen (Eds.), *Psychoneuroimmunology* (pp. 475–493). San Diego: Academic Press.

Mountz, J. D., Wu, J., Cheng, J., & Zhou, T. (1994). Autoimmune diseases: A problem of defective apoptosis. *Arthritis & Rheumatism, 37*(10), 1415–1420.

Mudge-Groud, C. L. (1992). *Immunologic disorders.* St. Louis, MO: Mosby Year Book.

Nossen, J. C. (1993). Course and prognostic value of systemic lupus erythematosus disease activity index in Black Caribbean patients. *Seminars in Arthritis & Rheumatism, 23*(1), 16–21.

Petri, M., Howard, D., & Repke, J. (1991). Frequency of lupus flare in pregnancy: Johns Hopkins Lupus Pregnancy Center experience. *Arthritis & Rheumatism, 34,* 1538–1545.

Pistiner, M., Wallace, D. J., Nessim, S., Metzger, A. L., & Klineberg, J. R. (1991). Lupus erythematosus in the 1980's: A survey of 570 patients. *Seminars in Arthritis and Rheumatism, 12,* 55–64.

Repke, J. T., & Petri, M. (1991). Management of the pregnant lupus patient. *Maryland Medical Journal, 40,* 917–922.

Steinberg, A. (1994). Mechanisms of disordered immune regulation. In D. P. Stites, A. I. Terr, & T. G. Parslow (Eds.), *Basic and clinical immunology* (pp. 380–386). Norwalk, CT: Appleton & Lange.

Steinberg, L. (1993, September). Autoimmune disease. *Scientific American, 269*(3), 107–114.

Stevens, M. B. (1991). The clinical spectrum of SLE. *Maryland Medical Journal, 40,* 875–885.

Talal, N. (1987). The etiology of systemic lupus erythematosus. In D. J. Wallace & B. H. Hahn (Eds.), *Dubois' lupus erythematosus* (pp. 39–43). Philadelphia: Lea & Febinger.

Ziminski, C. M. (1991). Autoantibodies and SLE. *Maryland Medical Journal, 40,* 901–909.

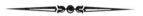

BOOKS AND ARTICLES

Atkinson, J. P. (1995). Some thoughts on autoimmunity. *Arthritis & Rheumatism, 38*(3), 301–305.

In this recent article, Atkinson reviews factors associated with autoimmunity such as sex hormones, drugs, genetic predisposition, and infections. Atkinson uses insulin dependent diabetes mellitus type 1 to show how genetic factors, immunodeficiency, and infection come together to induce it. The author discusses how an imperfect immune system, the wrong infection at the wrong time, and slight susceptibility can all induce autoimmunity.

Birney, M. H. (1991). Psychoneuroimmunology: A holistic framework for the study of stress and illness. *Holistic Nursing Practice, 5*(4), 32–38.

Birney's review of the link between stress and illness will satisfy the curiosity of most of those interested in the mind-body interaction. The author updates the older conceptions of the connection between psychosocial health and immunity, citing the recent identification of the direct innervation of the lymphatics in nerve fibers. The author explains that neuromodulation may occur through the conversion of electrical neurological signs into chemical immunological signals. The review is extensive and supplemented with interpretation of research findings, such as the suppressive effect of glucocorticoids, epinephrine, and norepinephrine on the immune cells.

Bootsma, H., Spronk, P., Derksen, R., de Boer, G., Wolters-Dicke, H., Hermans, J., Limburg, P., Gmelig-Meyling, F., Kater, L., & Kallenburg, C. (1995, June). Prevention of relapses in systemic lupus erythematosus. *The Lancet, 345,* 1595–1599.

Prednisone remains the drug of choice to treat moderate-to-severe SLE. Its use, however, has implications for women's health due to its side effects such as weight gain, osteoporosis, and increased risk for atherosclerosis. In this study, the researchers investigated whether or not relapses in SLE may be prevented by giving prednisone according to the rise in antibodies against double-stranded DNA (anti-dsDNA). The anti-dsDNA of 156 patients was measured and, when a rise was found, the patients were randomly assigned to prednisone and conventional treatment groups. Forty-six patients in the prednisone group received 30-mg prednisone added to their routine daily dose before returning the baseline in 18 weeks. At the end of the study, however, the cumulative oral prednisone doses of two groups did not significantly differ. The results showed the relapse rate was significantly higher among the conventional group than in the prednisone group. The study did not measure long-term morbidity and mortality. The overall decrease in disease activity, however, suggests less damage may have occurred in the prednisone group. The study implies that if timed according to biological indicators, prednisone can be used more efficiently.

Burckhardt, S., Archenholtz, B., & Bjelle, A. (1993). Quality of life of women with systemic lupus erythematosus: A comparison with women with rheumatoid arthritis. *Journal of Rheumatology, 20,* 977–981.

Very few studies have directly measured SLE patients' satisfaction with their lives. Especially frustrating to women with SLE has been the assumption that psychological disturbances are part of the picture of SLE but are not related to the disease itself. Aware of unexplored issues in SLE, Burckhardt, one of the few nurse-researchers of rheumatic diseases, and colleagues, examined the quality of life (QOL) of 50 SLE and 50 age-matched RA patients. To study the question indepth, the researchers used open-ended questions, the Quality of Life Scale (QOL-S), the Arthritis Impact Measurement Scales (AIMS), the Rheumatology Attitudes Index, and two measures of disease activity, the Ritchie Articular Activity Index (RITCHIE), and Systemic Lupus Activity Measure (SLAM). The results showed that although the SLE patients expressed more concerns about their disease state, there were no

differences between the two groups on the QOL-S. Moreover, both groups reported satisfaction with many aspects of their lives. Researchers, however, found that SLE patients were more concerned about their fatigue and inability to plan ahead. They were also dissatisfied with their jobs, due to the lack of understanding by their mates and supervisors. In addition, SLE patients expressed a feeling of uncertainty and lack of control over the disease. More significantly, no correlations were found between demographic variables, disease duration, drug therapy variables, and QOL.

Carr, R. I. (1986). *Lupus erythematosus: A handbook for physicians, patients and their families.* Washington, DC: Lupus Foundation of America.

Written for the lay public, this book is sophisticated enough for healthcare professionals to learn about the etiology, manifestations, diagnosis, and management of SLE. The chapter on pregnancy and lupus answers many questions including pregnancy-related complications such as deep vein and arterial clotting. Carr's book gives readers with the disease a sense of control over SLE. The book can be obtained from LFA, Inc. Bethesda, Maryland, or local LFA chapters. Also available in Spanish.

Fuller, C., & Hartley, B. (1991). Systemic lupus erythematosus in adolescents. *Journal of Pediatric Nursing, 6,* 251–257.

SLE in adolescent females presents special challenges to the individual, family, and healthcare professionals. The article presents a case history of a 14-year-old girl who is taking prednisone to control her arthritis, occasional grand mal seizures, and pericardial and gastrointestinal disturbances. Through this case study, the authors delineate how nursing care can be structured to promote four development tasks: developing a positive body image, establishing a sexual identity, achieving independence, and acquiring formal thought process. This article may be of use to practicing nurses, nursing students, young SLE patients, and their families.

Gladman, D. D. (1995). Prognosis and treatment of systemic lupus erythematosus. *Current Opinion in Rheumatology, 7,* 402–408.

The improvements made in the management of SLE are presented with support from research. In addition, the reasons behind increased survival, the national and international data for morbidity and mortality rates since 1955 are presented. While in the 1950s only 50 percent of the SLE patients survived beyond five years, survival exceeded 90 percent in the 1990s. The increased survival is limited primarily to the developed world. In India and the Caribbean, for example, 5-year survival remains 68 percent and 56 percent respectively. Factors that affect mortality are gender, age, and race. Being male, having a higher age at the onset of SLE, and being black all worsen the prognosis. The assessment of disease activity has become easier with the development of assessment tools such as the most commonly used Systemic Lupus Erythematosus Disease Activity Index (SLEDAI), and Systemic Lupus Activity Measure (SLAM). Gladman also covers outcome measures to describe prognosis, such as kidney and neurological involvement, and changes in general health status, including QOL issues. The current treatment modalities are also addressed.

Grossman, C. J. (1984). Regulation of the immune system by sex steroids. *Endocrine Reviews, 5*(3), 435–455.

This is required reading for anybody interested in autoimmunity and autoimmune disorders. A highly recognized researcher of the immune system and sex steroids, reviews the physiology of the immune system, the effects of gonadectomy, adrenalectomy, and sex hormones on T and B cell-mediated immunity with support from massive scientific data from animal research. Integrating his own research with findings of others, Grossman reviews

studies in various mammalian species which demonstrate that the immune response in females is greater than that observed in males. For example, female Swiss Albino mice develop a greater number of antibodies to bovine serum albumin than do males. In female rats, estrogen appears to regulate the synthesis of uterine IgA and IgG, suggesting the reasons behind the observed increase in Ig levels in pregnancy. Moreover, data show that *in vitro,* the female hormone estradiol draws significant immune response from the culture of normal thymocytes. Research on the effect of the male hormones, androgens, on cell-mediated immunity, and antibody production indicates that male mice with high androgen sensitivity have lower levels of IgM and IgG_2, than female mice. Also, progesterone treated monkeys have lymphocytopenia and lymphocytosis, a decrease in hemoglobin and hematocrit levels and increased skin homograft survival, showing the immunosuppressive effects of progesterone. Moreover, there is a significant depression of cell-mediated immune response among pseudopregnant rabbits. This frequently cited article consolidates a vast and divergent body of research on sex steroids with the researcher's own works and interpretation.

Ginsburg, K. S., Wright, E. A., Larson, M. G., Fossel, A. H., Albert, M., Schur, P. H., & Liang, M. H. (1992). A controlled study of the prevalence of cognitive dysfunction in randomly selected patients with systemic lupus erythematosus. *Arthritis & Rheumatism, 35,* 776–781.

A decline in cognitive skills, which remains poorly delineated, is of particular concern to women with SLE. A sample of 49 randomly selected patients with SLE and 40 patients with RA were given neuropsychological tests with the following instruments: Associate Learning, Switching Attention, Continuous Performance, Associate Recall, Hand Eye Coordination, Pattern Comparison, Pattern Memory, the Stroop Color and Word Test and the Symptoms Checklist-90R. Using multiple linear regression analysis, the researchers found that SLE patients had poorer performance than RA patients on the tests of attention and visuospatial ability independent of age, education, and steroid use. In general, SLE patients showed more symptoms of cognitive difficulty. Moreover, the researchers found that self-reported cognitive difficulty correlated with objective performance. These findings have implications for the QOL of SLE patients as decline in the cognitive ability contributed to distress and impaired functioning.

Harvey, C. J., & Verkland, T. (1990). Systemic lupus erythematosus: Obstetric and neonatal implications. *Nurses Association of the American Colleges of Obstetricians and Gynecologists, 1*(2), 177–185.

Pregnant women with SLE are at risk for fetal wastage, intrauterine growth retardation, intrauterine fetal demise, pregnancy-induced hypertension, and lupus flares. The authors discuss the nature of clot formation in pregnancy and indicate that the incidence of spontaneous abortion and fetal death is as high as 98 percent in some studies. The authors report that more than 20 percent of SLE cases are first diagnosed during pregnancy. The authors emphasize that intensive pregnancy care is necessary for women with SLE as worsening kidney, lung, heart, hematological, skin, and joint conditions may be observed in 16 percent to 60 percent of SLE patients. The authors also report that the minimum risk for neonatal lupus ranges from 3 percent to 32 percent. However, some forms of neonatal lupus may be transient. There is a very informative discussion on the clinical features and variations of neonatal lupus.

Joyce, K., Berkebile, C., Hastings, C., Yarboro, C., & Yocum, D. (1989). Health status and disease activity in systemic lupus erythematosus. *Arthritis Care and Research, 2*, 65–69.

Very few studies examined the relationship between disease activity and health status

in SLE. Studies as such are needed to describe the impact of disease on QOL, an increasing area of concern to Americans with chronic and terminal diseases. In this study, 45 SLE patients completed the Arthritis Impact Measurement Scale (AIMS) and were examined by a rheumatologist to document the clinical features of the disease according to the Clinical Activity Index (CAI). The results showed that there was a significant correlation between the CAI and AIMS indicating a relationship between disease activity and health status. For example, the total CAI was significantly correlated with physical activity, pain, and depression subscales of health status. Also, the total score for health status (AIMS), significantly correlated with mucocutaneous, musculoskeletal and general features of CAI. More important was the significant correlation between musculoskeletal aspects of disease and pain.

Lahita, R. G. (1990). Sex hormones and the immune system—Part 1. *Baillieres Clinical Rheumatology, 4*, 1–12.

This article, rich in scientific evidence, shows the interaction between the immune system and sex steroids. Lahita, internationally recognized researcher, author, educator of rheumatoid diseases, and a specialist in SLE, reviews data showing that the immune system is regulated in part by sex steroids. Lahita using both his and other investigators' data shows that the regulation of the immune system is steroid-hormone dependent and that this regulation affects humans in health and disease. According to the body of research presented, the immune function is critical to the process of reproduction and the delivery of a healthy baby. Lahita shows that sexual dimorphism exists in regard to the immune response of men and women as sex hormones produce immunologically active cytokines. Lahita reviews research showing the influence of estrogens, progesterone, and androgens on immune response, and the variation seen in the lymphocyte count of men and women: normal women have a higher number of T helper (they intensify immune response) and a lower number of T suppressor (they suppress immune response) cells. Moreover, while estrogens increase the secretion of reactive IgG, androgens have the opposite effect. By contrast, progesterone, the female hormone necessary for preparation for pregnancy, increases the suppressor T cells, which, in turn, suppresses immune response to a variety of antigens.

Lash, A. A. (1993). Systemic lupus erythematosus: Part 2. Diagnosis, treatment modalities, and nursing management. *MEDSURG Nursing*, 2(5), 375–385.

This article provides a comprehensive review of the etiology, pathophysiology and treatment, and nursing care of SLE patients and their families. Pathophysiological changes in all body systems are detailed with support from clinical research. The American Rheumatism Association's (ARA) criteria for diagnosis of SLE is presented along with a comprehensive discussion of nonpharmacological and pharmacological treatments. There is a case study that applies the content to the nursing process. There are several tables that list specific manifestations of organ involvement. A conceptual model that emphasizes self-care is presented.

Lash, A. A. (1993). Why so many women? Part 1. Systemic lupus erythematosus. *MEDSURG Nursing*, 2(4), 259–264.

This review article discusses in detail the influence of gender-based sex hormones on the prevalence of SLE and other autoimmune disorders among women. The article reviews animal and human research related to immune reactivity and details how estrogens depress the activities of suppressor T cells and thereby allow B cell antibody production to go unchecked. The article concludes with the identification of the areas that await nursing research such as QOL in SLE and the self-care needs of SLE patients and families.

Lash, A. A. (1996). Anticancer drugs for noncancer diseases. *MEDSURG Nursing*, 5(3), 177–184, 190.

An increasing body of evidence shows that drugs used for treating cancer successfully control and slow the progress of immune-mediated disorders such as RA and SLE. However, the use of anticancer drugs for noncancer diseases differs significantly from their use in cancer. When used to treat autoimmune disorders, dosaging is reduced to once daily, 2 to 3 times a week or even once a month. Also in treating autoimmune disorders, anticancer drugs are taken for extended periods of time, from several months to several years. The article provides scheduling and dosaging information as well as consolidating the massive research on the therapeutic effects of anticancer drugs, such as purine analogues (azathioprine), alkylating agents (cytoxan, neosar), and folic acid antagonists (methotrexate), on autoimmune disorders.

Lash, A. A. (in review). Quality of life in systemic lupus erythematosus: A pilot study. *Applied Nursing Research*.

This study examined the impact of SLE on QOL of 37 SLE patients using two QOL instruments, Sickness Impact Profile (SIP), and Arthritis Impact Measurement Scale 2 (AIMS2), and demographic variables. The results showed that SLE affected all areas scientists consider essential for QOL. The areas most affected were alertness behavior, recreation, pastime, sleep and rest, home management, social interaction, and emotional balance. Of all the demographic variables included, only age and marital status had an impact on QOL with SLE: those older and those living alone had poorer QOL.

Legun, L. A. (1990). Systemic lupus erythematosus during pregnancy. *Journal of Obstetric, Gynecologic and Neonatal Nursing 19*, 304–310.

This article discusses the reciprocal relationship between pregnancy and lupus. Legun's review shows that of those patients with SLE before pregnancy, 25 percent to 50 percent experience lupus flares during pregnancy. She states that risk for flares, renal damage, and poor fetal outcomes can be minimized when patients are in clinical remission for six months before pregnancy. Legun discusses the mechanism of the production of lupus anticoagulant and how the antibody causes thrombosis. Her discussion includes pre-eclampsia, hypertension, renal complications, and the effects of SLE on the fetus and infant.

Liang, M., Socher, S. A., Larson, M. G., & Schur, P. H. (1989). Reliability and validity of six systems for clinical assessment of disease activity in systemic lupus erythematosus. *Arthritis & Rheumatism, 32*, 1107–1118.

This is an important investigation for researchers and clinicians. The authors tested six tools for their validity and reliability in defining and evaluating SLE. The tested tools were the following: the Rope System, the National Institute of Health System, the New York Hospital for Special Surgery System, the British Isle Lupus Assessment Group (BILAG) Scale, the Toronto Disease Activity Index (SLE-DAI), and the systemic Lupus Activity Measure (SLAM). Twenty-five patients with a range of disease activity were evaluated by two physicians on two occasions approximately one month apart. The BILAG, SLEDAI, and SLAM had the best inter-visit and inter-rater reliability. Convergent validity among all instruments was high with correlation score of $r = .81$ to .97. In addition, all instruments correlated highly with the physicians' clinical impressions of the disease but less well with their evaluation of disease severity. However, disease severity scores correlated less well between self-reports and physician assessments, $r = .49$ to .69 and self-reported severity values were lower than the means from physicians. The BILAG, SLEDAI, and SLAM appeared to have better psychometric properties than the other instruments.

McKinney, P. S., Ouellette, S. C., & Winkel, G. H. (1995). The contribution of disease activity, sleep patterns, and depression to fatigue in systemic lupus erythematosus. *Arthritis & Rheumatism, 38*, 826–834.

Fatigue, a debilitating symptom of SLE, remains understudied. In this investigation, 48 women with SLE and 27 from the general population were assessed to describe lupus fatigue multidimensionally using the Piper Fatigue Scale (PFS), the Systemic Lupus Activity Measure (SLAM), the Center for Epidemiological Studies Depression Scale (CESD) and the Sleep Symptom Questionnaire (SSQ). The results showed that women with SLE reported greater overall fatigue than did the control group. The SLE group also reported longer sleep latency and total sleep time without showing significant differences on depression scores. Researchers indicated that women with SLE considered fatigue a problem only when it became chronic. The researchers also proposed a fatigue path model that may be tested by other researchers.

Nossent, J. C. (1993). Course and prognostic value of systemic lupus erythematosus disease activity index in Black Caribbean patients. *Seminars In Arthritis & Rheumatism, 23*(1), 16–21.

The significance of this research lies in its use of SLEDAI and black Caribbean patients to determine the course and prognosis of SLE. Since it has been shown that SLE has a more aggressive course in black patients with higher morbidity and mortality rates, this study makes a significant contribution to SLE patient care. A total of 68 patients (12 percent were male) were included in the ten-year study and the mean age at the time of diagnosis was 34.5. Nossent found that 78 percent of the SLE patients had already developed lupus nephritis at the time the study was undertaken. This rate is at the upper limits of reported frequencies. The initial average SLEDAI scores were 13 where initial scores of greater than 10 indicate high disease activity and poor prognosis.

In addition, 46 percent of patients reached maximum disease activity 3 months after diagnosis of SLE while other researchers reported no disease activity in 50 percent of patients for 10 years. Morbidity was not a predictor of survival, but patients with high maximum disease activity had more exacerbations. Survival among black Caribbean patients was much lower than the reported 10-year survival rate of 90 percent. Nossent reported that infection caused half of the deaths, often in patients with SLEDAI scores of 15. More importantly, high weighted average SLEDAI predicted poor survival in black Caribbean patients. Nossent suggested that socioeconomic status and patient compliance may be factors as they were inversely related to morbidity in previous studies. The researcher reported that SLEDAI was an effective and practical tool to follow disease activity although it had a poor prognostic value.

Petri, M., Howard, D., & Repke, J. (1991). Frequency of lupus flare in pregnancy: Johns Hopkins Lupus Pregnancy Center experience. *Arthritis & Rheumatism, 34,* 1538–1545.

This study was conducted to determine whether pregnancy was associated with an increased rate of SLE flares in 37 women with 40 pregnancies. The results showed that the flare occurred in 27 of the pregnancies. Flares presented were constitutional symptoms, renal, skin, and joint involvements. Three pregnancies associated with flares ended in spontaneous abortion. One pregnancy associated with flare resulted in preterm birth and perinatal death. In addition to the 27 flares that occurred during pregnancy, 7 flares occurred during the first 2-month postpartum period.

Petri, M., Lakatta, C., Magder, L., & Goldman, D. (1994). Effect of prednisone and hyroxycholoroquine on coronary artery disease risk factors in systemic lupus erythematosus: A longitudinal data analysis. *American Journal of Medicine, 95,* 254–259.

Preventing and treating heart disease in women is an important issue in women's health. This investigation by well-known SLE researchers examines the relationship between drug treatment and risk factors for coronary heart disease in SLE patients. The results showed that increasing prednisone intake by 10 mg a day was associated with an increased cholesterol level of 7.5 mg/dl. By contrast, the use of hydroxychloroquine (plaquenil) was associated with cholesterol levels of 8.9 mg/dl. It is known that some patients increase their drug dose when they feel worse. This study shows that drug treatment in SLE may contribute to the risk for atherosclerosis, and, so drugs must be taken strictly as prescribed.

Tan, E. M., Cohen, A. S., Fries, J., Masi, A. T., McShane, D. J., Rothfield, N. F., Schaller, J. G., Talal, N., & Winchester, R. J. (1982). The revised criteria for the classification of systemic lupus erythematosus. *Arthritis & Rheumatism, 25,* 1271.

SLE remains a difficult disease to diagnose. In 1982, the ARA published a report for the classification of SLE. This criteria has been widely used for diagnosis and management of the disease as well as for clinical research. The criteria for SLE is 96 percent sensitive and 96 percent specific when tested with SLE and control patients. It has been shown to have good discriminating power against RA, scleroderma, dermato/polymyositis but not to the rest of the rheumatic diseases presented on Table 8.1. It is extremely important for healthcare professionals and patients with the SLE to be familiar with this criteria.

Wallace, J. D. (1995). *The lupus book.* New York: Oxford University Press.

This is an excellent book written for the lay public by a prominent researcher, author, and teacher of rheumatology. The book explains all aspects of lupus in understandable language. The role of sex hormones, ultraviolet light, overactive lymphocytes, and genetics in inducing SLE, and drug treatment are presented. In terms of genetics, if one's mother has SLE, a woman has 10 percent chance to develop the disease, in contrast to a 2 percent chance for men.

Wallace spends considerable time discussing the connection between the nervous system and the behavioral changes, an area of great interest to women with SLE. The most common change is in the cognitive function, characterized by confusion, fatigue, memory impairment, and difficulty articulating thoughts. Patients may experience headaches, visual disturbances, seizures, excessive sleepiness, aseptic meningitis, tremors, numbness, paralysis, stroke, and psychosis. The underlying reason for nervous system involvement is due to vasculitis (inflammation) of the brain's blood vessels.

In terms of marriage and sex, Wallace states SLE does not affect sexual functions and fertility. However, within five years of the diagnosis, nearly half of SLE patients are divorced. Wallace believes this arises from partners not being open with each about the nature of SLE. For example, fatigue control is an important part of the symptoms which sometimes may interfere with social life. Wallace emphasizes that the sooner the patients develop adequate coping mechanisms and social support, the better individuals and families will deal with the disease. He recommends spouses become part of any decision related to the therapy and become informed about the manifestations of the disease and side-effects of the drugs used.

Wallace writes that about 90 percent of the SLE patients are treated with anti-inflammatory, antimalarial and immunosuppresive drugs along with glucocorticosteroids. All of these drugs have significant side effects such as weight gain and osteoporosis.

Wallace, D. J., & Hahn, B. H. (Eds.). (1993). *Dubois' lupus erythematosus.* Philadelphia: Lea & Febinger.

Written by 53 specialists, this book includes 62 chapters with over 8,000 references. It includes basic science research in relation to immune responses such as the mechanisms of auto-antibody production, pathogenesis, and clinical manifestations. The treatment modalities of SLE are superbly covered. The book would be of the greatest use to practicing rheumatologists, nurses, and researchers of rheumatology.

Ward, M. M., Pyun, E., & Studenski, S. (1995). Long-term survival in systemic lupus erythematosus: Patient characteristics associated with poorer outcomes. *Arthritis & Rheumatism, 38,* 274–283.

The researchers present the results of a study with a cohort of 408 SLE patients followed at Duke University. The study showed better overall survival rate for whites than blacks, younger than older, and female than male patients. A significant finding for nursing was the influence of socioeconomic status that was a factor for blacks. It has been shown in other studies that when socioeconomic status was controlled, blacks and whites had similar survival. Therefore, this study implies if socioeconomic variables can be manipulated, the reported higher morbidity and mortality among black SLE patients can be decreased.

Chapter 9

The Management of Hypertension in Women

Lynne T. Braun

Beth A. Staffileno

Kathleen Potempa

Hypertension, or high blood pressure (BP), is itself a disease, and is also a risk factor for other cardiovascular diseases, namely coronary heart disease (CHD) and stroke. According to the Third National Health and Nutrition Examination Survey (NHANES III), as many as 43 million Americans have elevated BP, defined as a systolic blood pressure (SBP) of 140 mm Hg or greater and/or a diastolic blood pressure (DBP) of 90 mm Hg or greater, or are taking antihypertensive medication (Burt et al., 1995). Hypertension is the most prevalent type of cardiovascular disease (CVD) and, in 1993, claimed the lives of 37,520 Americans. Although one out of every four American adults has high BP, 35 percent are unaware that they have it. Furthermore, 44 percent of those individuals with known high BP are either taking no medication or inadequate medication (American Heart Association [AHA], 1995). Hypertension remains a significant health problem in the United States, since the sequelae of this disease are observed in the heart, blood vessels, brain, eyes, and kidneys, in the forms of myocardial infarction (MI), heart failure, widespread vascular (blood vessel) disease, stroke, retinal abnormalities leading to blindness, and kidney failure.

As a major contributor to excess morbidity and mortality, hypertension is at least as significant in women as in men. The incidence of high BP is more common in young adult and middle-aged males than females, but thereafter the reverse is true. Hypertension occurs more frequently in older women compared to older men (Joint National Committee [JNC], 1993). Typically, SBP increases to age 70 or 80, and DBP increases to age 50 or 60 when it tends to plateau or decrease slightly. Between the ages of 30 and 70, the rise in SBP is notably steeper in women compared to men (approximately 1 to 9 mm Hg greater for women), (Burt et al., 1995; Byyny, 1995). Women aged 60 years and older are particularly affected by elevations in SBP. This is referred to as isolated systolic hypertension (ISH), which occurs in approximately 30 percent of older women and has been linked with an increased risk for CVD (Systolic Hypertension in the Elderly Program [SHEP], 1991, 1993).

In the final 1992 mortality report, hypertension-related deaths for women were 58 percent of the total compared to 42 percent for men (AHA, 1995), suggesting that women are at greater risk for developing sequelae of elevated BP. In general, women have not been included to the same extent as men in observational studies and clinical trials; therefore, less information is available regarding hypertension in women and associated CVD risk factors (Douglas et al., 1992; Eaker et al., 1993). The relative importance of hypertension as a risk factor and the magnitude of its effects may differ in women compared to men.

Reports from large population-based studies indicate that women are more aware of their hypertension than men (76 percent and 63 percent, respectively). In addition, women were more likely than men to have their hypertension treated (61 percent and 44 percent, respectively) and controlled (28 percent and 19 percent, respectively) (Burt et al., 1995). Both gender and racial differences were observed in the Atherosclerosis Risk in Communities Study, which evaluated levels of hypertension awareness, treatment, and control in 15,739 individuals, aged 45 to 64 years (Nieto et al., 1995). Hypertension was more prevalent among blacks than whites and in older rather than younger participants. Slightly more blacks were aware of their hypertension than whites; however, the reverse was true with respect to treatment and control. Once hypertension was identified, only 61 percent of blacks had their BP adequately controlled, compared to 73 percent of whites. Hypertension awareness, treatment, and control were greater for women compared to men; however, the differences were greater for blacks.

These statistics show that women, in general, are more aware of having hypertension and are more likely to treat and control it compared to their male counterparts; however, a greater percentage of women suffer from the complications of hypertension. These disturbing circumstances require an aggressive, multifaceted approach to managing hypertension in women. This approach must include prevention of hypertension in high-risk women; an overall cardiovascular risk appraisal, and reduction of risk factors that may co-exist with hypertension; lifestyle modifications that contribute to BP reduction; and pharmacologic therapy when indicated.

CLASSIFICATION OF BLOOD PRESSURE

The current classification of BP for adults aged 18 years and older is displayed in Table 9.1. In 1993, the Joint National Committee on Detection,

Table 9.1
Classification of Blood Pressure for Adults 18 Years and Older[a]

Category	Systolic (mm Hg)	Diastolic (mm Hg)
Normal[b]	<130	<85
High Normal	130–139	85–89
Hypertension[c]		
Stage 1 (mild)	140–159	90–99
Stage 2 (moderate)	160–179	100–109
Stage 3 (severe)	180–209	110–119
Stage 4 (very severe)	≥210	≥120

From Joint National Committee. (1993). The fifth report of the Joint National Committee on Detection, Evaluation, and Treatment of High Blood Pressure (JNCV). *Archives of Internal Medicine, 153*(2) 154–183.

[a] These definitions apply to adults who are not taking antihypertensive drugs and who are not acutely ill. When systolic and diastolic blood pressures fall into different categories, the higher category should be selected to classify the individual's blood pressure status. Isolated systolic hypertension is defined as a systolic blood pressure of 140 mm Hg or more and a diastolic blood pressure of less than 90 mm Hg and staged appropriately.

[b] Optimal blood pressure with respect to cardiovascular risk is less than 120 mm Hg systolic and less than 80 mm Hg diastolic. However, unusually low readings should be evaluated for clinical significance.

[c] Based on the average of two or more readings taken at each of two or more visits after an initial screening.

Evaluation, and Treatment of High Blood Pressure classified BP based upon the impact of risk. The risks associated with hypertension increase progressively with higher levels of SBP or DBP (Stage 1 through Stage 4). The risk of death from CHD is 2.45 times greater for individuals with SBP between 140 and 159 mm Hg (Stage 1 Hypertension) (Neaton, Kuller, Stamler, & Wentworth, 1995). Similarly, when MacMahon et al. (1990) evaluated the results of nine investigations that followed the outcome of untreated hypertensive individuals for an average of 10 years, a significant association between DBP and stroke and CHD events (i.e., heart attacks) emerged. Differences of 5 mm Hg, 7.5 mm Hg, and 10 mm Hg lower DBP were associated with 34 percent, 46 percent, and 56 percent fewer strokes and 21 percent, 29 percent, and 37 percent fewer CHD events. Therefore, the higher the BP, the greater the risk of stroke and CHD events; and both SBP and DBP contribute to an increased risk.

The classification scheme for BP includes the term "high-normal" (SBP 130–139, DBP 85–89). Individuals with BPs within this range are at increased risk for developing definite hypertension and its associated risks compared to those individuals with lower BP (Stamler, Stamler, & Neaton, 1993). Therefore, targeted interventions (evaluation of the entire cardiovascular risk profile, education, and lifestyle modifications) should be initiated when high-normal BP is detected.

Hypertension may also be classified by cause. In 90 percent to 95 percent of cases of hypertension, the cause is unknown. This is referred to as primary or essential hypertension. Generally, primary hypertension may be initiated and maintained by one or more of the following mechanisms: an increase in sympathetic nervous system activity; excess sodium intake; renal sodium retention; a defect in sodium transport at the cellular level; an increase in intracellular calcium; an increase in renin and angiotensin II; an alteration in baroreceptor function; ineffective insulin; exposure to stress and/or greater reactivity to stress; and hereditary factors which may encompass one or more of the above (Kaplan, 1994). Primary hypertension cannot be cured; however, it can be adequately controlled and does require lifetime treatment. Most often, the exact mechanisms promoting elevated BP cannot be delineated in a given individual, which substantiates the rationale for a multifaceted approach to treatment.

Secondary hypertension (5 percent to 10 percent of cases) is hypertension resulting from some other condition. Generally, when the underlying problem is corrected, BP normalizes. The following types of secondary hypertension are unique to women: fibromuscular hyperplasia, a form of kidney disease often seen in younger women, which causes thickening of arteriolar smooth muscle; estrogen therapy in oral contraceptives, which may require some women to discontinue this form of birth control; and pregnancy-induced hypertension, which increases the risk of morbidity and mortality for both mother and baby (Healy, 1995).

RISK FACTORS
FOR HYPERTENSION

Certain characteristics or behaviors (risk factors) increase an individual's chance of having hypertension. Specific references to women are provided when information is available.

Family History of Hypertension

Primary hypertension tends to occur within families. A person with two or more first-degree relatives (parents or siblings) with hypertension before age 55 has almost a fourfold greater risk of developing hypertension before age 50 (Williams et al., 1991).

Age and Gender

In the United States, BP, particularly SBP, tends to increase with age. Based on a 30-year follow-up period in the Framingham Study, older people with hypertension (ages 65 to 94 years) have greater rates of cardiovascular disease (Levy & Kannel, 1988). Hypertension exists in over 70 percent of women who are over 65 years of age; therefore, in the older population, women are more likely than men to have hypertension (Wenger, 1995).

Race/Ethnicity

Adult blacks have higher BP levels overall, and therefore, a greater prevalence of hypertension than whites. Puerto Ricans, Cuban- and Mexican-Americans are also more likely to have hypertension than Anglo-Americans (Kaplan, 1994; AHA, 1995). Furthermore, over 50 percent of the white women in the United States and almost 80 percent of the black women older than 45 years of age have hypertension, with the disease notably more severe in black men and women (Wenger, 1995). Compared to whites, black individuals acquire hypertension at an earlier age. The 1992 death rates were 6.3 (age-adjusted per 100,000 population) for white males, 29.3 for black males, 4.7 for white females, and 22.5 for black females (AHA, 1995).

Excess Dietary Sodium

Diets in nonprimitive cultures, such as ours, contain several times the daily adult sodium requirement; however, only about half of the population will develop hypertension. This suggests that the BPs of certain individuals are more sensitive to dietary sodium, and along with heredity and other environmental factors, contributes to an elevated BP. Many studies have observed significant correlations among the amount of salt intake, level of blood pressure, and frequency of hypertension. In general, when hypertensive individuals ingest a sodium-restricted diet, their BP falls (Kaplan, 1994).

Alcohol Intake

In contrast to the well-publicized vasodilatory effect of small amounts of alcohol, chronic consumption in moderate to heavy amounts has a vasopressor effect. Three or more drinks per day is associated with a significant increase in BP (Shaper, Wannamethee, & Whincup, 1988).

Obesity

Women who are obese, defined as at least 20 percent or more of their ideal body weight, develop hypertension four times more frequently than nonobese women of similar background (Carlson, Eisenstat, & Ziporyn, 1996). Furthermore, data from the Framingham study (Kannel et al., 1986) showed that obesity is particularly significant as a predictor of cardiovascular risk among women. Obesity is associated with insulin resistance, resulting in decreased uptake of glucose into skeletal muscle, and reduced muscle blood flow. These effects are particularly observed in persons with the "android" pattern or abdominal obesity. The waist to hip circumference ratio in women should not exceed 0.8.

Physical Inactivity

In general, habitual physical activity is associated with lower BP and lower cardiovascular risk. The relationship holds even greater significance for women compared to men. In a study of women aged 50 to 89 years, the time at which hypertension is most prevalent among women, rates of hypertension were significantly lower in women engaged in light, moderate, or heavy physical activity compared to sedentary women (Reaven, Barrett-Conner, & Edelstein, 1991).

Stress

People exposed to repeated stressors tend to develop hypertension more frequently than nonstressed counterparts. For example, studies have observed greater rates of hypertension among air traffic controllers compared to nonprofessional pilots, men with excessive job strain, and individuals in a low socioeconomic class. Hypertension is also associated with feeling a greater intensity of anger and hostility, suppressing rather than expressing anger, and remaining emotionally stressed for a longer period of time (Kaplan, 1994).

MANAGEMENT OF HYPERTENSION IN WOMEN

Evaluation

Evaluation of women with confirmed hypertension (three elevated BP measurements separated by one-week intervals) should include a clinical examination directed at the following questions: (1) Is the diagnosis primary or secondary hypertension? (2) Is target organ damage present? (3) What additional cardiovascular risk factors are present? (JNC, 1993).

History. A family history of cardiovascular and related disorders is obtained: hypertension, coronary artery disease (CAD) (especially CAD known to occur prior to menopause), stroke, peripheral vascular disease, diabetes, and lipid disorders. Specific information about the elevated BP is obtained, such as known duration of elevated BP, levels of BP (in physician's office, at home), any previous treatment of hypertension (medications and lifestyle measures), response to treatment, and side effects of medications. Details of a woman's personal history must include current age, age of onset of menses, current status of menses (date of last menstrual period, regularity of periods, cycle length, duration of periods, discomfort with menses), history of hysterectomy, age of onset of menopause, symptoms of menopause, treatment of symptoms, use of hormone replacement therapy (HRT), and the details of any medical problems/illnesses (past or present). The medical history should target the presence of symptoms of cardiovascular, cerebrovascular, and renal diseases and diabetes.

A thorough history of lifestyle behaviors should be solicited, including body weight changes, smoking (age of initiation, duration of habit, packs per day), illicit drug use, physical activity habits (leisure-time and during work), and regular performance of stress-reduction techniques (yoga, relaxation exercises, etc.). A dietary assessment is made, including sodium intake (foods high in sodium, added salt during cooking and at the table), alcohol use (types of alcoholic beverages consumed and number of drinks per day or week), and intake of cholesterol and saturated fats. Psychological and environmental factors that may influence blood pressure are assessed, such as marital status, number of children, family environment, employment status, work environment, and educational level. A complete history of all prescribed and over-the-counter medications is obtained, especially medications that may affect BP—oral contraceptives, nonsteroidal antiinflammatory drugs (NSAIDs), nasal decongestants and cold remedies, cyclosporine, erythropoietin, and antidepressant medications (JNC, 1993).

Primary or Secondary Hypertension.   The physical examination seeks to rule out the presence of a secondary form of hypertension. For example, abdominal bruits may be indicative of renovascular hypertension; delayed or absent pulses in the femoral arteries and decreased BP in the legs compared to the arms usually indicates co-artation of the aorta; tachycardia, tremors, sweating, pallor, and orthostatic hypotension may be signs of pheochromocytoma. When physical findings point to a secondary form of hypertension, additional diagnostic procedures will be performed to confirm the diagnosis. However, for most individuals, elevated BP is the result of primary hypertension, and lifestyle and medication management must be initiated.

Target Organ Damage.   The hypertension evaluation must determine the presence and severity of target organ damage. The extent of target organ damage is an indirect measure of the severity of hypertension. A fundoscopic examination is performed to observe for arteriolar narrowing, arteriovenous nicking, hemorrhages, exudates, or papilledema. The neck is examined for carotid bruits, distended veins, or an enlarged thyroid. The heart is examined for abnormalities, such as a displaced point of maximal impulse, precordial heave, presence of a third or fourth heart sound, murmur, or irregular rhythm. The abdomen is also examined for bruits, masses, enlarged kidneys, or abnormal aortic pulsations. The extremities are assessed for diminished or absent peripheral pulses, bruits, and edema. Finally, a complete neurologic assessment is performed. Routine laboratory and diagnostic testing includes urinalysis; complete blood count; fasting blood glucose; blood chemistry, including urea nitrogen, creatinine, potassium, calcium, uric acid, and cholesterol; fasting lipid and lipoprotein profile (triglycerides, high-density lipoprotein cholesterol—HDL, low-density lipoprotein cholesterol—LDL); and electrocardiogram (ECG).

Cardiovascular Risk Profile.   Hypertension management in women must include a comprehensive assessment of risk factors for hypertension (as described above), and those additional factors related to cardiovascular disease/stroke in general. The complete cardiovascular risk profile includes family history of hypertension, CAD, stroke, or diabetes; patient's age, race, and ethnicity; levels of SBP and DBP; dietary sodium intake; alcohol intake; smoking history; height and body weight; waist to hip ratio; total cholesterol, triglycerides, HDL, LDL; presence of left ventricular hypertrophy on

ECG; blood glucose and presence of diabetes; physical activity habits; and level of personal stress.

Although not all cohort studies examining cardiovascular risk factors have included women, those that have included women have shown that both genders have similar cardiovascular risk factors. However, these studies also indicate that certain risk factors influence women differently than men. When a woman's cardiovascular risk profile is ascertained, a comprehensive and aggressive plan can be instituted to control or eliminate risk factors and promote cardiovascular health.

In addition to the risk factors for hypertension described above, smoking, lipid disorders, and diabetes deserve special comment as they pertain to coronary disease in women. Currently, 23 percent of American women aged 18 and older smoke cigarettes (AHA, 1995). Smoking increases the risk of MI three-fold, even for postmenopausal women. Smoking is associated with an earlier age of menopause, an average of two years; therefore, CVD will occur earlier in women who smoke (Wenger, 1995). Data from the Nurses' Health Study (Willett et al., 1987) show that the number of cigarettes smoked correlates with the risk of fatal CHD, nonfatal MI, and angina. However, smoking cessation is associated with a 24 percent reduction in death from CVD in women within two years of quitting smoking (Kawachi et al., 1993). Many women smoke for weight control; therefore, smoking cessation programs must include dietary and exercise interventions to prevent the associated weight gain (Wenger, 1995).

In 1993, approximately 50 percent of women in the United States had elevated cholesterol levels (at least 200 mg/dl) (AHA, 1995). Premenopausal women have higher levels of HDL and lower levels of LDL compared to similarly aged men. Elevated total cholesterol and LDL are prominent features of the postmenopausal years, with greater increases in white women compared to black women (Wenger, 1995). The presence of high triglycerides appears to be a stronger risk factor for women compared to men (Eaker et al., 1993), and when combined with low HDL and elevated LDL, a woman's risk for CAD is greatly increased.

Diabetes is a more potent risk factor for women than for men. Even when diabetes is present in premenopausal women, the cardioprotective effect of estrogen is negated (Wenger, 1995). In the Nurses' Health Study (Manson et al., 1991), maturity-onset diabetes was associated with a three to seven times greater risk of cardiovascular events. Diabetes tends to occur in concert with other risk factors, such as lipid abnormalities, hypertension, and obesity, which together, amplify a woman's risk (Wenger, 1995).

Lifestyle Modifications

Lifestyle modifications are nondrug strategies for lowering BP and promoting cardiovascular health. The Fifth Report of the Joint National Committee on Detection, Evaluation, and Treatment of High Blood Pressure recommends lifestyle modifications as a definitive or adjunctive first step therapy for hypertension (JNC, 1993). The American Heart Association (AHA) also advocates lifestyle modifications by encouraging behaviors that are conducive for health-related benefits (AHA, 1995).

Lifestyle modifications are usually implemented for at least three to six months after an elevation in BP has been confirmed (either as high-normal BP or definite hypertension). Individuals with elevated BP need to be monitored closely because: (a) they may or may not need pharmacologic therapy, and (b) they unequivocally need counseling regarding lifestyle modifications that can reduce their BP. Nondrug therapy may be favorable, because antihypertensive drug therapy can amount to 70 percent to 80 percent of total expenditure for treating hypertension (JNC, 1993). Undesirable effects from antihypertensive drug therapy include metabolic disturbances (i.e., exacerbation of lipid disorders and glucose intolerance), interference with quality of life (i.e., fatigue, depression, and sexual disturbances), and financial burdens. The impact of increasing costs for newer antihypertensive agents may be particularly troublesome for elderly women who have limited income and medical insurance. Along with the potential for drug-related side effects, drug therapy often involves a period of trial and error before finding the best drug (or combination of drugs) to achieve adequate BP control. This contributes to additional medical expenses and loss of time in treating hypertension. Lifestyle modifications can be implemented for primary prevention of hypertension in a high-risk individual, or as definitive or adjunctive therapy for women with confirmed hypertension. Although lifestyle modifications alone may be insufficient to normalize BP, the amount of drug therapy required may be lessened.

Lifestyle modifications that are specific for hypertensive individuals include reducing excess body weight; engaging in regular physical activity, limiting dietary sodium intake to 110 mmol/day (2.4 g of sodium or 6 g of NaCl); consuming alcohol moderately (no more than 1 ounce/day which is equivalent to 2 usual portions of wine, beer, or spirits); stop smoking; restricting consumption of saturated fat; increasing dietary potassium intake from fresh fruits and vegetables; adequate intake of calcium and magnesium or supplement if deficient; and using relaxation strategies for stress reduction (JNC, 1993; Kaplan, 1994).

Although many women know what they need to do in order to take care of themselves, there are several barriers that prevent them from adopting a more healthful lifestyle. Many times women feel they are given too much conflicting information concerning healthful behaviors. When counseling women, it is important to provide information that is consistent and empirically based. In addition, some women find it difficult and/or inconvenient to follow a particular regimen. It will be helpful to encourage women to be an active participant in developing lifestyle modifications that are realistic and feasible. Last, some women fail to understand that health benefits can occur from small lifestyle changes rather than the preconceived "all or nothing" proposition. A small reduction in weight and fat intake is better than no reduction. Similarly, exercising for 15 minutes a day is better than not exercising at all. Making changes in eating, drinking, smoking, and exercise habits (no matter how small they may be) will reduce the risk for CVD and contribute to a more healthy lifestyle for women.

Diet and Weight Reduction.   Reducing excess weight (even as modest as 5 or 10 pounds) and adhering to a healthy diet are two important interventions for lowering BP and reducing cardiovascular risk. Changing old habits into healthy new ones may not be easy at first; therefore, a woman must be encouraged to set realistic goals and start out small. For instance, rather than attempting a fad diet, she would be more successful to aim for a gradual weight loss of ½ to 1 pound per week. Specific heart-healthy diet information includes the following:

- Overall, choosing low-fat foods is beneficial because they are lower in total calories (foods high in fat are high in calories), and low-fat foods can also help reduce serum cholesterol levels. Selecting fresh fruits, fresh vegetables, grains and beans (i.e., apples, broccoli, brown rice, pasta, and oatmeal) is a healthier choice compared to fast foods, processed foods, and snack foods (i.e., fast foods, sausage, cold cuts, and cookies). A great start to healthier eating would be to add or substitute 1 piece of fruit per day instead of choosing a cookie or a donut. The amount of fat content per serving can easily be determined by: reading the food label and finding the number of grams of fat; taking that number and multiplying it by 9 (this is the number of calories from fat); on the food label locate the number of total calories per serving and divide the number of fat calories by the number of total calories per serving; and multiply that number by 100. The final result is the percentage calories from fat.

- Extra calories and fat can also be reduced when preparing meals. Simple ways to leave out fat when cooking include trimming visible fat off meat; removing skin from poultry; baking or broiling foods without butter; and substituting vegetable oils (such as olive oil, sunflower oils, or canola) for lard, coconut oil, or palm oil. In addition, use flavorful spices or seasonings (such as, fresh herbs, lemon juice, vinegar, or mustard) instead of rich sauces (creams, cheese, and butter). Nonfat yogurt can be substituted for mayonnaise, 2 egg whites can be substituted for 1 whole egg, and ground turkey breast can be substituted for ground beef. Check food labels for the amount of total fat, saturated fat, and cholesterol per serving. Learning to cut back on saturated fats (such as meats and whole milk dairy products) will reduce calories and cholesterol.

- Sodium intake is another dietary factor that can elevate BP. One of the best ways to reduce the intake of sodium is by reading labels to avoid high-sodium ingredients (i.e., soy sauce, baking soda or powder, monosodium glutamate [MSG], and brine). Sodium is often added to foods for flavoring, and as a preservative. Subsequently, most processed foods are high in sodium (i.e., canned soups, cheese, lunch meats, and canned vegetables). To avoid too much sodium, select healthier food products that are labeled low-sodium/low-salt, plain frozen foods, or fresh foods whenever possible. To add cooking flavor, use herbs, pepper, garlic, lemon, and spices as a substitute for salt. Also, when eating out it is easy to ask for food to be prepared with little or no salt.

Moderation of Alcohol Intake.   Consuming alcohol in large amounts not only raises BP, but also may contribute to high triglycerides. In addition, alcohol contributes to extra calories. Women should be advised to limit alcohol to no more than 1 ounce per day. An ounce of alcohol is equivalent to: two 4-ounce glasses of wine, two 12-ounce beers, or two single shots of 100-proof liquor. Drinking alcohol in moderation is best for healthy lifestyle habits. For instance, substitute the second or third glass of alcohol with a glass of flavored seltzer water or juice.

Smoking Cessation.   Breaking old smoking habits is difficult for many smokers, but making a commitment to stop smoking is the first step to a healthier lifestyle. Some helpful steps to quit smoking include: set a quit smoking date; throw away cigarettes, ash trays, cigarette lighters; avoid tempting smoking situations (i.e., bars, parties, and break rooms); include friends and family for support during the quitting process; overcome an urge to smoke by engaging in fun activities; and after several smoke-free days, a special treat or reward is warranted. Weight gain can be avoided by becoming more physically active and eating low-fat/low-calorie snacks (such as fresh fruits, low-fat popcorn, and low-fat pretzels).

Stress Reduction.   The best approach to successful stress management is learning to manage stress in a healthy manner. For instance, stress can be reduced by engaging in some mode of physical activity (taking a walk), visualizing a peaceful scene (a beautiful picture of a sunset), deep breathing (slow, rhythmic diaphragmatic breathing), avoiding stressful situations (avoiding rush hour traffic), and finding realistic solutions to problems. Talking with friends and/or support groups can also be a good source for relieving stress.

Increased Physical Activity.   Increased physical activity will improve BP and cholesterol, and it is an important element of weight management. Some helpful hints for starting an exercise regimen include choosing a type (or mode) of physical activity that is enjoyable as well as convenient and accessible; scheduling time to exercise by making it a priority of daily routines; exercising slowly and gradually increasing the intensity (difficulty), duration (time), and frequency (amount) of exercise sessions per week; exercise with a friend or participate in a structured exercise class; varying exercise routines in order to avoid boredom and to avoid injury by using different muscles; and if a few days of exercising are missed, don't give up on the routine.

Women over the age of 50 or with known or suspected CAD should have an exercise test prior to the initiation of a vigorous exercise program (one in which the exercise intensity is greater than 60 percent capacity), (American College of Sports Medicine, 1995). However, moderate-intensity physical activity is encouraged for all healthy women and women with an elevated risk for CAD, as long as they are without symptoms. An example of moderate-intensity activity is brisk walking (3–4 mph or 1.5–2 miles in 30 minutes), and should be done at least five days per week.

Often women find it difficult to find a 30- or 40-minute block of time to exercise. However, some simple steps to take to start incorporating physical activity into daily routines include walking whenever possible, taking stairs rather than waiting for an elevator, taking a 10-minute work break and walk briskly, engaging in household chores and gardening, golfing without a cart, walking in place or doing stretches while talking on the telephone. The goal is to incorporate more movement into daily routines; therefore, focus on moving even if it is only for a few minutes.

The changes necessary for the adoption of a healthier lifestyle may seem overwhelming for women at first (especially if there are several old habits to break). An important strategy is to set realistic goals for each day and each week. Focusing on one lifestyle modification at a time is important. For example, initiating dietary restrictions and smoking cessation at the same time is usually unsuccessful. Positive feedback and reinforcement for every success (no matter how small it is) is imperative to insure adherence in a program of lifestyle modifications.

Until women are fully educated about hypertension, and perceive themselves at risk for developing CHD, they will be less likely to adopt preventive strategies for healthier lifestyles. Therefore, women of all ages need to be counseled about CVD risk factors. Interventions for hypertension and CHD need to be implemented across the lifespan in women. Although lifestyle modifications alone may not be sufficient to control elevated BP, they will provide multiple benefits with minimal expense and minimal risk.

Drug Therapy

Overall, drug therapy for hypertension clearly reduces the rates of cardiovascular morbidity (stroke, coronary events, heart failure) and mortality

(JNC, 1993). For Stages 1 and 2 hypertension, drug therapy should be initiated if BP remains at or above 140/90 after three to six months of lifestyle modifications, especially in women with additional CVD risk factors and/or target organ damage. Initial therapy is the use of a single drug (monotherapy), generally a diuretic or beta blocker (see Table 9.2), since clinical trials have documented a reduction in CVD morbidity and mortality with these drugs. Alternative first-choice drugs include calcium channel blockers, angiotensin converting enzyme (ACE) inhibitors, alpha$_1$-receptor blockers, and the alpha-beta blocker. Various factors must be considered in drug selection for a given individual, such as other diseases/conditions a woman may have, the cost of medication, side effects, and drug-drug interactions (JNC, 1993).

Drug therapy is absolutely required for Stages 3 and 4 hypertension. Although some women may respond adequately to only one drug, many require the addition of a second or a third drug if BP control is not achieved after a short period of time. Supplemental antihypertensive agents include direct vasodilators, central-acting alpha$_2$-agonists, and peripheral-acting adrenergic blockers. Table 9.2 describes the action of each antihypertensive drug category.

The presence or absence of certain characteristics, diseases, or conditions in women assist the healthcare provider in selecting the appropriate drug. For example, black women tend to respond better to diuretics and calcium channel blockers than to beta-blockers or ACE inhibitors (JNC, 1993). If a hypertensive woman has sustained an MI, certain beta blockers (those without sympathomimetic activity) are preferred, because they offer a cardioprotective effect and have been shown to reduce mortality after MI. If a woman has a lipid disorder, the use of diuretics and beta blockers requires special monitoring, because these drugs have adverse effects on the lipid profile. Similarly, diuretics and beta blockers are used with caution in diabetics, because both types of drugs may worsen glucose tolerance and beta blockers mask the symptoms of and prolong the recovery from hypoglycemia. The drug of choice for pregnancy-induced hypertension is methyldopa, and ACE inhibitors are contraindicated (JNC, 1993).

Several large clinical trials of antihypertensive treatment show that women often receive less benefit than men. In the Hypertension Detection and Follow-up Program, mortality was reduced by 27.8 percent in black women receiving the stepped-care approach, a reduction in mortality greater than men; however, a small (2.5 percent) increase in mortality occurred in white women. The Medical Research Council Trial showed a 26 percent increase in CVD mortality in treated women (predominantly white) compared with a 15 percent decrease for men. An 18 percent reduction in cardiovascular mortality was observed in treated women compared to a 47 percent reduction in men in the European Working Party on High Blood Pressure in the Elderly Trial. The Systolic Hypertension in the Elderly Program, however, showed a similar reduction in stroke events for both treated

Table 9.2
Categories of Antihypertensive Drugs

Drug Category	Mechanisms of Action

First Choice Drugs
Diuretics
   Thiazides most common,
   i.e., Hydrochlorothiazide
	Act directly on kidneys to promote sodium and water excretion; reduce plasma volume; long-term, decrease arteriolar resistance

Beta Blockers
   i.e., Propranolol, Atenolol,
   Metoprolol, Pindolol
	Decrease the force of myocardial contraction and heart rate; decrease renin activity

ACE Inhibitors
   i.e., Captopril, Benazepril,
   Enalapril, Lisinopril
	Block the formation of angiotensin II; promote vasodilation; decrease aldosterone, thus reduce sodium and water retention

Calcium Channel Blockers
   i.e., Diltiazem, Verapamil,
   Nifedipine, Isradipine
	Block the inward movement of calcium into arterioles, causing arteriolar dilation

Alpha$_1$-Receptor Blockers
   i.e., Prazosin, Doxazosin,
   Terazosin
	Interfere with postsynaptic alpha$_1$-receptors, arteriolar dilation

Alpha-Beta Blocker Labetalol	Same mechanisms as beta blockers and alpha$_1$-receptor blockers

Supplemental Drugs
Central Alpha$_2$-Agonists
   i.e., Clonidine,
   Guanfacine, Methyldopa
	Stimulate alpha$_2$-receptors in the brain that inhibit efferent sympathetic activity (to the heart, kidneys, and the arteries)

Peripheral-Acting
Adrenergic Blockers
   i.e., Guanethidine,
   Reserpine
	Inhibit catecholamine release from neuronal storage sites or deplete tissue stores of catecholamines; promote vasodilation

Direct Vasodilators
   i.e., Hydralazine,
   Minoxidil
	Act directly to dilate blood vessels, primarily arteries

Adapted from JNC (1993).

men (33 percent) and women (36 percent) over 60 years of age (Kaplan, 1995).

Many reasons have been suggested for the gender differences in treatment outcomes. Women in these trials may have a lower risk for CVD events, and the risks of drug therapy may outweigh the benefits. The excess mortality in white women, in particular, may be related to a steep drop in BP leading to cardiovascular complications. Given that the onset of hypertension is often earlier for black women, they may derive a greater benefit from drug treatment (Anastos et al., 1991; Kaplan, 1995).

More information is needed to create a treatment algorithm tailored to women. Given the potential risks and adverse effects of antihypertensive drug therapy, the lowest dose for adequate BP control should be selected. Vigorous attempts at lifestyle modifications must be made, initially for Stages 1 and 2 hypertension, and during the course of treatment for all stages of hypertension. With successful lifestyle changes, drug dosage and/or number of antihypertensive drugs may be reduced. Once BP is stabilized, women should be followed every 3-6 months. Self-monitoring and recording of BP is encouraged. The drug regimen should be as simple and cost-effective as possible. Women must be guided to discuss side effects and personal concerns so that adherence to the treatment regimen is maintained.

Hormone Replacement Therapy and Hypertension

Given the known hypertensive effects of high doses of estrogen in oral contraceptives, there are concerns that the smaller doses in hormone replacement therapy (HRT) might also raise BP. However, this was not the case in the Postmenopausal Estrogen/Progestin Interventions (PEPI) Trial (Writing Group, 1995). In the PEPI Trial, postmenopausal women were randomized to one of four different estrogen/progestin regimens (one of which was unopposed conjugated equine estrogen) or placebo. Blood pressure did not significantly differ among the five treatment groups, although SBP rose slightly during the second and third years in all groups including placebo. Furthermore, many of the estrogen/progestin regimens provided improvement in the lipid profile (increased HDL and decreased LDL) and decreased fibrinogen levels, thus reducing cardiovascular risk. All active treatments modestly increased triglycerides, however, compared to placebo.

The presence of hypertension is not a contraindication to postmenopausal HRT, which has been shown to improve a woman's cardiovascular risk profile into the eighth decade of life (Manolio et al., 1993). However, because a rise in BP has occurred in a few women after initiating HRT, all women undergoing HRT, especially hypertensives, should have their BP monitored more frequently (JNC, 1993). The decision to institute HRT for an individual woman must include consideration of post-menopausal symptoms, cardiovascular risk status, potential benefits regarding osteoporosis and cardiovascular risk, and the potential risks regarding uterine and breast cancer (Wenger, 1995).

Implications for Practice, Education, Research, and Health Policy

Hypertension screening and risk factor assessment must occur in community settings where women congregate, such as schools, churches, clubs, community centers, supermarkets, pharmacies, and all healthcare sites, particularly women's health practices. Given that women perceive their risk of cancer as much greater than that of heart disease and stroke, women must be helped to understand the significant potential for death and disability from untreated hypertension and other CVD risk factors. In addition to promoting lifestyle modifications for BP control among known hypertensives, health professionals should encourage these strategies for primary prevention among women who are most likely to develop hypertension, including women with high-normal BPs, a family history of hypertension, and/or other risk factors.

Health professionals and interested lay individuals must work together with community/professional organizations to insure the environmental supports necessary for healthy lifestyles, such as informative food labels, heart-healthy menu selections in restaurants, and safe hiking and biking trails (JNC, 1993). Furthermore, legislators must be urged to make research funding for cardiovascular diseases, such as hypertension, heart disease, and stroke, a national priority. Although CVD is the number one killer in the United States, cancer and AIDS funding exceeded CVD funding by 2 to 2.5 to 1 in 1995 (National Institute of Health, 1995).

Given that women are underrepresented in clinical research, they should be encouraged by their healthcare providers to participate in research related to hypertension in women. Hypertension research should be targeted at identifying efficacious treatments for women. Specifically, do women respond differently to lifestyle modifications compared to men? What lifestyle modifiers are most effective for BP control in women? What are the relationships among personality, behavioral features, stress and BP in women, and how will this knowledge influence hypertension management? Can hypertension be prevented in women? Which strategies will insure the greatest adherence to hypertensive management regimens in women? What is the efficacy and side effects of the different antihypertensive drug categories in women? More research is also needed to assess the treatment of hypertension among various ethnic/racial groups. Do responses to antihypertensive medications vary among age-specific and ethnic/race-specific female groups? Finally, does HRT have a role in hypertension management?

REFERENCES

American College of Sports Medicine (ACSM). (1995). *ACSM's guidelines for exercise testing and prescription.* Baltimore: Williams & Wilkins.

American Heart Association (AHA). (1995). *Heart and stroke facts: 1996 statistical supplement.* Dallas: American Heart Association.

Anastos, K., Charney, P., Charon, R. A., Cohen, E., Jones, C. Y., Marte, C., Swiderski, D. M., Wheat, M. E., & Williams, S. (1991). Hypertension in women: What is really known? *Annals of Internal Medicine, 115*(4), 287–293.

Burt, V. L., Whelton, P., Roccella, E. J., Brown, C., Cutler, J. A., Higgins, M., Horan, M. J., & Labarthe, D. (1995). Prevalence of hypertension in the U.S. adult population: Results from the third National Health and Nutrition Examination Survey, 1988–1991. *Hypertension, 25*(3), 305–313.

Byyny, R. L. (1995). Hypertension in the elderly. In J. Laragh & B. M. Brenner (Eds.), *Hypertension: Pathophysiology, diagnosis, and management* (pp. 227–251). New York: Raven Press.

Carlson, K. J., Eisenstat, S. A., & Ziporyn, T. (1996). *The Harvard guide to women's health.* Cambridge, MA: Harvard University Press.

Douglas, P. S., Clarkson, T. B., Flowers, N. C., Hajjar, K. A., Horton, E., Klocke, F. J., LaRosa, J., & Shively, C. (1992). Exercise and atherosclerotic heart disease in women. *Medicine and Science in Sports and Exercise, 24*, S266–S276.

Eaker, E. D., Chesebro, J. H., Sacks, F. M., Wenger, N. K., Whisnant, J. P., & Winston, M. (1993). Cardiovascular disease in women. *Circulation, 88*(4, Pt. 1), 1999–2009.

Healy, B. (1995). *A new prescription for women's health.* New York: Viking Penguin.

Joint National Committee V. (1993). The fifth report of the Joint National Committee on Detection, Evaluation, and Treatment of High Blood Pressure. *Archives of Internal Medicine, 153*(2), 154–183.

Kannel, W. B., Neaton, J. D., Wentworth, D., Thomas, H. E., Stamler, J., Hulley, S. B., & Kjelsberg, M. O. (1986). Overall and coronary heart disease mortality rates in relation to major risk factors in 325,348 men screened for the MRFIT. *American Heart Journal, 112*(4), 825–836.

Kaplan, N. M. (1994). *Clinical hypertension.* Baltimore: William & Wilkins.

Kaplan, N. M. (1995). The treatment of hypertension in women. *Archives of Internal Medicine, 155*(6), 563–567.

Kawachi, I., Colditz, G. A., Stampfer, M. J., Willett, W. C., Manson, J. E., Rosner, B., Hunter, D. J., Hennekens, C. H., & Speizer, F. E. (1993). Smoking cessation in relation to total mortality rates in women. A prospective cohort study. *Annals of Internal Medicine, 119*(10), 992–1000.

Levy, D., & Kannel, W. B. (1988). Cardiovascular risks: New insights from Framingham. *American Heart Journal, 116*(1, Pt. 2), 266–272.

MacMahon, S., Peto, R., Cutler, J., Collins, R., Sorlie, P., Neaton, J., Abbott, R., Godwin, J., Dyer, A., & Stamler, J. (1990). Blood pressure, stroke, and coronary heart disease: Part 1. Prolonged differences in blood pressure: prospective observational studies corrected for the regression dilution bias. *The Lancet, 335*(8692), 765–774.

Manolio, T. A., Furberg, C. D., Shemanski, L., Psaty, B. M., O'Leary, D. H., Tracy, R. P., & Bush, T. L. (1993). Association of postmenopausal estrogen use with cardiovascular disease and its risk factors in older women. *Circulation, 88*(5, Pt. 1), 2163–2171.

Manson, J. E., Colditz, G. A., Stampfer, M. J., Willett, W. C., Krolewski, A. S., Rosner, B., Arky, R. A., Speizer, F. E., & Hennekens, C. H. (1991). A prospective study of maturity-onset diabetes mellitus and risk of coronary heart disease and stroke in women. *Archives of Internal Medicine, 151*(6), 1141–1147.

National Institute of Health. (1995). NIH Research Finding: FY 1995 Current Dollars. Washington DC: DHHS.

Neaton, J., Kuller, L., Stamler, J., & Wentworth, D. (1995). Impact of systolic and diastolic blood pressure on cardiovascular mortality. In J. Laragh & B. Brenner (Eds.), *Hypertension: Pathophysiology, diagnosis, and management* (pp. 127–144). New York: Raven Press.

Nieto, F. J., Alonso, J. A., Chambless, L. E., Zhong, M., Ceraso, M., Romm, F. J., Cooper, L., Folsom, A. R., & Szklo, M. (1995). Population awareness and control of hypertension and hypercholesterolemia, the atherosclerosis risk in communities study. *Archives of Internal Medicine, 155*(10), 677–684.

Reaven, P. D., Barrett-Connor, E., & Edelstein, S. (1991). Relation between leisure-time physical activity and blood pressure in older women. *Circulation, 83*(2), 559–565.

Shaper, A. G., Wannamethee, G., & Whincup, P. (1988). Alcohol and blood pressure in middle-aged British men. *Journal of Human Hypertension, 2*(2), 71–78.

Stamler, J., Stamler, R., & Neaton, J. D. (1993). Blood pressure, systolic and diastolic, and cardiovascular risks. *Archives of Internal Medicine, 153*(5), 598–615.

Systolic Hypertension in the Elderly Program Cooperative Research Group. (1991). Prevention of stroke by antihypertensive drug treatment in older persons with isolated systolic hypertension: Final results of the Systolic Hypertension in the Elderly Program (SHEP). *Journal of the American Medical Association, 265*(24), 3255–3264.

Systolic Hypertension in the Elderly Program Cooperative Research Group. (1993). Implications of the Systolic Hypertension in the Elderly Program. *Hypertension, 21*(3), 335–343.

Wenger, N. (1995). Hypertension and other cardiovascular risk factors in women. *American Journal of Hypertension, 8*(12, Pt. 2), 94S–99S.

Wenger, N. K., Speroff, L., & Packard, B. (1993). Cardiovascular health and disease in women. *New England Journal of Medicine, 329*(4), 247–256.

Willett, W. C., Green, A., Stampfer, M. J., Speizer, F. E., Colditz, G. A., Rosner, B., Monson, R. R., Stason, W., & Hennekens, C. H. (1987). Relative and absolute excess risks of coronary heart disease among women who smoke cigarettes. *New England Journal of Medicine, 317*(21), 1303–1309.

Williams, R. R., Hunt, S. C., Hasstedt, S. J., Hopkins, P. N., Wu, L. L., Berry, T. D., Stults, B. M., Barlow, G. K., Schumacher, M. C., & Lifton, R. P. (1991). Are there interactions and relations between genetic and environmental factors predisposing to high blood pressure? *Hypertension, 18*(3, Suppl. 1), I-29–I-37.

Writing Group for the PEPI Trial. (1995). Effects of estrogen or estrogen/progestin regimens on heart disease risk factors in post-menopausal women. *Journal of the American Medical Association, 273*(3), 199–208.

⟶⟩●⟨⟵

ABSTRACTS

Anastos, K., Charney, P., Charon, R. A., Cohen, E., Jones, C. Y., Marte, C., Swiderski, D. M., Wheat, M. E., & Williams, S. (1991). Hypertension in women: What is really known? *Annals of Internal Medicine, 115*(4), 287–293.

The purpose of this review article was to determine whether information in the medical literature was sufficient to guide treatment in hypertensive women. Epidemiologic surveys and clinical trials of antihypertensive therapy were examined. Surveys indicate that women have a greater risk of cardiovascular complications of hypertension compared to men. Clinical trials demonstrate a benefit of medication therapy for black women, however a clear benefit has not been observed for white women. In fact, some studies imply that treatment of white women may be harmful. Therefore, current guidelines are inadequate for the treatment of hypertensive women, and additional research is necessary.

Ascherio, A., Hennekens, C., Willett, W. C., Sacks, F., Rosner, B., Manson, J., Witterman, J., & Stampfer, M. J. (1996). Prospective study of nutritional factors, blood pressure, and hypertension among US women. *Hypertension, 27*(5), 1065–1072.

This study examined the relation of nutritional factors and blood pressure. A semiquantitative food frequency questionnaire was administered to 41,541 U.S. female nurses, aged 38 to 63 years, who were without known hypertension, cancer, or other cardiovascular disease. During the study period (1984 to 1988), 2,526 women reported a diagnosis of hypertension. In this cohort of women, age, body weight, and alcohol intake were significant predictors of hypertension. Notably, there was an inverse relationship of calcium, dietary fiber, potassium, and magnesium among women who did not report the development of hypertension during the study period.

Devine, E., & Reifschneider, E. (1995). A meta-analysis of the effects of psychoeducational care in adults with hypertension. *Nursing Research, 44*(4), 237–245.

The purpose of this meta-analysis was to determine the effects of education and psychosocial support (psychoeducational care) among adults with hypertension. A total of 102 studies were included in the analysis. Although several limitations in the research base were identified, distinct types of psychoeducational care were found to be effective in reducing BP. Beneficial effects were noted with education, self-monitoring of BP/medications, and mobilizing psychosocial supports. Further research is needed to evaluate the effects of psychological care on weight, anxiety, and relaxation on BP.

Greendale, G., Bodin-Dunn, L., Ingles, S., Haile, R., & Barrett-Conner, E. (1996). Leisure, home, and occupational physical activity and cardiovascular risk factors in postmenopausal women. *Archives of Internal Medicine, 156*(4), 418–424.

The purpose of this cross-sectional study was to examine the associations between self-reported leisure, home, and occupational physical activity and cardiovascular risk factors. Baseline data from the Postmenopausal Estrogen/Progestins Intervention Trial (PEPI) were analyzed in 851 women aged 45 to 65 years. Although SBP did not significantly change among the various types of physical activity, positive benefits were noted among other cardiovascular risk factors (HDL-C, insulin, and fibrinogen). A positive increase in HDL-C was noted with moderate ($P < .001$) and heavy ($P = .004$) leisure activities compared to inactive and light leisure activity. Furthermore, leisure activity was inversely associated with levels of insulin ($P = .001$) and fibrinogen ($P = .02$). These results underscore the importance of lifestyle modifications and the cardiovascular risk profile in women.

Iso, H., Shimamoto, T., Yokota, K., Sankai, T., Jacobs, D., & Komachi, Y. (1996). Community-based education classes for hypertension control. *Hypertension, 27*(4), 968–974.

This 1.5 year community-based study examined the effects of a hypertension control program in Japanese men and women aged 35 to 69 years. Subjects were randomly assigned to an intervention group (4 education classes in the first 6 months and 4 classes during the following year) or to a control group (2 education classes). Education classes focused on lifestyle modifications such as, reducing dietary sodium, sugar, and alcohol intake, increasing milk intake, and increasing physical activity through brisk walking. At the end of 1.5 years, the need for antihypertensive medication was less for the intervention group compared to the control group (9 percent versus 24 percent, respectively). There was a 5 to 6 mmHg reduction in mean SBP for the intervention group at 6 months and 1.5 years compared to the control group ($P < .05$). There was a greater reduction in sodium and alcohol intake and a greater increase in milk consumption in the intervention group compared to the control group ($P < .08$, $P < .04$, $P < .01$, respectively). Additionally, more individuals developed the habit of taking brisk walks. Between the 2 groups, there were no significant changes in DBP or BMI. These data suggest that nonpharmacologic interventions are beneficial in reducing SBP.

Kanai, H., Tokunaga, K., Fujioka, S., Yamashita, S., Kameda-Takemura, K., & Matsuzawa, Y. (1996). Decrease in intra-abdominal visceral fat may reduce blood pressure in obese hypertensive women. *Hypertension,* 27(1), 125–129.

This intervention study examined the effects of a low-calorie diet on blood pressure and fat distribution. Twenty-six Japanese women, aged 31 to 73 years, with a mean BP of 112 +9 mmHg and mean BMI of 33.7 +3.1 kg/m^2 followed a 1,200 kcal/day diet for 12 weeks. A relationship between the visceral/subcutaneous (V/S) fat ratio and SBP ($r = .58$, $P < .01$) and DBP ($r = .41$, $P < .05$) was observed prior to starting the diet. After diet, there was a mean weight reduction of 9.4 +kg as well as significant reductions in both SBP ($P < .001$) and DBP ($P < .001$). Notably, changes in the V/S ratio were correlated more strongly with changes in BP rather than changes in body weight or other anthropometric parameters. These data suggest that an in-

crease in visceral fat/subcutaneous fat may be linked to the pathogenesis of hypertension in this population of women.

Kaplan, N. M. (1995). The treatment of hypertension in women. *Archives of Internal Medicine,* 155(6), 563–567.

This is a review article that discusses the prevalence, consequences, and treatment of hypertension in women. A greater number of women than men in the United States are hypertensive, which relates to women living longer than men and the high prevalence of hypertension among the elderly. The rise in hypertension after menopause may reflect an increase in blood volume, and is often associated with obesity. Lifestyle modifications may significantly benefit hypertensive women, especially since women appear to receive less benefit from antihypertensive drug therapy. The use of estrogen in hormone replacement therapy usually does not raise blood pressure; therefore, this valuable therapy should not be withheld because of the presence of hypertension.

Manson, J., Willett, W., Stampfer, M., Colditz, G., Hunter, D., Hankinson, S., Hennekens, C., & Speizer, F. (1995). Body weight and mortality among women. *New England Journal of Medicine,* 333(11), 677–685.

This study examined the association between BMI (Body M Index) and overall mortality and mortality from specific causes. A cohort of 115,195 U.S. women, aged 30 to 55 years, who were participating in the Nurses' Health Study were followed for 16 years. During this time, 4,726 deaths were identified (881 from CVD, 2,586 from cancer, and 1259 from other causes). The prevalence of hypertension, diabetes, and elevated cholesterol were 2 to 6-fold among overweight women (defined as BMI > 29.0) compared to leaner women (BMI < 19.0). An inverse relationship was noted between BMI and smoking status. Notably, alcohol consumption, HRT, and regular physical activity were more common among leaner women. These data indicate that body weight is a determinant of CVD risks and mortality among this cohort of women.

Midgley, J., Matthew, A., Greenwood, C., & Logan, A. (1996). Effect of reduced dietary sodium on blood pressure: A meta-analysis of randomized trials. *Journal of American Medical Association, 275*(20), 1590–1597.

The practice of restricting dietary sodium intake to prevent or treat hypertension remains controversial. Therefore, a meta-analysis was performed to evaluate the effect of restricting dietary sodium on BP in hypertensive and normotensive individuals. A total of 56 randomized-control trials (28 hypertensive and 28 normotensive) using a dietary sodium intervention, measures of urinary sodium excretion, and monitoring both SBP and DBP were included in the analyses. Overall, BP was reduced with sodium restriction with a greater reduction observed in older hypertensives compared to normotensives. When dietary sodium intake was restricted to 100 mmol/d, hypertensive trials showed a reduction in SBP of 3.7 mmHg ($P < .001$) and DBP of 0.9 mmHg ($P = .09$) compared to normotensive trials which showed a reduction in SBP of 1.0 mmHg ($P < .001$) and DBP of 0.51 mmHg ($P = .56$). Overall, the magnitude of BP response was greater for older hypertensives (mean age of 45 years or older) compared to younger hypertensives.

Rauramaa, R., Vaisanen, S., Rankinen, T., Penttila, I., Saarikoski, S., Tuomilehto, J., & Nissinen, A. (1995). Inverse relation of physical activity and apolipoprotein Al to blood pressure in elderly women. *Medicine and Science in Sports and Exercise, 27*(2), 164–169.

This cross-sectional study evaluated the relation of habitual physical activity, diet, and lipoproteins in a cohort of 202 Finnish women, aged 60 to 69 years. Among the women not taking antihypertensive medications, those more physically active (5 or more times/week) had significantly lower DBP compared to those less active (2 or less times/week) ($P < .007$). Additionally, HDL-C and apolipoprotein (the major protein of HDL) were inversely associated with SBP. These data suggest that the frequency of physical activity is associated with improved BP and lipoproteins.

Seidell, J., Verschuren, M., van Leer, E., & Kromhout, D. (1996). Overweight, underweight, and mortality: A prospective study of 48,287 men and women. *Archives of Internal Medicine, 156*(9), 958–963.

The purpose of this study was to evaluate the relationship between BMI and all-cause mortality and cause-specific mortality. A cohort of 48,287 Dutch men and women, aged 30 to 54 years were followed for an average of 12-years. Overall, total mortality was greater among obese men (BMI > 30 kg/m^2) and underweight men (BMI < 18.5 kg/m^2) but not in women. Approximately 65.6 percent men and 47.1 percent women were smokers. An inverse association was noted between the percentage of smokers and BMI, where as the percentage of hypercholesterolemic and hypertensive individuals increased sharply as BMI increased. The combination of risk factors (smoking, hypercholesterolemia, and hypertension) increased with increasing obesity and was more common among men than women, 7.6 percent and 2.4 percent, respectively. Hypertension increased progressively with obesity. Among women, hazard ratios for CHD increased nearly 3-fold with increases in BMI.

Part IX

Mental Health/Illness

Chapter 10

Suicide Morbidity and Mortality in Latina Youth: Prevention Opportunities

Janet Grossman
Claudia Cotes

The rate of self-reported suicide attempts for Latina* high school students was the highest of all gender and ethnic groups in a national survey (Kann et al., 1995). In addition, although the greatest risk for completed suicide is for white males, the suicide mortality rate for minority youth (e.g., African-American and Latino), has increased significantly since 1980 (Centers for Disease Control [CDC], 1995). Given the increased risk for suicide in Latina youth combined with the sociodemographic risk factors for the Latino population as a whole and its underutilization of

This work was supported in full by a grant to the Community Action for Youth Survival project from the Ronald McDonald Children's House Charities. Claudia Cotes was supported in full as a Minority Medical Student Clinical Fellow by the American Academy of Child and Adolescent Psychiatry. We gratefully acknowledge Erin Hynes, Janet Bryant, and Kesanet Gebrekidan for their assistance in the preparation of this manuscript.

* The term Latina will be used to indicate females; the term Latino will be used to indicate males or the people. Many authors who are cited use other terminology (i.e., Hispanic) and their terms will be used and explained throughout the text.

health and mental health services, there is an urgent need to address the issue of suicide and prevention efforts within a culturally relevant context. This chapter explores this need and recommends preventive approaches. Much of this chapter is the product of collaboration between the co-investigators of an adolescent suicide prevention project targeting minority youth and a Latina medical student's project in a minority fellowship. It is beyond the scope of this chapter to discuss suicide in minority youth in general or in Latino youth.

LATINO-AMERICAN CULTURE AS CONTEXT

The issue of suicide in Latina youth must be understood within the context of the Hispanic-American culture. The Hispanic-American population is the second largest and fastest growing minority population at 22.4 million persons or 9 percent of the population. Hispanics in the United States represent 20 different countries. The largest group of Hispanics in the United States are Mexican (60 percent), Puerto Rican, and Cuban (Earls, Escobar, & Manson, 1990). Geographic location is important for access to native country; proximity enables easier access to native country and its support systems. For example, Mexican-Americans living in the southwest have easier access to support systems and ties in Mexico, as compared to Puerto Rican or Cuban populations. Acculturation refers to the psychosocial changes occurring when individuals from one culture come in contact with another. There is conflicting data about whether suicide rates in immigrant populations are lower in those groups who maintain strong ethnic identification and ties, as compared to those who have rapid assimilation, such as adolescents.

Sociodemographic factors and societal conditions, such as economic instability or deprivation, social disintegration, racial and ethnic discrimination, interpersonal violence, criminal behavior, family mental illness, family instability, and abuse are associated with depression and suicidal behavior. These conditions increase the pressure on vulnerable groups, such as immigrant families and adolescents (Diekstra & Garneefski, 1995; Ruiz, 1995). Several authors have described cultural values in the Latino community, such as familism, fatalism, Catholicism, and traditional gender roles. Cultural values in the Latino communities can be protective or increase the risk factor. They are frequently the source of conflict between Latino adolescents and their parents (Heacock, 1990).

There are also sociodemographic characteristics and cultural values that are barriers to utilization of mental health services; both need to be considered in developing a prevention approach and mental health services for Latinas. For example, coverage for mental health is specific to each employer. A majority of Latinos work for employers who do not provide healthcare coverage. In fact, Hispanics and African-Americans comprise 50 percent of the uninsured population; being uninsured decreases the use of health and mental health services and delays treatment. Children in uninsured, low income families have the lowest number of health visits, and Hispanics, in particular, have the least access to healthcare and the poorest healthcare. Both of these factors increase the risk of morbidity and mortality. Other factors that affect utilization of mental health services include language barriers, cultural values regarding mental health treatment, transportation barriers, and provider insensitivity (Ruiz, 1995).

There is a high rate of Hispanics entering the healthcare system through the emergency departments in public sector institutions (Ruiz, 1995). If Latina adolescents seek any healthcare, it is most likely through the emergency department. Therefore, nontraditional medical settings, such as emergency departments, should be targeted for suicide prevention among Latina youth.

SUICIDE MORTALITY AND MORBIDITY IN LATINA YOUTH

The information on risk factors, correlates of suicide, and suicidal behaviors comes from several sources, including analyses of national mortality data, population-based psychological autopsy studies by specific geographic areas, population-based surveys, and studies of clinical populations (Moscicki, 1995).

Suicide Mortality

The National Center for Health Statistics (NCHS) of the Centers for Disease Control and Prevention is the federal government's principal vital and health statistics agency and the major source of information on death from suicide (Potter, Powell, & Kachur, 1995). The mission of the NCHS is to provide data that will guide actions and policies to improve the health of the American people. However, these data have not been specific to Latino populations (Centers for Disease Control & Prevention [CDCP], 1995; Shaffer, Gould, & Hicks, 1994). The data are divided by gender and by race, white, black, and other, none of which specifically identify Hispanics. The category termed "other" comprises all those races that are not considered black or white, including Hispanics. Within the other group, the rates are variable.

For example, American Indian males have rates higher than white males, and Hispanic males of all ages have rates lower than white and black males.

The NCHS data show that violence accounted for 75 percent of deaths in youth ages 15 to 24 in 1993. The majority of violent deaths were due to accidents, with homicide and suicide following as the next leading causes of violent death in this age group. In contrast, medical illness comprised the next seven causes of death, accounting for the remaining 25 percent of deaths in youth ages 15 to 24. A total of 4,849 persons ages 15 to 24 died by suicide in 1993; this amount is more than the total of all those who died by the seven medical illnesses combined (NIMH, 1996).

In fact, youth suicide has reached epidemic proportions. In 1993, the rate of suicide for youth ages 15 to 19 was 10.9/100,000. The rate of suicide for this age group has more than quadrupled over the four decades from 1950 to 1990, rising from 2.7/100,000 population in 1950 to 11.1/100,000 population in 1990 (Kachur, Potter, James, & Powell, 1995). Although suicide is rare in children, the rates for 10- to 14-year-olds have increased 120 percent from 1980 to 1992. However, the rate for 10- to 14-year-olds remains low, 1.7/100,000 in 1992 (CDC, 1995).

Regional Mortality Studies in Minority Youth.   Although there are no available national data for Latino adolescents per se, regional mortality studies may provide data on suicide deaths among minority youth. Psychological autopsy studies represent one form of regional study that might be useful in examining minority youth suicide completions. However, many of these studies do not include minority youth. The studies were primarily conducted in the early and mid-1980s, when the majority of adolescent suicide deaths, as reported by coroners, were Caucasian. Recruitment of parents of minority youth for these studies was difficult. For example, minority families often labeled the death a homicide, and language barriers hampered the efforts to interview Latino families (Clark & Grossman, personal communications, 1995). Many of these studies are limited because the ethnic makeup of the participants is not described at all. This was the case in psychological autopsy studies done by Brent, Perper, Kolko, & Zelenak (1988) and Shaffer (1988). If minorities are included, they are most likely African-American. For example, in two psychological autopsy studies of youth, over 90 percent of the victims were Caucasian, and the remaining were African-American (Brent, Perper, Moritz, Allman, et al., 1993; Shaffi, Carrigan, Wittinghill, & Derrick, 1985). The composition of these studies underscores the issue of ethnicity of nonparticipants.

Two psychological autopsy studies did include minority youth and the findings were consistent with Shaffer's findings that the rate of suicide in minority males is increasing (Shaffer et al., 1994). The first study, specifically examined Latino youth in Miami. A total of 23, 13- to 19-year-olds committed suicide in Miami over an 18-month period (January 1988 to June

1989). Fourteen (61 percent) of the victims were Latinos; this number considerably exceeded the proportion of Latinos (46 percent) in Dade county. All of the Latinos were immigrant youth, and only three of the victims were female (Queralt, 1993).

The second, more recent psychological autopsy study was carried out between 1990 and 1995 and included consecutive cases of suicide committed by adolescents ages 15 to 19 in three Chicago area counties over a five-year period. A significant portion of the suicide deaths in Chicago over this time period were minority youth, including Latinos. This investigation revealed an unusual phenomenon of peer-witnessed suicides in a portion of the minority males (Clark, personal communication, 1995; Rigsbee, Goebel, DiCanio, & Clark, 1993). In both studies, the Latino victims were primarily male and the preferred method of suicide was a firearm. Although completed suicide in Latinos is increasing, it remains higher in Caucasian males (CDC, 1995).

Gender, Ethnicity, and Suicide.   Gender is the best predictor of suicide mortality. Gender differences in suicide are influenced by culture and nationality, age, social class, employment, personal relationships, method, and mental disorders (Canetto & Lester, 1995). Canetto and Lester also describe how misclassification and underreporting of female suicides, compared to male suicides, distorts mortality data. There are regional and social class differences in suicide mortality by gender. In some societies where women have low status, female suicide mortality rates are higher than male suicide rates.

Internationally, most countries report their deaths to the World Health Organization (WHO). Based on these data, the overall rate of female-to-male suicide is 1:2; however, there are Asian and Papua New Guinea populations in which female deaths exceed male deaths (Canetto & Lester, 1995; Lester, 1988; WHO, 1969–1991). In a comparison of international rates, the rates for females in the majority of Latin countries were low (Canetto & Lester, 1995). In the United States, although there are no national suicide mortality data on Hispanics, there are regional data which provide some comparison to the international data. In 1984, vital statistics were kept for Hispanics in 15 states; these states represented approximately 45 percent of the Hispanic population. Hispanics had the lowest rates of suicide mortality; however, 15- to 24-year-old Hispanics had the highest rates among Hispanics (Earls, Escobar, & Manson, 1990).

Over the past 40 years in the United States, the completed suicide rates for all adolescents ages 15 to 19 have varied by age and gender. White youth commit suicide more often than non-whites, that is, black and other (Shaffer et al., 1994). Although the rate for 15- to 19 -year old females of other races remains low, there was a 67 percent increase from the 1980 rate of 3/100,000 to the 1992 rate of 5/100,000 (CDC, 1995). Reporting bias has an effect on the data on suicide in minority populations; for example, under-reporting of Latino youth with a non-Hispanic surname can occur.

Male adolescents have traditionally had the highest suicide rate and are at the greatest risk for suicide. Completion rates were over four times greater for adolescent males than adolescent females in 1993 (Ryland & Kruesi, 1992). The rate for white males peaked in 1988. Following this peak, the rate for white males stabilized below that peak. The female rate remained stable at a low rate compared to males.

The rate for minority youth males has increased since 1965 (Shaffer et al., 1994). There has been a significant increase in suicides of minority youth. Specifically the suicide rate for African-American males increased 165.3 percent from 1980 to 1992 (CDC, 1995). The greatest increase in the minority youth rate is in urban areas.

Method and Suicide.   Choice of method is the strongest predictor of outcome. Males are more likely to choose lethal methods, and females are more likely to choose methods that provide for discovery and recovery from injuries. Females are also more likely to seek help and communicate distress to potential caregivers. Canetto and Lester (1995) assert that choice of method is not the only determinant of outcome; consideration must be given to availability, familiarity, and cultural acceptability. For example, dying may be considered more masculine and thus more acceptable for males than for females. Males are also more likely to carry a weapon than females; thus, excluding firearms in the home, guns are more accessible and familiar to males (Kann et al., 1995).

Approximately 61 percent of all persons who die by suicide use firearms. Although firearms are the most common method used by both men and women, it is used by a far greater number of men. Firearms are the major method used by adolescent suicide victims, accounting for approximately 60 percent of these deaths (Kachur et al., 1995). Firearms are a highly lethal method—self-inflicted firearm injuries result in death almost 90 percent of the time. The increased availability of firearms in American homes has been identified as the major reason for both the rise in adolescent suicides and the rise in adolescent firearm suicides. The presence of firearms in the home increases the risk of suicide for both genders, regardless of whether the adolescent has a psychiatric disorder and the firearm is locked in storage (Brent et al., 1988; Brent, Perper, Moritz, Baugher, Schweers, & Roth, 1991). Although males are more likely to use firearms than females, increasingly firearms are the major choice of method for both adolescent males and females.

Suicide rates vary geographically, with the highest suicide rates being in rural areas and the western states. Higher rates in the west appear to result from higher firearm suicide rates. Firearm suicides are strongly correlated with overall suicide rates in most states. Ingestion is the most common method used in suicide attempts and is used most frequently by females. Adolescents ingest prescriptive drugs, over-the-counter drugs, or some combination.

Suicide Morbidity in Latina Youth

Adolescent suicide attempts have been studied by surveillance of emergency department visits of adolescent attempters, surveys of health risk behaviors, and clinical studies of suicide attempters. Latino youth are underrepresented in clinical studies of attempters because of their low utilization of clinical services and previous lower suicide rates than Caucasians.

Youth age 15 to 19 years in a primarily Caucasian sample had a suicide attempt rate higher than any other age group seen in an emergency department surveillance of suicide attempts in Cobb County, Georgia (Birkhead, Galvin, Meehan, O'Carroll, & Mercy, 1993). In a state-wide surveillance of suicide-related visits of youth to emergency departments in Oregon, the attempt rate was 120.7/100,000 for Latino youth, a rate lower than that of African-Americans, Caucasians, and Native Americans (CDC, 1995). In surveying risk behaviors in a nationwide study of high school students, the frequency of suicide risk behaviors in Latinas was consistently higher than the group in general, other gender and ethnic groups and Latino males specifically. The self-reported rate of suicide attempt for the Latinas was 19.7 percent as compared to a rate of 8.6 percent for the overall rate (Kann et al., 1995).

There have also been regional and local studies comparing depression and suicidal ideation between adolescents in the Hispanic and white communities and between male and female adolescents. The studies have overwhelmingly found that females are more likely to have depressive symptoms and suicidal behavior than are males. They have also found that Hispanics are more likely to have depressive symptoms and suicidal ideations than are Caucasians (Roberts & Chen, 1995).

At North Central Bronx Hospital, suicide attempts by Latinas represented more than 25 percent of all patients admitted to the hospital for suicidal behavior, whereas Latinas account for only 1.4 percent of the community. This community, although predominantly Latino and African-American, also includes substantial numbers of several other ethnic adolescent groups. This local ethnic diversity makes the high incidence of suicide among urban Latina adolescents all the more striking (Razin et al., 1991).

Limitations of Studies of
Suicidality in Latinas

Several methodological issues limit our understanding of suicidality in Latinas. Sampling is limited by underrepresentation of undocumented aliens and various methods of determining ethnicity. The social stigma associated with suicide within the Latino community may reflect reporting bias. There is also little comparative research on suicide in native and immigrant Latino populations and very little psychological autopsy data on Latina youth. In some studies, instruments used to determine if a person is depressed or if they have suicidal ideations were primarily developed for adults. In studies that include Latino youth, the findings may not be segmented by cultural group and Latino subjects may not be included in the analysis because they comprise a small number in the sample (Garrison, McKeown, Valois, & Vincent, 1993; Roberts & Chen, 1995; Smith, Mercy, & Warren, 1985; Sorenson & Golding, 1988).

Risk Factors for Suicide in Latinas

A framework for risk factors for adolescent suicide can assist in understanding both the contribution of various risk factors and identifying areas for prevention efforts (Ryland & Kruesi, 1992). Moscicki (1995) provides an epidemiologic framework for risk factors of both completed and attempted suicide including psychiatric, biological, familial, and situational risk factors. The co-occurrence of proximal and distal risk factors is associated with the greatest risk of suicide (Henricksson, Hillevi, Marrunen, & Isometsa, 1993).

Psychiatric Risk Factors. Psychiatric disorders are the major risk factor for youth suicide; however, the majority of adolescents with mental disorders do not die by suicide. Psychological autopsy studies have revealed that approximately 90 percent of all adolescent suicides are associated with psychiatric disorders. These disorders include affective disorders (most often depression and less often manic-depressive illness), conduct disorders or antisocial personality disorders, and substance abuse disorders (Brent et al., 1988, 1993b; Martunnen et al., 1991; Shaffer et al., 1988; Shaffi et al., 1985). Depression, substance abuse, and aggressive behavior have also been found to differentiate suicidal from nonsuicidal youth (Andrews & Lewinsohn, 1992; Garrison et al., 1993). Co-occurrence, having more than one disorder, or symptoms of another psychiatric disorder and prior suicide attempts also increase risk for attempts and completion (Brent et al., 1988; Shaffer, 1988; Shaffi et al., 1985). In the 1991 Youth Risk Survey, half of the Latinas who reported an attempt in the prior year reattempted in the same year.

Biological Risk Factors. Biological factors, may play a role in suicide attempts and completion and are currently being studied in adolescents. These studies include serotonin brain tissue of adolescent suicide victims (Arango et al., 1990) and neurotransmitter metabolites in spinal fluid of suicide attempters (Kruesi et al., 1992). Adolescents with epilepsy, AIDS, and diabetes have been shown to be at increased risk for suicide (Callahan,

Clark, Grossman, & Donoghue, 1995; Golston, Kovacs, Ho, Parrone, & Stiffler, 1994).

Familial Risk Factors. Familial risk factors include sharing biological vulnerability, sharing an adverse family environment and interaction of these factors (Moscicki, 1995). Family psychiatric disorders can be a risk factor for adolescent suicide and are significantly higher in frequency in both adolescents who die by suicide and suicidal inpatients compared to controls (Brent et al., 1993a). Evidence for genetic factors come from studies of adults, such as studies of a familial tendency for impulsivity (Roy, Segal, Centerwall, & Robinette, 1991). Family environments, such as those with absent father, violence and abuse, and family discord, are associated with risk for attempted suicide by youth (Andrews & Lewinsohn, 1992; CDC, 1995; deWilde, Kienhorst, Diekstra, & Wolters, 1991; Shaffi et al., 1985).

Situational Risk Factors. Many situations, including interpersonal conflict, loss, and external stressors, occur in close proximity to a suicidal act by an adolescent (Brent et al., 1993b). These situations by themselves do not cause a suicide, but in combination with other risk factors, such as a psychiatric disorder, may create the conditions that lead to a suicide (Moscicki, 1955). The presence of a firearm in the home is one of the strongest risk factors for adolescent suicide (Brent et al., 1988, 1991). Incarceration or exposure to suicidal behavior of a family member, peer, or the media in an adolescent who is already depressed or suicidal may serve as a situational risk factor (Moscicki, 1955).

Risk Factors in Latinas. Suicide is a complex phenomenon, determined by multiple factors intersecting at a point in the life of an individual. Edwin Shneidman, who is known as the Father of Suicidology, because of his early work in the field in Los Angeles, describes the elements that determine suicide as the following: biological, cultural, sociological, intrapsychic, interpersonal, intrapersonal, logical, conscious, unconscious, philosophical, and environmental elements. Because multiple and complex factors lead to suicide, an interaction of these risk factors may account for increases in the suicide rates in minority youth; however, there are no widely accepted explanations. Gender, culture, family, economics, migration, socialization, violence and depression interact and place many Latinas at high risk for suicide (Shaffer et al., 1994).

Suicide Prevention
in Latinas

Several major policy groups, communities, conferences, and programs have formed to respond to the crisis of youth suicide by identifying significant issues in youth suicide and addressing appropriate responses by society and researchers. The guidelines and recommendations of these groups have served to guide community, school, policy, and research efforts in youth suicide prevention. Examples of exemplary efforts include the Secretary's Task Force on Youth Suicide, the LivingWorks Program in Canada, the New Jersey Adolescent Suicide Prevention Project, and the Washington State Plan for suicide prevention. Only recently have such efforts begun to address the issues of suicide in minority youth and the need for suicide prevention efforts targeted toward minority youth.

Traditionally, the mental health approach to youth suicide has focused on the identification and treatment of persons with mental disorders. These efforts have not reached Latino youth. Although this approach remains the cornerstone of youth suicide prevention, there has been recognition of the variety of factors contributing to youth suicide and, thus, an expansion of the conceptualization of youth suicide and intervention (DHHS, 1992).

Recently youth suicide has been viewed as a significant public health problem, rather than solely a mental health problem. Prevention was labeled as the number one health priority for the 1990s. The Year 2000 National Health Objectives set by the Public Health Service provide objectives for improving the health of the nation in the next century, including reversing the rising trend in youth suicide. Specifically, these objectives aim to reduce suicide to no more than 8.2/100,000 in youth 15 to 19; to reduce by 15 percent the incidence of injurious suicide attempts among adolescents aged 14 to 17; and to reduce by 20 percent the proportion of people who possess weapons that are inappropriately stored and therefore dangerously accessible (U.S. Department of Health and Human Services [DHHS], 1992).

Consistent with these objectives, the Centers for Disease Control has taken on the task of developing a preventive foci for intentional injuries, including suicide. CDC developed a resource guide to describe the rationale and evidence for the effectiveness of various youth suicide strategies and to identify model programs that incorporated these different strategies. The eight suicide strategies included: School Gatekeeper Training, Community Gatekeeper Training, General Suicide Education, Screening Programs, Peer Support Programs, Crisis Centers and Hotlines, Means Restriction, and Intervention After a Suicide. Five recommendations were made in regard to programs: (1) new and current suicide prevention programs link closely with professional mental health resources in the community, (2) programs should avoid a single prevention strategy, (3) underused strategies should be incorporated into current programs, (4) suicide prevention efforts need to be expanded for young adults 20 to 24 years of age, and (5) evaluation efforts need to be incorporated into all new and existing suicide prevention programs (CDC, 1992).

A recent report by the Institute of Medicine Committee reviews the mental health intervention spectrum for mental disorders: prevention, treatment, and maintenance. Prevention is commonly used for those interventions occurring before the onset of a disorder and are classified as universal, selective, or indicated. High risk groups and culturally diverse populations have been targeted for prevention research (National Academy of Sciences, 1994). Since Latinas are underserved, this chapter focuses heavily on prevention.

Universal preventive interventions are targeted to the general public or entire populations group, not identified on the basis of individual risk. Selective preventive interventions are targeted to individuals or subgroups of the population whose risk of developing mental disorders is significantly higher than the norm. Indicated preventive interventions are targeted to high-risk youth who are identified as having minimal but detectable signs or symptoms, or biological markers, indicating predisposition for the mental disorder but not meeting the diagnostic criteria (National Academy of Sciences, 1994). Table 10.1 provides a list of other preventions/preventive interventions for Latina youth, consistent with experts' proposed targeted efforts (Berman & Jobes, 1991). Three examples of preventive interventions will also be discussed.

Youth Suicide Prevention for Latinas in Nontraditional Settings

Given that the Latino population underutilizes health and mental health services and large numbers of Latinas have early school drop out, emergency departments and junior high school are important target settings for suicide prevention in Latinas. Three model programs in these settings will be described.

Emergency Department Intervention with Latina Suicide Attempters. Few interventions have been developed for suicidal adolescents. Families of suicidal adolescents tend to have poor compliance with treatment recommendations. There is a need for cost-effective, short-term family interventions which focus on coping and problem solving skills (Rotheram-Borus, Piacentini, Miller, Graae, & Castro-Blanco, 1994). These authors have developed systematic family intervention for high-risk adolescents and measured the impact of these interventions, including a large controlled investigation of two family interventions for adolescent suicide attempters. The investigators evaluated an emergency-based program to improve outpatient treatment adherence during follow-up treatment with Latina adolescent suicide attempters from disadvantaged families (Rotheram-Borus et al., 1996). Staff training and new emergency room procedures were implemented to provide the specialized treatment.

Suicide attempters received either a standard or specialized ER Program and then the Standardized Family Therapy (SNAP) in outpatient,

Table 10.1
Suicide Prevention/Intervention Strategies for Latina Youth

	Universal Preventive Intervention	Selective Preventive Intervention	Indicated Preventive Intervention
Prevention	• School-based clinics • School drop-out prevention • Teen pregnancy education • Violence prevention	• Depression screening by school nurse • Psychoeducation for parents • Community outreach • Protective services for abused youth and their mothers • Caregiver training in Latino communities in identification and referral of children	• Parent education to restrict lethal means • Services for illegal families • Parent education about affective illness • Substance abuse intervention • Hotlines for Latino youth
Treatment			• Means Restriction education • Community outreach • Culturally sensitive mental health services • Caregiver training • Home-based family intervention • Family systems interventions • Cognitive-behavioral groups • Promotion of family interaction with church or community social activities
Maintenance			• Psychotherapy for depression • Psychiatric treatment • Localized community mental health services • Depression screening in local health clinics

with follow up at 3, 6, 12, and 18 months. The specialized ER program consisted of a structured family therapy session with a bilingual family therapist who was a liaison for the family with emergency and outpatient staff. A soap opera type videotape was used, portraying the experience of two adolescent attempters in the videotape, in order to educate the family about ER procedures, adaptive coping, and follow-up treatment. The therapist then helped the family plan for suicide-eliciting situations, set outpatient treatment goals, and make a contract. The adolescents were then referred to the Adolescent Suicidal Disorders Clinic for Standardized Family Therapy (SNAP), a six session behavioral and cognitive structured protocol to learn positive family problem solving (Rotheram-Borus et al., 1994).

School-Based Clinics for Urban, Minority Youth. Adolescents have high rates of health problems, underutilize health settings, and have failed to improve their healthcare over the last decade (Walter, Vaughan, Armstrong, Krakoff, Tiezzi, & McCarthy, 1995). Although schools are considered a natural and significant site for the delivery of mental health services to youth, these services have not been widely implemented (Ring-Kurtz, Sonnichsen, & Hoover-Demsy, 1995). Walter et al. (1995) describe school-based health clinics in junior high schools serving predominantly disadvantaged Hispanic students. The program included outreach services through such methods as health screening and risk surveys. Mental health problems, including suicide and depression, were the predominant presenting complaints. These authors advocate that school mental health services be based on a principle that mental health is a normal and desirable developmental goal.

School-based programs can provide assessment, prevention, and intervention services for youth and their families, as part of a health clinic or specialized mental health clinic or services (Ring-Kurtz et al., 1995). Programs for Latina youth could include cognitive-behavioral approaches for Latinas identified as high risk for depression. Given the high frequency of adolescent-parent conflict focused on acculturation issues, family systems interventions could also be used. This approach may provide alternative solutions and prevent crises, such as suicide attempts by Latinas. In the event of a suicide attempt by a Latina youth, school-based mental health services may be more agreeable to parents than outpatient treatment.

Three-Step Intervention for Parents of Latinas At-Risk for Suicide. One prevention strategy aimed at addressing known or suspected risk factors is "Means Restriction" (CDC, 1992). Means Restriction is the suicide prevention strategy of restricting access to lethal means of suicide, such as firearms and medications in the home. The rationale for the means restriction suicide prevention programs is that adolescents whose access to lethal means of committing suicide is restricted, may be more likely to switch methods of suicide, perhaps to a method that is less lethal.

Means restriction has the potential of decreasing suicides even if it does not decrease the incidence of suicide attempts (See CDC, 1992, p. 147 for a review of this strategy). Moreover, there is growing evidence that means restriction may prevent some suicides altogether. Evidence for the effectiveness of this method has been described in relation to the restriction of cooking gas, barbiturates, carbon monoxide, and firearms. The CDC described means restriction as a "promising but underused strategy," underscoring the need for systematic programs and evaluation of outcomes. Although some suicide prevention strategies have been targeted for certain subgroups of youth (for example, runaways), there has been little effort to adapt suicide prevention strategies to ethnic groups.

The Three-Step Intervention for Parents of Suicidal Adolescents is targeted at health professionals. A brochure provides a simple intervention that health professionals use with parents and caretakers of adolescent suicide attempters or those at high risk (Kruesi, Hirsch, & Grossman, 1996). The three-step intervention, based on the public health approach of injury prevention, is intended to be delivered to parents/caretakers of adolescent suicide attempters or those at high risk. The steps include:

1. Inform the parents that their adolescent is at risk for suicide and why you think so. For example, in the case of an adolescent who has made a previous attempt by overdose: "Adolescents who have made a suicide attempt are at risk for another attempt."

2. Tell parents they can reduce the risk of suicide by getting medications and firearms out of the house. Ingestion of household medications is the most common method used by adolescent females who attempt suicide. Adolescents who overdose on medication often take more than one medication. Alcohol is often a facilitator of suicide. "The risk of suicide doubles if a firearm is in the house, even if the firearm is locked up." The parents must understand the importance of removing access to a firearm. Tell parents this even if they don't presently own a firearm.

3. Educate parents about different ways to dispose of, or at the very least, limit access to medications and firearms. During the intervention, offer parents your assistance with this process. A parent can safeguard the home environment by removing all medications except those being actively used. If removal is not possible, it is strongly recommended that all prescription medications, as well as over-the-counter medications and alcoholic beverages be locked up in the house. Adults taking medication daily should carry it with them to limit their child's access. A number of police departments are willing to help with the disposal of firearms. Ideally, the health professional should know the policies and procedures of their local police departments regarding firearm disposal prior to the delivery of the intervention.

This intervention can be implemented in schools, emergency departments, outpatient and inpatient child mental health services, pediatric settings, and other services for high risk youth. Parents/caretakers of depressed, suicidal, acting out, or addicted Latina youth should be instructed about how to restrict these methods. Means restriction specific for Latina youth needs to target prescription drugs and over the counter medications.

Multicultural Framework in Prevention Services

All services directed at reducing depression and suicide in Latina youth need to be contextualized in the Latino culture. The multicultural framework provides guidelines for this approach. In the multicultural framework, culture includes ethnicity and sociocultural contexts, such as age, race, gender, education, and economics (Breunlin, Schwartz, & MacKune-Karrer, 1992). Culture influences all levels of systems, including individuals, families, schools, and communities. There are multiple sociocultural contexts, and families and caregivers share cultural similarities and differences.

Each sociocultural contact between families and caregivers triggers opportunities and constraints. A session with the parents of a student and a health caregiver offers the opportunity for each party to learn about the adolescent and for the caregiver and parents to share a concern for this adolescent and a commitment to keep the adolescent alive. To be effective, the caregiver needs to consider the following questions: (1) What is the culture of this family? (2) What is my own culture? (3) Where do they differ? (4) How are they the same? (5) How can we elicit family members' cooperation, given their culture? (6) How do I monitor my own beliefs so they do not become a hindrance to engaging this family?

Consider the following example: A student at high risk for suicide is a 17-year-old, Catholic, Latina whose parents are immigrants with college degrees in business and literature. In contrast, the caregiver is a 30-year-old, Caucasian, Baptist female whose parents were farmers. The caregiver is aware that in the Latino community, persons who are depressed, anxious or suicidal are often referred to as the "nervous type" and depression in women is often covered up. The parents may report, "In our community we don't go to shrinks. We go to the local healer or the parish priest." In the family meeting, the parents learn Latinas have the highest rate of youth suicide attempts in the United States and are at high risk for reattempting suicide in the same year without intervention. The caregiver provides a referral to the local Catholic hospital for mental health services for the adolescent, a setting more consistent with these parents' belief system.

IMPLICATIONS

Youth suicide mortality data underscores the need for intensifying prevention efforts targeting minority youth, youth ages 10 to 14 years, and lethal methods (CDC, 1995). Although limited in number, the national and regional studies of suicide morbidity in adolescents suggest that Latina youth are at significant risk for suicide morbidity and depression. More systematic research is needed on suicide risk and prevention efforts in Latinas (National Academy of Science, 1994). Given the evidence of suicide risk in Latina youth, qualitative studies are needed with suicidal Latina youth and their families to understand the meanings and acceptability of the suicidal behavior.

Prevention efforts must be sensitive to the interface between cultural and social variables on one hand and risk and protective factors on the other hand, that must fit in that community and be owned and supported by that community (National Academy of Science, 1994). Primary prevention approaches should include the gender cultures of suicide, thus assessing and focusing on the meanings and acceptability of suicide within Latina youth (Canetto & Lester, 1995).

Latina youth are a high risk group for suicide attempts. They are most likely to overdose on medication. Adolescent-parental conflict related to traditional cultural values may trigger these attempts. Culture needs to be addressed as part of the drama of depression and suicide in Latina youth and as a crucial focus of prevention endeavors (Alarcon, 1995). School and emergency department settings should be targeted for such efforts using cultural-specific psychoeducation and counseling for Latinas and their families. Rotheram-Borus and her colleagues have developed extensive training materials for prevention and intervention with suicidal youth and their families, including culturally specific materials. Emergency department staff, school health staff, and community workers in the Hispanic community need to be trained in these approaches.

At the policy level, uninsured, underserved and poorly served Latinas need to have increased opportunities for equal access to healthcare, in order that early screening and intervention can prevent the cycle of depression and the tragedy of suicide.

REFERENCES

Alarcon, R. D. (Ed.), (1995, September). *The psychiatric clinics of North America: Cultural psychiatry, 18*(3), 1–679.

Andrews, J. A., & Lewinsohn, P. M. (1992). Suicidal attempts among older adolescents: Prevalence and co-occurrence with psychiatric disorders. *Journal of the American Academy of Child Psychiatry, 31,* 655–662.

Arango, V., Ernsberger, P., Marzuk, P. M., Chen, J. S., Tierney, H., Stanley, M., Reis, D. J., & Mann, J. (1990). Autoradiographic demonstration of increased serotonin 5-HT (2) and B-adrenergic receptor binding sites in the brain of suicide victims. *Archives of General Psychiatry, 47,* 1038–1047.

Berman, A., & Jobes, D. (1991). *Adolescent suicide assessment and intervention.* Washington, DC: American Psychological Association.

Birkhead, G., Galvin, V., Meehan, P., O'Carroll, P., & Mercy, J. (1993). The emergency department in surveillance of attempted suicide: Findings and methodologic considerations. *Public Health Reports, 108,* 323–331.

Brent, D., Perper, J., Allman, C., Moritz, G., Wartella, M., & Zelenak, J. (1991). The presence and accessibility of firearms in the homes of adolescent suicides: A case-control study. *Journal of the American Medical Association, 266*(21), 2989–2995.

Brent, D., Perper, J., Kolko, D., & Zelenak, J. (1988). The psychological autopsy: Methodological considerations for the study of adolescent suicide. *Journal of the American Academy of Child and Adolescent Psychiatry, 27*(3), 362–366.

Brent, D., Perper, J., Moritz, G., Allman, C., Friend, A., Roth, C., Schweers, J., Balach, L., & Baugher, M. (1993a). Psychiatric risk factors for adolescent suicide: A case-control study. *Journal of the American Academy of Child and Adolescent Psychiatry, 32*(3), 521–529.

Brent, D. A., Perper, J. A., Moritz, G., Baughner, M., Roth, C., Balach, L., & Schweers, J. (1993b). Stressful life event, psychopathology, and adolescent suicide: A case control study. *Suicide and Life Threatening Behavior, 23*(3), 179–187.

Bruenlin, D. C., Schwartz, R. C., & MacKune-Karrer, B. (1992). *Metaframeworks: Transcending the models of family therapy.* San Francisco: Jossey-Bass.

Callahan, J., Clark, D. C., Grossman, J. A., & Donoghue, E. (1996). *Prototypes of adolescent suicide.* Manuscript in revision.

Canetto, S. (1994). Gender issues in the treatment of suicidal individuals. In A. Leenaars, J. Maltsberger, & R. Neimeyer (Eds.), *Treatment of suicidal people* (pp. 115–126). Bristol, PA: Taylor & Francis.

Canetto, S., & Lester, D. (1995). Gender and the primary prevention of suicide mortality. In M. M. Silverman & R. W. Maris (Eds.), *Suicide prevention: Toward the year 2000* (pp. 58–69). New York: Guilford Press.

Centers for Disease Control & Prevention. (1995, April 28). Fatal and nonfatal suicide attempts among adolescents—Oregon, 1988–1993. *Morbidity and Mortality Weekly Report, 44*(16), 312–323.

Centers for Disease Prevention & Epidemiology, Oregon Health Division. (1993, September 7). *Adolescent Suicide, 42*(18).

Centers for Disease Control. (1992). *Youth suicide prevention programs: A resource guide* (pp. 147–151). Atlanta, GA: National Center for Injury Prevention and Control.

Centers for Disease Control. (1995). Suicide among children, adolescents, and young adults—United States, 1980–1992. *Morbidity and Mortality Weekly Report, 44*(15), 289–291.

deWilde, E., Kienhorst, I. C. W. N., Diekstra, R. F. W., & Wolters, W. H. G. (1991). The relationship between adolescent suicidal behavior and life events in childhood and adolescence. *American Journal of Psychiatry, 149*, 45–51.

Diekstra, R., & Garneefski, N. (1995). On the nature, magnitude, and causality of suicidal behaviors: An international perspective. In M. Silverman & R. Maris (Eds.), *Suicide prevention: Toward the year 2000.* New York: Guilford Press.

Earls, F., Escobar, J. & Manson, S. (1990). Suicide in minority groups: Epidemiologic and cultural perspectives. In S. Blumenthal & D. Kupfer (Eds.), *Suicide over the life cycle: Risk factors, assessment, and treatment of suicidal patients* (pp. 127–134). Washington, DC: American Psychiatric Press, Inc.

Garrison, C. Z., McKeown, R. E., Valois, R. F., & Vincent, M. L. (1993). Aggression, substance use, and suicidal behaviors in high school students. *American Journal of Public Health, 83*, 179–184.

Golston, D. B., Kovacs, M., Ho, V. Y., Parrone, P. L., & Stiffler, L. (1994). Suicidal ideation and suicide attempts among youth with insulin-dependent diabetes mellitus. *Journal of the American Academy of Child and Adolescent Psychiatry, 33*, 240–245.

Heacock, D. R. (1990). Suicidal behavior in black and Hispanic youth. *Psychiatric Annals, 20*(3), 134–142.

Henriksson, M. M., Hillevi, M. A., Marunnen, M. J., Isometsa, E. T., et al. (1993). Mental disorders and comorbidity in suicide. *American Journal of Psychiatry, 150*, 935–940.

Kachur, S., Potter, L., James, S., & Powell, K. (1995). *Suicide in the United States, 1980–1993.* Atlanta, GA: Centers for Disease Control and Prevention, National Center for Injury Prevention and Control, Violence Surveillance Summary Series, No. 1.

Kann, L., Warren, C. W., Harris, W. A., Collins, J. L., Douglas, K. A., Collins, M. E, Williams, B. I., Ross, J. G., & Kolbe, L. J. (1995). Youth risk behavior surveillance—United States, 1993. *Morbidity and Mortality Weekly Report, 44*(SS-1), 1–56.

Kruesi, M., Hibbs, E., Zahn, T., Keysor, C., Hamburger, S., Bartko, J., & Rapoport, J. (1992). A 2-year prospective follow-up study of children and adolescents with disruptive behavior disorders. *Archives of General Psychiatry, 49,* 429–435.

Kruesi, M., Hirsch, J., & Grossman, J. (1996). *Three step intervention for parents of suicidal adolescents* [Brochure]. University of Illinois at Chicago & Ronald McDonald House Charities.

Lester, D. (Ed.). (1988). *Why women kill themselves.* Springfield, IL: C.C. Thomas.

Malgady, R., Costantino, G., & Rogler, L. (1990). Culturally sensitive psychotherapy for Puerto Rican children and adolescents: A program of treatment outcome research. *Journal of Consulting and Clinical Psychology 58*(6), 704–712.

Moscicki, E. K. (1995). Epidemiology of suicide. *Suicide and Life Threatening Behavior, 25*(1), 22–35.

National Academy of Sciences. (1994). *Reducing risks for mental disorders: Frontiers for preventive research.* Washington, DC: National Academy Press.

National Institute of Mental Health. (1996). *Suicide facts.* Washington, DC: NIMH.

Payton, J. (1992). *School personnel fact sheets for youth risk survey 1991.* Chicago, IL: Department of Research, Evaluation and Planning.

Potter, L. B., Powell, K. E., & Kachur, S. P. (1995). Suicide perspective from a public health approach. *Suicide & Life Threatening Behavior, 25*(1), 83–84.

Queralt, M. (1993). Risk factors associated with completed suicide in Latino adolescents. *Adolescence, 112,* 831–850.

Razin, A., O'Dowd, A., Nathan, A., Rodriguez, I., Goldfield, A., Martin, C., Goulet, L., Scheftel, S., Mezan, P., & Mosca, J. (1991). Suicidal behavior among inner-city Hispanic adolescent females. *General Hospital Psychiatry, 13,* 45–58.

Rich, C. L., & Runeson, B. S. (1992). Similarities in diagnostic comorbidity between suicide among young people in Sweden and the United States. *Acta Psychiatrica Scandinavavia, 86,* 335–339.

Rigsbee, S., Goebel, A., DiCanio, P., & Clark, D. (1993). *Possible trends in adolescent suicide by firearm.* Suicide 93: Proceedings of the American Association of Suicidology, Denver, CO (82–84).

Ring-Kurtz, S., Sonnichsen, S., & Hoover-Demsy, K. (1995). School-based mental health services for children. In L. Bickman & D. Rog (Eds.), *Children's mental health services: Research, policy, and evaluation* (pp. 117–144). Thousand Oaks: Sage.

Roberts, R., & Chen, Y. (1995). Depressive symptoms and suicidal ideation among Mexican-origin and Anglo adolescents. *Journal of the American Academy of Child and Adolescent Psychiatry, 34*(1), 81–90.

Rotheram-Borus, M. J., Piacentini, J., Miller, S., Graae, F., & Castro-Blanco, D. (1994). Brief cognitive-behavioral treatment for adolescent suicide attempters and their families. *Journal of the American Academy of Child and Adolescent Psychiatry, 33*(4), 508–517.

Rotheram-Borus, M. J., Piacentini, J., VonRossem, R., Graae, F., Cantwell, C., Castro-Blanco, D., Miller, S., & Feldman, J. (1996). Enhancing treatment adherence with a specialized emergency room program for adolescent suicide attempters. *Journal of the American Academy of Child and Adolescent Psychiatry, 35*(5), 564–663.

Roy, A., Segal, N. L., Centerwall, B. S., & Robinette, C. D. (1991). Suicide in twins. *Archives of General Psychiatry, 48*, 29–32.

Ruiz, P. (1995). Assessing, diagnosing, and treating culturally diverse individuals: A Hispanic perspective. *Psychiatric Quarterly, 66*(4), 329–341.

Ryland, D. H., & Kruesi, M. J. P. (1992). Suicide among adolescents. *International Review of Psychiatry, 4*, 185–195.

Shaffer, D. (1988). The epidemiology of teen suicide: An examination of risk factors. *Journal of Clinical Psychiatry, 49*(9, Suppl.), 36–41.

Shaffer, D., Gould, M., & Hicks, R. (1994). Worsening suicide rate in black teenagers. *American Journal of Psychiatry, 151*(12), 1810–1812.

Shaffi, M., Carrigan, S., Wittinghill, J., & Derrick, A. (1985). Psychological autopsy of completed suicide in children and adolescents. *American Journal of Psychiatry 142a*, 1061–1064.

Silverman, M., & Felner, R. (1995). The place of suicide prevention in the spectrum of intervention: Definitions of critical terms and constructs. *Suicide & Life Threatening Behavior, 25*(1), 70–81.

Simoni, J., & Perez, L (1995). Latinos and mutual support groups: A case for considering culture. *The American Orthopsychiatric Association, 65*(3), 440–445.

Smith, J., Mercy, J., & Warren, C. (1985). Comparison of suicides among Anglos and Hispanics in five southwestern states. *Suicide and Life-Threatening Behavior, 15*(1), 14–26.

Sorenson, S., & Golding, J. (1988). Suicide ideation and attempts in Hispanics and non-Hispanic Whites: Demographic and psychiatric disorder issues. *Suicide and Life-Threatening Behavior, 18*(3), 322–333.

Spirito, A., Bond, A., Kurkjian, J., Devost, L., Bosworth, T., & Brown, L. (1993). Gender differences among adolescent suicide attempters. *Crisis, 14*(4), 178–184.

U.S. Department of Health and Human Services. (1990). *Healthy people 2000: National health promotion and disease prevention objectives* (DHHS Publication No. PHS 91-50212). U.S. Government Printing Office.

Walter, H., Vaughan, R., Armstrong, B., Krakoff, R., Maldonado, L., Tiezzi, L., & McCarthy, J. (1995). Sexual, assaultive, and suicidal behaviors among urban minority junior high school students. *Journal of the American Academy of Child and Adolescent Psychiatry, 34*(1), 73–80.

Walter, H., Vaughan, R., Armstrong, B., Krakoff, R., Tiezzi, L., & McCarthy, J. (1995). School-based health care for urban minority junior high school students. *Archives of Pediatric Medicine, 149*, 1221–1225.

World Health Organization. (1969–1991). *Statistics annual.* Geneva, Switzerland: Author.

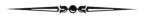

REVIEW OF LITERATURE

Several books and articles were chosen to reflect the current understanding of suicide in general and youth suicide, in particular. A Year 2000 monograph on suicide serves as a scholarly orientation to the field and review of current work. The international perspective offered is essential to address cultural-specific suicide prevention. Four articles were chosen to reflect three epidemiological sources on youth suicide: psychological autopsy, emergency department surveillance, and risk behavior surveys; these serve to underscore the issue of suicide in Latino youth. A book on cultural psychiatry emphasizes the importance of contextualizing interventions for mental health problems in ethnic groups. Finally literature is provided on several culturally-specific interventions in non-traditional settings for suicide prevention in Latina youth, including emergency department intervention, school-based health clinics, parent support groups and caregiver training.

Alarcon, R. D. (Ed.) (1995, September). *The Psychiatric Clinics of North America: Cultural Psychiatry, 18*(3) 1–679.

The field of cultural psychiatry is experiencing a renaissance, both in the United States and internationally. This is the first issue of *The Clinics* devoted entirely to the topic of cultural psychiatry. The volume comprehensively presents the current cultural concerns of psychiatry and emphasizes that cultural understanding is as important as biological factors. Specific to Latina youth is the article by Ruiz on the complexity of providing high-quality mental health services to ethnic populations. Recommended actions are offered. Manson's discussion of depression focuses on the need to move beyond diagnostic nomenclature. By considering the social contexts and social forces that shape a person's world, give meaning to interpersonal relationships, and life events, the mental health professional focuses on the process of inquiry and elicits the person's story of their illness. Kaslow, Celano, and Dreelin discuss the theoretical underpinnings and approaches of culturally informed and sensitive family therapy, and approaches to adapting and modifying current practices to enhance the cultural fit between intervention approach and the family.

Centers for Disease Control & Prevention. (1995, April 28). Fatal and non-fatal suicide attempts among adolescents—Oregon, 1988–1993. *Morbidity and Mortality Weekly Report, 44*(16), 312–323.

In 1987, the Oregon state legislature mandated that hospitals who treat youth ages 17 years or younger for suicide-related injuries report the attempt to the Oregon Health Division, Department of Human Resources and refer the youth for counseling. Oregon is the only state with a legal requirement for reporting suicide attempts and with a surveillance monitoring system. During the 1988–1993 period, a total of 3,783 attempts were reported in Oregon for youth 17 years old and younger—124 youth died; the major method used was firearms (64 percent). The ratio of attempts was 4 females to 1 male. The attempt rate was highest for the 15- to 17-year-old group. The primary method in attempts was overdose (75.5 percent), including the use of analgesics in almost half of the overdoses and laceration or stabbing. The most commonly reported reasons were family discord (59.4 percent), argument with a boyfriend or girlfriend (32.6 percent), and school-related problems (23 percent). Previous attempts were more common in those who reported sexual abuse, physical abuse, or substance abuse as the reason for the attempt.

Kann, L., Warren, C. W., Harris, W. A., Collins, J. L., Douglas, K. A., Colllins, M. E., Williams, B. I., Ross, J. G., & Kolbe, L. J. (1995). Youth risk behavior surveillance—United States, 1993. *Morbidity and Mortality Weekly Report, 44*(SS-1), 1–56.

In 1990, 1991, and 1993 the Centers for Disease Control and Prevention conducted the national Youth Risk Behavior Surveillance System, a study of health risk behaviors in American high school students in grades nine through twelve. In 1993, a total of 16,296 students in 24 states and nine local areas were interviewed using the Youth Risk Survey (YRS) covering six categories of risk behaviors including: intentional and unintentional injuries, tobacco, alcohol, and other drugs, sexual behaviors, dietary behaviors, and physical behaviors. The percentage of students reporting suicidal behavior in the past 12 months included: seriously considering suicide (24.1 percent), making a plan to attempt suicide (19 percent), attempting suicide (13.6 percent), and having injuries resulting from the attempt that required treatment by a doctor or a nurse (2.7 percent). Females were significantly more likely than males to report these behaviors in all categories. Hispanic females were significantly more likely to report considering suicide (34.1 percent), making a plan to attempt suicide (26.6 percent), and attempting suicide (19.7 percent) as compared to other female groups. Of Hispanic females, 5.5 percent reported making a suicide attempt requiring medical attention. Hispanic males with a suicide attempt rate of 7.4 percent, were significantly more likely to attempt suicide as compared to white males. These data are being used by school and health officials to improve school health policies and programs designed to reduce risks associated with leading causes of mortality and morbidity and measure achievement of national health and education objectives.

Roberts, R., & Chen, Y. (1995). Depressive symptoms and suicidal ideation among Mexican-origin and Anglo adolescents.

American Academy of Child and Adolescent Psychiatry, 34(1), 81–90.

There are limited data on suicidal behaviors among minority youth. The literature is conflicting regarding depression in minority youth. This study compares depressive symptoms, suicidal ideation and loneliness (2614) in non-Hispanic whites and Mexican-American adolescents; consisting of Mexican (1354) and Anglos (925) and the remaining other minorities. Females reported more depressive symptoms and suicidal ideation. Ten percent of the Anglos and 15 percent of the minority youth reported high levels of suicidal ideation. Mexican-American adolescents had 1:7 times the risk of depression and more thoughts of suicide as compared to Anglos. Mexican-American females were the most likely to report depressive symptoms. Loneliness was strongly associated with suicidal ideation. Depression was the most significant correlate of suicidal ideation, followed by loneliness. Increasing acculturation, defined as use of English, greatly decreased the risk of depression and suicidal ideation among adolescents of Mexican-American origin. Limitations of the study include the use of self report measures.

Rotheram-Borus, M. J., Piacentini, J., Von-Rossem, R., Graae, F., Cantwell, C., Castro-Blanco, D., Miller, S., & Feldman J. (1996). Enhancing treatment adherence with a specialized emergency room program for adolescent suicide attempters. *Journal of the American Academy of Child and Adolescent Psychiatry, 35*(5), 564–663.

Despite the clear indication for psychotherapeutic intervention following an adolescent suicide attempt, there are low rates of referrals and patient compliance. Differences in sociodemographic characteristics between families and health professionals are associated with incongruent social expectations and assumptions about mental healthcare. This manuscript describes a program to enhance positive interactions among family members. Emergency staff discuss realistic expectations with the families using a videotape and a brief family therapy session and contract for outpatient treatment. A consecutive series of 140 female adolescents, primarily Latina (88 percent), seen at the Columbia Presbyterian Medical Center between 1991-1994 for suicide attempts were included in the study and received the standard emergency care (the first 75) or the specialized program. All the adolescents were also referred to a six-session, standardized outpatient treatment program. Baseline data were collected in the emergency department and postdischarge using measures of depression, suicidality, impulsiveness, self-esteem, psychological distress of the adolescent and her mother, family relationships, attitudes toward treatment and treatment adherence. The subjects in the specialized treatment were more likely to attend their initial treatment session and complete treatment; however, their mothers attended fewer sessions than those in the standard treatment. Those subjects in the specialized group also had reduced depression and suicidality and their mothers had less symptoms, more positive attitudes toward treatment, and improved family perceptions. The authors raise issues related to other family characteristics that may have affected mothers' attendance and the impact of the parent's completion on drop out from treatment.

Silverman, M., & Maris, R. (1995). *Suicide prevention: Toward the year 2000.* New York: Guilford Press. This monograph is also *Suicide & Life-Threatening Behavior, 25*(1).

This monograph reviews the essential ingredients of suicide prevention, with a focus on epidemiology, modifiable risk and protective factors, theoretical and conceptual foundations of preventive interventions, specific settings for interventions, and identification of high risk populations. The title reflects the resurgence of interest in prevention of suicidal behaviors on an international level by the year 2000. Authored by international experts, the monograph provides practical guidelines and examples of interventions and techniques that currently work and techniques that are in the process of development and study. Specific to the issue of suicide in Latina youth are four chapters: Diekstra's international perspective addresses the question of why depressive disorders and suicide mortality are increasing among adolescents and young adults in the twentieth century. Cannetto and Lester address the interaction of gender and culture and the underreporting of suicidal behaviors in women. Kalafat and Elias focus on multidimensional, noncategorical prevention programs targeting at risk behaviors in school-based populations. Berman and Jobe offer a suicide prevention model of levels of intervention from primary through tertiary preventions, emphasizing preventing predisposing factors and strengthening protective factors.

Simoni, J., & Perez, L. (1995). Latinos and mutual support groups: A case for considering culture. *American Orthopsychiatric Association,* 65(3), 440–445.

Latinos have low utilization rates of traditional mental health services and traditional primary prevention programs. This may stem in part from incompatibility of psychological services with Latino cultural values and characteristics. Incorporating these values and ideals into mental health services for Latinos may improve utilization. This manuscript describes the development of elementary school-based mutual support groups for Latino parents. The groups were offered on a voluntary basis for low-income, recent immigrant Latino parents with limited education and little or no proficiency in English. The groups were designed to provide social support and mutual aid, and enhance school involvement and personal empowerment. The authors stress the need for the group facilitators to be knowledgeable about the particular subgroup of the community being targeted and the limitations of implementing programs across subgroups. Of six initial attempts, three groups were established. One group lasted four years and

developed other programs, including English programs. These types of groups could provide the opportunity to educate parents about youth depression and suicide and the need for intervention.

Suicide Prevention Training Programs. (1995). *Strengthening community: Fortaleciendo la comunidad: A suicide prevention workshop for the Latin American community.* Calgary, Alberta, Canada: Author.

This Trainer's Guide is intended to enhance the helping skills already available within the Latin American community. It was a joint effort of a group of professionals working in suicide prevention and social services for immigrants and members of the Latin American community in Calgary. The training was an effort to respond to the unique issues that place Latin immigrant groups at risk for suicide, the barriers that decrease their use of mainstream service, and the failure of suicide prevention programs to address culturally specific content. The efforts began in the Chilean community but then expanded to the broader Latin American community. The workshop was developed out of a sequential series of methods to gather information and test materials through literature review, interviews, an advisory group, and pilot workshops. The programs are based on the Latin community's natural way of learning and caring. The workshop is intended to be given in Spanish and the guide is a detailed description of how to implement and follow up the workshop. This is a unique resource from a well-established center and provides a blueprint for training school and community caregivers who have the potential to prevent suicide in Latina youth.

Walter, H., Vaughan, R., Armstrong, B., Krakoff, R., Tiezzi L., & McCarthy, J. (1995). School-based health care for urban minority junior high school students. *Archives of Pediatric Medicine, 149,* 1221–1225.

Adolescents, in general, and urban, minority adolescents, in particular, have high rates of physical and mental health problems and underutilize healthcare. School-based and school-linked programs are one approach to addressing these problems, although there has been little evaluation of these programs. This manuscript describes the use of four school-based health clinics by students in four junior high schools, serving predominantly Hispanic students (from Caribbean, immigrant families) in an economically disadvantaged and medically underserved district in New York. Sixty four percent ($n = 3723$) of the students used the clinic with parental consent, averaging 3.3 visits. The students were predominantly Hispanic (87 percent) and fairly evenly divided by gender and grade. The predominant presenting complaints (33 percent) were mental health problems, including depression and suicidal behavior, and 36 percent of the students were seen for mental health problems. Mental health services included diagnosis, psychosocial assessment, individual and group therapy, parent counseling and referral. Feasibility, acceptability, and effectiveness of these clinics are discussed. The authors stress the need to link the effectiveness of these clinics with decreased involvement in risky behaviors and positive impact on morbidity and mortality. This article makes a unique contribution because the majority of previous publications on school-based programs described those targeted toward African-American adolescents; however, the authors do not include any discussion of culturally-specific issues.

Part X

Drugs, Devices, and Therapeutic Interventions

Chapter 11

Pain Management in Women

Christine Miaskowski

Pain is a universal human experience that usually serves as a warning signal about some type of tissue injury. The phenomenon has several dimensions that must be evaluated in order to understand the human experience of pain. Ahles and colleagues (Ahles, Blanchard, & Ruckdeschel, 1983), as well as McGuire (1992) have described a multidimensional model of pain that includes a physiological dimension (e.g., the cause of the pain); a sensory dimension (e.g., location, intensity of the pain); an affective dimension (e.g., emotional responses to pain); a behavioral dimension (e.g., pain behaviors, ways of communicating about pain); a cognitive dimension (e.g., meaning of the pain); and a sociocultural dimension (e.g., ethnic differences, gender differences, family perspectives).

Until recently, little attention has been given to evaluating whether gender influences the human pain experience. Only a limited number of studies have been done to determine whether men and women experience pain differently or whether different pain management strategies are more efficacious depending on gender. This review describes the findings from research studies that evaluated gender differences in pain perception and analgesic responsiveness and discusses the implications of the study findings for education, practice, research, and health policy.

REVIEW OF EXISTING RESEARCH

Many of the studies that evaluated gender differences in responses to painful stimuli were conducted in an experimental laboratory setting. The majority of these studies attempted to determine if men and women have different pain thresholds and levels of pain tolerance. Pain threshold is defined as the minimum amount of stimulation that reliably evokes a report of pain in an individual. Pain tolerance is defined as the time that a continuous stimulus is endured by an individual or the maximally tolerated stimulus intensity that a person can endure. In an excellent article, Fillingim and Maixner (1995) present a careful analysis of the experimental laboratory studies using a variety of painful procedures including electrical and thermal stimulation, mechanical and pressure pain, cold pressor pain, and ischemic pain that have evaluated gender differences in responses to painful stimuli. In most of these studies, females exhibit lower pain thresholds and show less tolerance to most types of induced pain. Findings from the experimental pain studies are often interpreted to suggest that women are more sensitive to painful stimuli than men.

Why do men and women differ in their responses to painful stimuli? At least two explanations for the gender differences have been proposed. One physiological factor is the hormonal status of the individual. Fillingim and Maixner (1995) point out that the menstrual cycle is a factor related to pain perception. However, the pattern of the responses differs considerably across the studies done to date. Some studies have reported that women have greater pain sensitivity during the premenstrual phase, others at ovulation, some following menses, while other studies have reported no changes in pain sensitivity during the menstrual cycle. No definitive conclusions can be drawn about the effect of the menstrual cycle on women's pain sensitivity.

An additional psychosocial factor that has been proposed to explain the gender differences in pain threshold and tolerance is the gender of the person performing the experiments. Levine and De Simone (1991) found that men reported less pain in front of a female experimenter than a male experimenter. However, experimenter gender did not influence the responses of the female participants.

Most experimental pain studies have focused on an evaluation of the sensory dimension of the human pain experience. Attention has not been given to how the other dimensions [e.g., the meaning of the pain (cognitive dimension), the individual's level of anxiety (affective dimension)] interrelate with a person's gender to influence an individual's response to a painful stimulus. Women may be more sensitive to painful stimuli evoked in a laboratory setting. However, until additional factors that could contribute to the processing and perception of pain are evaluated, definitive conclusions about gender differences in pain responses cannot be drawn from the existing studies.

While experimental pain studies help elucidate some of the basic physiological principles that underlie gender differences in responses to painful stimuli, perhaps more relevant areas for discussion and investigation are the gender differences observed in a variety of clinically painful conditions, such as women's use of and response to analgesic drugs. The remainder of this review will focus on the research related to gender differences in clinical pain problems and the responses of women to analgesic medications.

Based on a series of epidemiological studies, several pain syndromes appear to have a specific gender distribution (Donohoe, 1996), including migraine headaches (F, 3:1); cluster headache (M, 8:1); trigeminal neuralgia (F, 2:1); rheumatoid arthritis (F, 3:1); and carpal tunnel syndrome (F, 2:1).

Data from three epidemiological studies suggest that women, in the general population, report a higher rate of abdominal pain (Adelman, Revicki, Magaziner, & Hebel, 1995), migraine headaches (Honkasalo, Kaprio, Heikkila, Sillanpaa, & Koskenvuo, 1993), and a variety of chronic pain problems (Andersson, Ejlertsson, Leden, & Rosenberg, 1993). In addition, the findings from a large clinical study that evaluated pain intensity measures in men and women following dental surgery for third molar extractions (Faucett, Gordon, & Levine, 1994), suggest that women report higher pain intensity scores than men.

Again, data from clinical studies suggest that women are more sensitive to painful stimuli and report pain problems more frequently than men. However, in order to understand and accurately interpret the data from the epidemiological and clinical studies, it is important to note that several reports indicate that women tend to report more symptoms than men and to seek healthcare more frequently than men. This trend appears to be consistent for pain problems as well as other health problems. Therefore, health professionals must evaluate whether there is increased prevalence of pain problems in females or whether there are gender differences in the reporting of a specific pain problem. In addition, data are needed on what factors influence men and women to report symptoms and seek an evaluation from a healthcare professional.

While data from experimental and clinical studies suggest that women have an increased sensitivity to painful stimuli, anecdotal reports and data from one qualitative study (Bendelow, 1993) suggest that both males and females believe that women have a better ability to cope with pain than men. Bendelow (1993) in his critique of the experimental pain studies points out that most of these studies were done with undergraduate student volunteers and little consideration was given to evaluating factors such as age, ethnicity, or socioeconomic status. In his study, participants were asked whether they thought there were any differences in the ability of men and women to cope with pain. Both males and females believed that women were better able to cope with pain than men. Bendelow raises numerous interesting points that need to be considered when trying to interpret the influence of gender on pain perception.

For example, a recurrent theme in the interview data is that both men and women express the view that the combination of female biology and the reproductive role serve to equip women with a "natural" capacity to endure pain, both physically and emotionally. In essence, both men and women believed that women were better able to cope with pain because they were somehow equipped by nature to cope with the pain of childbirth. In addition, participants expressed the view that childhood socialization actively discouraged emotional expression in boys and adult males. Both of these stereotyped perspectives influence how men and women perceive a painful condition as well as when and how they report a painful condition to a healthcare provider.

One important consideration in the gender biology of pain is whether gender differences in pain perceptions and responses affect the clinical management of pain. In other words, do healthcare professionals react to patients' self-reports of pain and provide analgesics based on these self-reports and responses to analgesics or do stereotypes and preconceived notions about gender roles and pain behaviors influence clinical practice?

Calderone (1990) evaluated the frequency with which pain and sedative medication was administered to male and female patients who were recovering from coronary artery bypass grafting. Male patients were administered pain medication significantly more frequently than female patients and female patients were administered sedative medication significantly more frequently than male patients. Numerous questions are raised by these findings. Additional clinical studies are needed to determine if women display different pain behaviors than men and whether male and female healthcare providers react differently to pain behaviors in female and male patients. In addition, since self-report of pain intensity is the "gold standard" assessment parameter, additional research is warranted to determine if gender differences exist in pain intensity ratings in males and females who undergo similar surgical procedures.

Perhaps an even more important question, from a clinical practice perspective, is whether the effectiveness of analgesic drugs differs in men and women. Only two studies have been published to date that evaluated for gender differences in responses to analgesic medications (Gear, Gordon, Heller, Paul, Miaskowski, & Levine, 1996; Gordon, Gear, Heller, Paul, Miaskowski, & Levine, 1995). In these studies, the analgesic effects of morphine and pentazocine were evaluated in patients who were experiencing moderate to severe pain following oral surgery for third molar (i.e., wisdom teeth) extractions. Morphine and pentazocine are classified as opioid analgesics. However, these two analgesics exert their effects through actions at two different opioid receptors. Morphine exerts its analgesic effect by activating mu-opioid receptors. Pentazocine produces analgesia by activating a different group of receptors, namely, kappa-opioid receptors.

In the first study (Gordon et al., 1995), no gender differences were found in the analgesic efficacy of morphine; however, pentazocine was found to produce significantly better analgesia in females as compared to males. In a second study (Gear et al., 1996), the same group of investigators confirmed their initial observations that pentazocine produced better analgesia in females as compared to males. In addition, the analgesic responses of females did not differ whether they were in the follicular or luteal phase of their menstrual cycle.

The findings from these two studies suggest that males and females respond differently to different types of opioid analgesics. The physiological basis for the differences in female responses to the kappa-opioid analgesic, pentazocine, is not known. It may be that a male-related hormone, such as testosterone, interacts negatively with the kappa-opioid analgesic, that a female-related hormone, such as progesterone or estrogen, might potentiate the action of the kappa-opioid analgesic, or that both interactions may occur. Additional studies are warranted to determine the optimal approaches to pain management for both males and females.

IMPLICATIONS FOR EDUCATION, PRACTICE, RESEARCH, AND HEALTH POLICY

One must conclude from the available evidence that the human experience of pain is undoubtedly influenced by gender. However, pain is an individual experience. This point must be emphasized repeatedly when healthcare professionals and consumers of healthcare are educated about pain management. Healthcare professionals need to rely on patients self-reports of pain intensity and adjust the doses of analgesic medications to achieve the best pain control with minimum side effects.

Findings from epidemiological studies suggest that certain pain problems are more common in women than in men. These trends need to be confirmed in large-scale epidemiological studies. Studies need to be conducted in different cultures where male and female roles and role socialization around pain management differ.

Additional research is warranted on gender differences in physiological, psychological, and behavioral responses to pain. Careful attention needs to be given to determining if gender differences exist in responses to different types of acute and chronic pain. Research studies are needed that utilize both qualitative and quantitative methods. Further research is needed to understand the interrelationships between how males and females cope with pain and their physiological, psychological, and behavioral responses to pain.

Perhaps the most intriguing area for future research is identifying the mechanisms underlying gender differences in responses to analgesic medications. Perhaps when we understand the gender biology governing analgesic responsiveness, we will be able to tailor pain treatments to gender.

REFERENCES

Adelman, A. M., Revicki, D. A., Magaziner, J., & Hebel, R. (1995). Abdominal pain in an HMO. *Family Medicine, 27,* 321–325.

Ahles, T. A., Blanchard, E. B., & Ruckdeschel, J. C. (1983). The multidimensional nature of cancer-related pain. *Pain, 17,* 277–288.

Andersson, H. I., Ejlertsson, G., Leden, I., & Rosenberg, C. (1993). Chronic pain in a geographically defined general population: Studies of differences in age, gender, social class, and pain localization. *The Clinical Journal of Pain, 9,* 174–182.

Bendelow, G. (1993). Pain perceptions, emotions and gender. *Sociology of Health & Illness, 15*(3), 273–294.

Calderone, K. L. (1990). The influence of gender on the frequency of pain and sedative medication administered to postoperative patients. *Sex Roles, 23*(11/12), 713–725.

Donohoe, C. D. (1996). Evaluation of the patient in pain. In S. D. Waldman & A. P. Winne (Eds.), *Interventional pain management* (pp. 73–84). Philadelphia: W.B. Saunders.

Faucett, J., Gordon, N., & Levine, J. D. (1994). Differences in postoperative pain severity among four ethnic groups. *Journal of Pain and Symptom Management, 9*(6), 383–389.

Fillingim, R. B., & Maixner, W. (1995). Gender differences in the responses to noxious stimuli. *Pain Forum, 4*(4), 209–221.

Gear, R. W., Gordon, N. C., Heller, P. H., Paul, S., Miaskowski, C., & Levine, J. D. (1996). Gender differences in analgesic response to the kappa-opioid pentazocine. *Neuroscience Letters, 205,* 207–209.

Gordon, N. C., Gear, R. W., Heller, P. H., Paul, S., Miaskowski, C., & Levine, J. D. (1995). Enhancement of morphine analgesia by the GABA-B agonist baclofen. *Neuroscience, 69*(2), 345–349.

Honkasalo, M. -L., Kaprio, J., Heikkila, K., Sillanpaa, M., & Koskenvuo, M. (1993). A population-based study of headache and migraine in 22,809 adults. *Headache, 33,* 403–412.

Levine, F. M., & De Simone, L. L. (1991). The effects of experimenter gender on pain report in male and female subjects. *Pain, 44,* 69–72.

McGuire, D. B. (1992). Comprehensive and multidimensional assessment and measurement of pain. *Journal of Pain and Symptom Management, 7,* 312–319.

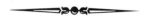

Adelman, A. M., Revicki, D. A., Magaziner, J., & Hebel, R. (1995). Abdominal pain in an HMO. *Family Medicine, 27,* 321–325.

The purpose of this study was to describe the prevalence of abdominal pain in a health maintenance organization (HMO) population. A total of 6,199 members of an HMO participated in a telephone interview about the occurrence of abdominal pain and related healthcare in the past year. Women in this study were more likely than men to have abdominal pain in the past year (30 percent versus 23 percent) and to have had more than three episodes of abdominal pain in the past year (22 percent versus 14 percent). In addition, among those individuals who reported abdominal pain, women were more likely than men to have seen a physician for abdominal pain in the past year (41 percent versus 33 percent). Women who reported that their abdominal pain was related to their menses were excluded from the data analysis.

One of the major limitations of this study is that the data were obtained from participants' recall of abdominal pain over the past 12 months. The higher prevalence of abdominal pain in women may be explained by women having a better recall of their health status than men. In addition, the authors point out that more research is needed to evaluate for gender differences in the severity, frequency, duration, and extent of interference with daily activities that are associated with abdominal pain complaints.

Andersson, H. I., Ejlertsson, G., Leden, I., & Rosenberg, C. (1993). Chronic pain in a geographically defined general population: Studies of differences in age, gender, social class, and pain localization. *The Clinical Journal of Pain, 9,* 174–182.

This large scale epidemiological study of 1,806 individuals who were randomly selected from two Swedish primary healthcare districts sought to establish basic epidemiological data on the extent of chronic pain (i.e., pain of greater than 3 months duration) in a general population. The survey was conducted by means of a mailed questionnaire that obtained information on pain symptoms including location, intensity, and duration of the pain, and the impact of the pain on the person's functional capacity. No differences were found in the overall prevalence of chronic pain in women (55.5 percent) and men (54.9 percent). However, some interesting gender differences were found in the location of the pain problems and the severity of the pain. Women reported pain in multiple locations more often than men. The mean number of pain sites among those reporting chronic pain was 2.75 for women, compared with 2.28 for men. In addition, women reported higher prevalence rates for chronic pain in the neck, shoulder, forearm, hip, and hand. The maximum pain intensity was reported by more women (23.6 percent) than men (16 percent). Women over 65 years of age reported pain more often than men of the same age. The findings that women report more severe pain and multiple pain complaints is consistent with previous studies. However, the lack of gender differences in the overall prevalence of pain problems conflicts with findings from previous studies. The authors provide no explanation for these differences.

This study evaluated chronic pain problems in a general population rather than evaluating pain prevalence rates among individuals who have sought medical treatment for a painful condition. Additional epidemiological research, in the general population, is warranted to better define the scope and the magnitude of chronic pain problems among the general population of men and women.

Bendelow, G. (1993). Pain perceptions, emotions and gender. *Sociology of Health & Illness, 15*(3), 273–294.

This research is one of the few qualitative evaluations of the effects of gender on pain perception. The study explored the relationships between perceptions of pain and various social characteristics of the individual, with a special focus on the influence of gender on the perception of pain. An emphasis was placed on trying to understand the meaning of the "lay" understanding of the phenomenon of pain. The study was conducted in two phases. In phase I, participants were asked to complete a questionnaire that was designed to examine their beliefs about health, illness, and pain and discover themes that would be examined in more depth through interviews with a subsample of the participants. A total of 107 men and women completed the questionnaire. In phase II, a total of 11 men and 11 women were interviewed in more detail.

One of the major findings from the questionnaire data was that significantly more women than men thought that anxiety, fear, and depression affected their perception of pain. In fact, twice as many men as women did *not* complete the items on the questionnaire that evaluated the impact of emotions on the individual's perception of pain. This finding suggests that men may dwell more on the physiological dimension of the pain experience and tend to ignore the psychological dimension of the pain experience.

An additional finding from this study is that 66 percent of the females and 33 percent of the males believed that women were better able to cope with pain than men. As one woman explained, "Women are made to suffer pain because we have periods and childbirth. Whatever the social climate, women end up child-rearing therefore they don't have the 'privilege' of giving in to pain and sickness" (p. 286). This theme requires additional investigation to determine exactly what is meant. Does this mean that women require less analgesics? Does it mean they tolerate higher levels of pain before they complain or seek healthcare? How do the findings from this study fit with the data that suggest that women report more painful symptoms than men? All of these questions need to be explored with male and female participants drawn from the general population.

Another finding that may contribute to the gender differences in pain perception is the way children are socialized to think of pain. Boys are actively discouraged from expressing emotions and adult males reported that they felt an obligation to display stoicism. The role of socialization around pain may affect how men and women behave when they are in pain, particularly around male as compared to female healthcare providers.

The results of this study suggest that we cannot rely simply on epidemiological techniques or psychophysiological measures to evaluate for gender differences in response to painful stimuli. Various aspects of the multidimensional model of pain need to be evaluated before definitive conclusions can be made about the gender biology of pain.

Calderone, K. L. (1990). The influence of gender on the frequency of pain and sedative medication administered to postoperative patients. *Sex Roles, 23*(11/12), 713–725.

The author of this paper hypothesized that women are perceived as being more emotionally labile than men and therefore are more apt to exaggerate complaints of pain than men. Therefore, women may be taken less seriously and receive less postoperative pain medication than men and may, in fact, receive more sedative medication to inhibit their expressive behavior. The purpose of the study was to examine whether the frequency of pain and sedative medications administered to postoperative coronary artery bypass patients differs according to patient gender.

The medical records of 30 male and 30 female patients were reviewed. Male and female patients were matched on age, number of coronary artery grafts, and the locations of the graft donor sites. The frequency of pain and sedative medication administered to these patients from 12 hours postop to 72 hours postop were evaluated. The results revealed that male patients were administered pain medication significantly more frequently than female patients and that the female patients were administered sedative medication significantly more frequently than male patients.

While the findings from this study are compelling, several factors need to be considered when evaluating the study findings. An evaluation of the frequency of pain medication administrations is not sufficient to make decisions about the adequacy of the postoperative pain management. Health providers need to evaluate self-reports of pain intensity and assess the efficacy of the prescribed analgesics. This study could have been strengthened by evaluating male and female patients self-reports of pain intensity and their responses, over time to various doses of postoperative pain medication. In addition, a qualitative evaluation of the nurses' perceptions of the pain experience of male and female patients is needed to elucidate some of the complex issues surrounding the expression of pain behaviors and healthcare professionals responses to male and female populations.

Faucett, J., Gordon, N., & Levine, J. D. (1994). Differences in postoperative pain severity among four ethnic groups. *Journal of Pain and Symptom Management, 9*(6), 383–389.

A variety of sociocultural factors (e.g., gender, ethnicity) may influence an individual's perception of pain. Very few studies have attempted to evaluate the influence of gender or ethnicity on patient's self-reports of pain intensity. However, numerous stereotypes exist regarding the responses of different ethnic groups to pain. This study represents a large-scale clinical investigation of young adults reports of pain intensity following third molar (i.e., wisdom teeth) extractions. Data were obtained from 543 patients who underwent third molar extractions using a standard operative procedure by the same surgeon. The results of this study demonstrate that the women reported significantly higher pain intensity scores (mean = 44.33) than men (mean = 34.55 on a 0 to 100 mm visual analogue scale) regardless of ethnic group. These findings are similar to those observed in studies using experimental painful stimuli. However, this study did not evaluate gender differences based on the women's phase in the menstrual cycle. In addition, other variables that may have influenced the participant's pain ratings (e.g., level of anxiety, extent of preoperative preparation) were not evaluated.

Fillingim, R. B., & Maixner, W. (1995). Gender differences in the responses to noxious stimuli. *Pain Forum, 4*(4), 209–221.

This article provides an excellent review of the studies done in an experimental laboratory setting, to determine if there are gender differences in responses to a variety of painful stimuli. Based on the experimental evidence, the authors conclude that females exhibit greater sensitivity to painful stimuli than males. The authors propose a theoretical model that includes several physiological and psychological factors that may be involved in modulating the gender differences observed in experimental pain studies. The model can be used and further tested to determine the extent to which it explains gender differences in pain responses.

Definitive conclusions about gender differences in responses to painful stimuli cannot be made until attention is paid to the multiple dimensions of the pain experience and evaluations are done for both acute and chronic pain problems. Factors that need to be evaluated include the gender of the experimenter, the women's phase in the menstrual cycle, the affective state of the individual, and the physiological responses of a given gender to painful stimuli (e.g., changes in heart rate and blood pressure). Laboratory and clinical research is needed to identify the mechanisms and physiological consequences of the gender differences in response to pain.

Gear, R. W., Gordon, N. C., Heller, P. H., Paul, S., Miaskowski, C., & Levine, J. D. (1996). Gender differences in analgesic response to the kappa-opioid pentazocine. *Neuroscience Letters, 205,* 207–209.

The purpose of this study was to confirm findings from a previous study (see Gordon et al., 1995) that pentazocine produces greater analgesia in females than in males and to determine if a woman's phase in the menstrual cycle significantly effects the level of analgesia produced in females. The study utilized a model of postoperative dental pain (i.e., patients who underwent oral surgery for third molar extractions). Gender differences in analgesic responses to pentazocine were evaluated using a repeated measure, analysis of variance. In a separate analysis, in order to test for differences in the analgesic effectiveness of pentazocine during different phases of the menstrual cycle, females were subdivided into two groups according to the number of days after the onset of menses. The analgesic responses of the females undergoing surgery within ten days of the onset of menses were compared to those undergoing surgery more than ten days after the onset of menses. The results of the study indicate that the analgesic efficacy of pentazocine was greater in females as compared to males, but that females did not differ in their analgesic responses according to the phase of the menstrual cycle.

Gordon, N. C., Gear, R. W., Heller, P. H., Paul, S., Miaskowski, C., & Levine, J. D. (1995). Enhancement of morphine analgesia by the GABA-B agonist baclofen. *Neuroscience, 69*(2), 345–349.

In this study, using a model of postoperative dental pain (i.e., patients who underwent oral surgery for third molar extractions), gender differences in the amount of analgesia produced by morphine and pentazocine were evaluated. The results of the study demonstrated that morphine (which produces its analgesic effect at the mu-opioid receptor) was equally effective in males and females. However, pentazocine (which produces its analgesic effect at the kappa-opioid receptor) produces better analgesic effects in females as compared to males. The mechanisms underlying these gender differences in analgesic responses between the two different opioid agonists remain unclear.

Honkasalo, M. -L., Kaprio, J., Heikkila, K., Sillanpaa, M., & Koskenvuo, M. (1993). A population-based study of headache and migraine in 22,809 adults. *Headache, 33,* 403–412.

The purpose of this paper was to describe the distribution, prevalence, and frequency of headaches with and without migrainous features, in a sample of Finnish adults. Participants were asked to complete a questionnaire about headache frequency and the nature of the headache attacks. Based on pre-established criteria, participants were classified as having headaches without migrainous features or headaches with migrainous features.

In this study, migraine headaches were reported four times more often by women than by men. However, the frequency of headache occurrences over a twelve-month period did not differ between the two groups. In this study, gender differences in the intensity of the migraine headaches or concomitant symptoms were not evaluated. Another interesting finding from this study that corroborates the findings from previous studies is the association of migraine headaches with menstrual cycle. According to the few studies that have been carried out with children, migraine prevalence appears to be similar between the two genders or somewhat higher in boys as compared to girls. After the onset of puberty, the gender ratio changes. In the present study, the proportion of women with migraine who suffered from headaches once a month was high, showing a clear decrease after menopause.

A lower percentage of women reported nonmigrainous headaches. However, the frequency of nonmigrainous headaches was higher in women (i.e., almost twice as often) as compared to men. Again the severity of the headaches and the impact of the headaches on the ability of women and men to function were not evaluated.

Part XI

Economics, Ethics, Policy, Legislation

Chapter 12

Battered Women and Their Children

Jacquelyn Campbell
Barbara Parker

This chapter builds on our two prior reviews of nursing research on battered women and their children (Campbell & Parker, 1992; Campbell & Parker, in press) to make policy recommendations in the field. It is important to make research-based health policy recommendations regarding intimate partner (domestic) violence. The battering of female partners and the resultant health effects on women and their children is clearly an area where there is sufficient nursing research upon which to base these policy recommendations.

Our two prior reviews used qualitative and quantitative data from published nursing research studies. We defined a nursing research study as one with at least one nurse author and/or published in a nursing journal and/or using a nursing theory and/or testing a nursing intervention identified from a Medline search through 1995. Additional articles were identified by hand searching the four primary adult violence specific journals in the field (*Journal of Family Violence, Journal of Interpersonal Violence, Violence and Victims, Violence Against Women*) and making oral solicitations at Nursing Network on Violence Against Women International (NNVAWI) meetings.

These reviews are widely available. The complete critical review upon which this chapter is based were published in those volumes. In addition, there are three other partial reviews of nursing research on battering (Campbell, 1995; Campbell, Anderson, & Fulmer, 1993; Campbell, Harris, & Lee, 1995; Campbell & Parker, 1992).

This chapter begins with an overall summary of the findings from the two prior reviews plus a methodological evaluation of the state of the science in nursing research on intimate partner violence. We then describe battering of female partners as a clinical problem along with its physical and mental health consequences, offering definitions, as well as incidence and prevalence estimates. The last section presents a series of specific health policy recommendations along with the nursing (and other disciplines) studies upon which they are based. Suggestions are made for further research essential to more definitively address those policy issues. There are other policy recommendations that could have been made related to the field of domestic violence, but we chose to address those which have nursing research support or those that are critical to the healthcare system response to domestic violence. Finally, the policy recommendations are summarized along with a discussion of the role of nursing in policy formulations in the area of female partner abuse, and the need for policy-related nursing research.

REVIEW OF NURSING RESEARCH

Nursing research has made a substantial contribution to the body of knowledge on battered women and their children in general, especially in the area of abuse during pregnancy. Nursing's contribution has been primarily in the area of women and children's responses (physical, mental, and behavioral) to battering rather than causation (with the exception of the early identification of risk factors by Parker & Schumacher, 1977). The contribution of nursing was considered noteworthy because of its activist and/or feminist (woman-centered) assumptions and stance. To substantiate that conclusion, there was evidence of (a) close collaboration with shelters and advocates for abused women, (b) particular concern for the safety of women and their children in both interventions and research endeavors (e.g., Parker et al., 1990), (c) a general concern for the empowerment of women as part of the research process as well as in the use of research results, (d) inquiry into battered women and their children's strengths as well as problems, and (e) an assumption that the locus of responsibility for battering was both the individual perpetrator and our societal structures and attitudes that facilitate or fail to sufficiently sanction or prevent the battering of female partners (Campbell & Parker, in press). For example, a group of nursing studies has documented the significant strengths of battered women, indications of normal processes of grieving and recovering, leaving battering relationships as a process, and cultural and social support influences on responses to battering (Campbell, 1989; Hoff, 1990; Landenburger, 1989; Ulrich, 1991).

ABUSE DURING PREGNANCY

The accumulation of nursing research in the area of battering during pregnancy has been particularly noteworthy and has made the most substantial contribution of any discipline to the knowledge base in that area. The early nursing studies of abuse during pregnancy importantly established that there were significant proportions of women abused during pregnancy (e.g., Helton, McFarlane, & Anderson, 1987). Nursing research has documented a higher prevalence of abuse during pregnancy (16 percent to 17 percent) than other studies probably because of the use of primarily face-to-face nurse conducted interviews using an appropriate screen (the Abuse Assessment Screen rather than research specific instruments), (McFarlane, Bullock, et al., 1989). Few risk factors for abuse during pregnancy were found other than abuse prior to pregnancy, but depression, anxiety, and substance abuse were identified as correlates (Campbell, Poland, Waller, & Ager, 1992; McFarlane & Parker, 1996). The more recent studies of abuse during pregnancy have investigated the dynamics of such abuse (Campbell, Oliver, & Bullock, 1993), relative prevalence amongst three major ethnic groups (McFarlane, Parker, Soeken, & Bullock, 1992), the prevalence of abuse during adolescent pregnancy (Parker, McFarlane, & Soeken, 1994) and the deleterious outcomes, including lower birthweight, of this form of violence against women (McFarlane, Parker, & Soeken, 1996; Parker et al., 1994).

OTHER HEALTHCARE SETTINGS AND PROBLEMS

Nursing research has generated significant knowledge about the health consequences of abuse in numerous health settings. Studies have documented significant prevalence of abused women in a variety of healthcare settings (emergency, primary care, prenatal) with a range of physical and mental healthcare problems correlated with the abuse (e.g., chronic pain, depression) and a general lack of identification by healthcare professionals (Campbell & Parker, 1991). Noteworthy physical health problems found across studies (both population based and clinical) are headaches, backaches, STD risk, and sleeping problems (Eby et al., in press; Ratner, 1993, 1995). Descriptive clinical studies have suggested important health-related effects, such as neurological problems, hypertension, and urinary tract infections (Campbell & Alford, 1989; Pliska et al., 1994; Rodriguez, 1993; Vavaro, 1992).

In the area of mental health consequences, findings from nursing research supported by other research include the link between abuse during pregnancy and substance abuse (Campbell et al., 1992; McFarlane et al., 1996). This relationship was supported and further explicated in samples of nonpregnant women (Eby, Campbell, Sullivan, & Davidson, 1995; Ratner, 1993). Depression has also been substantiated as a significant mental health problem of battered women (Campbell, Kub, Belknap, & Templin, 1996). Battered women, especially those sexually abused, were also found to have low self-esteem (e.g., Campbell, 1989a, 1989b; Mahon, 1981; Trimpey, 1989).

Marital rape and homicide risk are two other areas that are addressed in nursing investigations. Forced sex in battering relationships was documented as having important physical and mental health ramifications, including low self-esteem and unintended pregnancy (Campbell et al., 1995; Weingourt, 1990). The issue of homicide of battered women as a preventable problem was first published in the healthcare literature by Campbell (1981) who has continued to work to develop identifiable risk factors that can be assessed in the healthcare system (Campbell, 1995).

There has also been inquiry into cultural effects on women's responses to battering (e.g., Torres, 1987, 1991), including an examination of the psychometric properties of an instrument to measure severity and frequency of wife abuse (the ISA, now PASP, PASNP) in an African-American population (Campbell et al., 1995).

METHODOLOGICAL ISSUES

In spite of these strengths, there were also serious shortcomings in some nursing studies in terms of relatively small sample sizes and unsophisticated methodologies. Another serious gap is that there are no published studies actually testing nursing interventions; however, there are almost no valid evaluation studies from social service (including shelter and advocacy), criminal justice or the healthcare system testing interventions from any discipline (NRC, in press). Landenburger (1989) used grounded theory to develop a theory of entrapment and recovery from an abusive relationship that was later extended as a basis for clinical nursing intervention that is yet to be tested (Campbell, Ulrich, Campbell, Torres, Sheridan, Landenburger, & Humphreys, 1993; Landenburger, 1993). Vavaro (1995) has also begun to explore another nursing intervention based on self-efficacy theory. The most exciting development is that a three-year prospective study testing an intervention for abused pregnant women was completed in 1996, the results of which will soon be available (Parker, McFarlane, Reel, Silva, & Soeken).

The only published experimental intervention study in the nursing literature is a test of a training program for emergency room nurses that showed a significant increase in appropriate identification and documentation of battered women in the experimental group (Tilden & Shepard, 1987). This remains the only experimental study from any discipline showing the efficacy of training in any setting and is supported by other discipline pre- and postintervention (quasi-experimental) studies (e.g., McLeer & Anwar, 1989).

Nursing research on the children of battered women is relatively sparse (as is true in other fields) but includes a documentation of these youngsters having more health problems than other children (Kerouac, Taggart, Lescop, & Fortin, 1986; Westra & Martin, 1981), and beginning investigations of how both the mothers and the children try to take care of each other (Humphreys, 1995).

FUTURE DIRECTIONS

Another problem in the direction of nursing research to date has been the paucity of tests or application of nursing (or other) theories (with exceptions of Campbell, 1989; Humphreys, 1995), and a lack of studies that systematically document the kinds of health problems battered women have compared to other women and how and if battering compromises appropriate use of healthcare services. However, many of the study findings were corroborated by findings from other disciplines. Battered women's perception that professionals provide less than adequate care in healthcare settings has been documented by researchers in other disciplines (e.g., Kurz, 1989) and supported by attitude studies showing paternalistic and somewhat blaming attitudes of nurses, although less than physicians (King & Ryan, 1989; Rose & Saunders, 1986; Shipley & Sylvester, 1986). These studies of nursing attitudes and practices about abuse taken as a whole suggest that nurses are underutilized as a resource for battered women and although perceived as more helpful than not, too often use a medical rather than empowerment model approach to intervention. Additionally, training is needed to improve their knowledge, attitudes, and behavior regarding battered women. One study (Attala, Oetker, & McSweeney, 1995) indicates that the prevalence and effects of abuse among nursing students in one midwestern city are similar to the prevalence among American women overall, suggesting the need for nursing faculty to be alert for signs of abuse among students.

In order to further advance the body of nursing knowledge about battered women and their children, the strengths of nursing research should be continued and advanced. These include attention to culture and ethnicity, the use of both qualitative and quantitative data, a strong clinical grounding, and advocacy positions. Longitudinal, comparison group, and large sample studies are needed, especially those that further develop and test midrange nursing theory and/or further document and investigate health consequences of abuse for both mothers and children and/or build on existing nursing research. Most critical is the need for the testing of nursing interventions with battered women and their children, interventions that draw on research findings and formulated theory to demonstrate the value of nursing care in making the healthcare system both a form of sanctuary and a secondary as well as tertiary prevention site in the field of abuse.

POLICY RECOMMENDATIONS BASED ON NURSING RESEARCH

The first group of recommendations relate to when and how screening for intimate partner violence should occur in healthcare settings.

Recommendation #1
Routine Universal Screening of Women

All women coming to a healthcare setting for any reason should be routinely screened for abuse. Findings from both abuse during pregnancy studies and other health-related studies suggest that universal screening of all women (including adolescents) for intimate partner abuse at *each* healthcare system encounter needs to become routine nursing practice. Routine assessment is necessary for the following reasons: (a) the presence or absence of abuse changes over time (e.g., changes in pregnancy status, lifespan changes) (Campbell et al., 1994; Gielen, O'Campo, Faden, Kass, & Xue, 1994; McFarlane et al., 1992), (b) battered women experience a variety of physical and mental health problems (most often *without* injury) (Bekkemeier et al., in press; Goldberg & Tomlanovich, 1985; Ratner, 1993), and (c) there are no personal or demographic characteristics (risk factors) that can identify women more likely to be abused (Hotaling & Sugarman, 1990; Page-Adams & Dersch, in press) or likely to continue in battering relationships (Campbell et al., 1994).

As healthcare delivery moves into primary care settings, there is a concomitant need for universal screening (at least for those under 60) and interventions for abuse of women in those settings. Research has demonstrated in some studies (Druckman et al., 1992; McCauley et al., 1995) and suggested in others (e.g., Kerouac et al., 1986; Rodriguez, 1989) links between abuse and other primary care level problems such as chronic irritable bowel syndrome, headaches, and hypertension.

In emergency department settings, many hospital protocols direct the nurse to screen all women (or patients) presenting with trauma for domestic violence. Yet because of the nursing research (replicated in other studies) that shows abused women more often coming to the emergency department (ED) with other kinds of complaints (noticeably chronic pain), ED screening should also be performed with all women presenting with *any* problem (Goldberg & Tomlanovich, 1985; Pliska et al., 1994).

Another group of policy recommendations are related to specific nursing clinical settings or particular kinds of abuse. Those related to abuse during pregnancy and maternal child health settings are described next.

Recommendation #2
The Abuse Assessment Screen (AAS)
Should Be Used for Screening for
Domestic Violence in Healthcare Settings

Since pregnancy is one time that women are routinely interacting with the healthcare system, screening is especially relevant. Suggested protocols including an assessment screen (English and Spanish version) are published in a module published by the March of Dimes and available from local March of Dimes affiliates (McFarlane & Parker, 1995). This publication includes the Abuse Assessment Screen (AAS), developed by the Nursing Research Consortium on Violence and Abuse. The test retest reliability of the AAS has been measured at 83 percent to 100 percent (Soeken, Parker, McFarlane, & Lominak, 1996). Significant criterion related validity ($p < .001$) has been established for the AAS with scores compared to scores from the Conflict Tactics Scale, Index of Spouse Abuse and the Danger Assessment (Soeken et al., 1996). The AAS does not have a copyright and publications note that readers are encouraged to copy and use the instrument.

Because of the frequency of sexual assault in battering relationships, there are a series of recommendations that take into account the interface between nursing and women's sexuality in a variety of settings.

Recommendation #3
All Women Coming to Family Planning Centers
(e.g., Planned Parenthood) Should Be
Routinely Screened for Intimate Partner
Violence with Interventions Provided for
Women Reporting Abuse

Nursing as well as other research indicates that 40 percent to 45 percent of physically abused women are also being forced into sex with resulting physical (e.g., STDs, vaginal and anal tearing) and emotional (low self-esteem) consequences specific to the sexual assault (Campbell, 1989; Campbell & Alford, 1989; Eby et al., 1995; Weingourt, 1989, 1992). There is also indication from nursing research of unintended pregnancy resulting from this form of abuse (Campbell, Pugh, Campbell, & Visscher, 1995), although more research is necessary in this area. Bullock and McFarlane and their colleagues (1989) also demonstrated that women could be successfully screened for abuse in Planned Parenthood settings. Further, it was indicated that face-to-face interviews were more successful than questions (the AAS) in a written history form, although both methods yielded significant disclosure of abuse. Weingourt (1990) has also described nursing interventions in mental health settings for women sexually abused by an intimate partner, although these interventions have not been tested. In family planning settings, a brief nursing intervention of thorough gynecological assessment and treatment for identified problems, counseling about increased STD and HIV/AIDS risk, referral to domestic violence specific services (criminal justice, shelter) as desired, safety planning, and follow-up appointments would be appropriate on site because the majority of these women may not be ready or able (in terms of transportation or other obstacles) to seek services elsewhere.

Recommendation #4
All HIV/AIDS Prevention Programs and STD Interventions Programs Should Include Careful Assessment and Interventions for Intimate Partner Abuse

According to the nursing research findings (especially Campbell & Alford, 1989; Eby et al., 1995; Ratner, 1993) described in the prior recommendation plus evidence from a public health study (Gielen et al., 1994), it is clear that battered women, especially those who are also sexually abused, are at increased risk for HIV/AIDS and other STDs. There are complex interactions related to this issue that need to be investigated further. There are some data-based indications that abusive men may be particularly reluctant to use condoms and/or that their sexual partners would be afraid to insist on condom use (Campbell et al., 1995; Eby et al., 1995). Other abusers, already prone to jealousy, may interpret a request for safe sex practices as meaning that the woman has been sexually promiscuous. In actuality, the reverse is more likely to be accurate. To place the onus of responsibility on women for men to use a condom is naive and demonstrates a lack of understanding of the sexually coercive experiences of many women.

Recommendation #5
Nursing Advocacy Is Needed to Urge Increased Resources Directed toward the Development of Vaginal HIV Virus Killing Agents

The basic development of these agents is already completed, but their progress to clinical trials has been relatively slow. NIH should be urged to complete clinical trials on these agents if pharmaceutical companies are not progressing as swiftly as possible. Because of violence and sexual autonomy issues, this could be the most significant advance in the prevention of the spread of HIV/AIDS to women, short of a vaccine.

Recommendation #6
Research Related to Domestic Violence Needs to Have Regard for Women's Safety and to Consider the Possibility of Violent Partner Repercussions

A recent investigation of HIV/AIDS in Africa determined that a third of the women who had tested positive were beaten by their husbands after they informed them of the test results, according to the researchers' directions. The possibility of domestic violence in situations involving research on women's health issues needs to be taken into account in Institutional Review Board deliberations.

Nursing researchers (Parker et al., 1990) have collaborated to publish a protocol of safety for domestic violence research that should be used as a starting point in designing such studies.

Recommendation #7
Nursing Assessment of Battered Women Should Include a Lethality Assessment

There is ample nursing and other discipline research to indicate that women are most at risk for homicide from an intimate partner and that her abuse is the major identifiable precursor of the homicide (e.g., Campbell, 1992, 1995). There is some indication (e.g., Wilson & Daly, 1993) that women are most at risk for homicide when they leave the battering relationship although this has not been definitively established. Although there are no domestic homicide risk factor lists with actual evidence of predictive validity, there are several that have been developed and published with widespread support for some sort of lethality assessment being conducted. The Danger Assessment (DA) was specifically designed for nursing and other healthcare system administration in order to increase battered women's awareness of the potential for homicide and thereby enhance their self-care agency (Campbell, 1989). The DA has some construct validity support and has been used widely in many different kinds of health settings and can be obtained either from the author or in a number of nursing publications (Campbell, 1995; Campbell & Humphreys, 1993).

Recommendation #8
Treatment for Depression and Other Psychological Problems Needs to Include Assessment and Interventions for Domestic Violence

In the only population-based mental health nursing study on intimate partner violence, Ratner (1994) found that abused women were significantly more depressed than nonabused women, as well as having more physical symptoms of stress, more anxiety and insomnia, alcohol abuse, and exhibiting more social dysfunction than those not abused, with physical violence having a stronger effect than psychological abuse in all aspects. Also supporting the above and other nursing research findings of depression in battered women (e.g., Attala et al., 1995; Campbell, 1989; Campbell, Pliska et al., 1994; Campbell et al., 1992), Campbell and associates (Campbell, Kub, Belknap, & Templin, 1996) found 39 percent of a volunteer community sample of 164 battered women in the moderate to severe or severe depression categories on the Beck Depression Inventory, categories considered indicative of a psychiatric diagnosis of severe depression. Based on this research, interventions in the healthcare system for depression, eating disorders, and substance abuse need to include domestic violence assessment and interventions. Conversely, community domestic violence intervention programs (e.g., shelters) need to also include routine screening for depression, eating disorders, and substance abuse.

Recommendation #9
Programs Addressing Child Abuse
(e.g., Hospital-Based Multidisciplinary Child
Abuse Teams, Child Protective Services, and
Family Preservation Programs) as Well as
Inpatient Nursing Care for Abused Children
Should Include Domestic Violence
Assessment and Intervention

Research has indicated a strong overlap between wife abuse and child abuse, with as many as 77 percent of couples with severe wife abuse also abusing a child (Straus & Gelles, 1990). There is indication from two small qualitative nursing studies (Campbell, Oliver, & Bullock, 1993; Campbell, Pugh, et al., 1995) and a larger multinational study of child homicide (Daly & Wilson, 1990) that children are at increased risk when the abusive partner is not the biological father. Programs in whole or in part that are designed to prevent or address child abuse (e.g., Family Preservation Programs, Healthy Mothers, Healthy Babies, hospital multidisciplinary child abuse teams) all need to assess mothers of the children abused or at risk for abuse for wife abuse and intervene accordingly. Programs such as AWAKE at Children's Hospital of Boston have been designed to specifically address the needs of abused mothers of abused children. Although not yet rigorously evaluated, there is preliminary indication that this program is helpful not only in protecting the abused mothers, but in also protecting the children (NRC, in press). Pediatric nurses should also provide assessment and interventions for domestic violence for the mothers of hospitalized abused children in hospitals where programs such as AWAKE do not exist.

Recommendation #10
Interventions for Victims of Domestic Violence
Should Avoid All Forms of "Victim Blaming,"
Be Focused on Empowering the Woman
and Her Children, and Emphasize the
Long-Term Goal of Living Without Violence

Healthcare professionals must recognize that the desired outcome of interventions in violent relationships is ending the violence, not necessarily ending the relationship. Frequently, interventions imply that the desirable outcome is for the woman to leave the abuser. This unstated belief is not only patriarchal and patronizing in its assumptions, but it also serves to distance and alienate us from the women in need of our assistance. Instead, interventions need to be developed to empower women to make decisions that are in the best interest of themselves and their children.

In fact, research suggests that the majority of battered women do eventually leave the violent relationship (Campbell et al., 1994). However, it is a *process* of leaving that often involves leaving and returning several times. Interventions need to interpret this leaving and returning as a normal process of testing alternatives (Landenburger, 1989, 1993; Ulrich, 1991). Often when a woman leaves she is actually testing the reaction of her children, family and friends and her ability to live independently. Some women report that before they are able to leave they must first be able to visualize a life without the abuser.

Nurses need to realize that women frequently experience considerable abuse after they leave, ranging from mild forms of harassment to serious property destruction, stalking, and physical violence (Campbell et al., 1996; Campbell, Torres, Ulrich, Sheridan, & Landenburger, 1993). Sheridan (Campbell et al., 1993) has developed an instrument to measure this harassment that has the potential to contribute significantly to our knowledge about this less understood aspect of violent relationships. In a recent analysis of longitudinal data from a community (not clinical or shelter) sample of 57 women, Sebbio, Campbell, and Soeken (1996) found that after three years, a greater proportion of those who had left the abusive relationship (14 of 18 or 77.7 percent) were still being battered by the original partner than those who had stayed (16 of 25 or 64 percent)! This is not to argue that battered women *should* stay. However, nurses should be aware of the continued abuse that often occurs if women do leave and their need for continued protection as well as the possibility that abusive relationships can become nonviolent (although this is not the usual pattern).

Healthcare professionals must also recognize that abused women in healthcare settings are often not seeking intervention for the abuse per se and early in the relationship often do not define themselves as abused or battered (Campbell et al., 1993; Landenburger, 1993). They often wish to maintain the relationship, frequently out of concerns for children, financial problems, love for the spouse, pessimism that she will find a better relationship, or a sense that the partner has other problems that are causing the abuse (e.g., substance abuse, unemployment) that can perhaps be solved (Lubinski, Board, & Campbell, 1995; Ulrich, 1991). Minority cultural groups also express concern that criminal justice or relationship dissolution solutions for domestic violence are destructive to their communities and families. Thus, nursing and the healthcare system should be proactive in designing interventions that promote the transformation of relationships so that they are not only nonviolent but noncontrolling. Evaluations of such programs as Woman Kind (Hadley, Short, Lesin, & Zook, 1995) that provide domestic violence interventions in the healthcare system should be encouraged and new nursing interventions developed and tested.

Recommendation #11
New and Innovative Interventions Are Needed That Seek to Transform Controlling and Potentially Violent Relationships into Nonviolent and Supportive Ones

Nursing (Campbell et al., 1994) and other discipline research (Fagan & Browne, 1994; Feld & Straus, 1989) support that abusive relationships *can* become not only nonviolent but also noncontrolling and nonemotionally abusive. Public health principles would predict that identifying and intervening with battering relationships *early* would increase our chances of successful relationship transformation. Such interventions must begin with confronting batterers with their potentially violent and controlling behaviors and making sure they take responsibility for their actions. However, such interventions would go beyond most current batterer treatment to address building healthy, loving and supportive relationships as well.

Recommendation #12
Future Research and Intervention Studies Should Incorporate the Special Needs of Children and Be Sensitive to the Issues of Abused Women as Mothers

Several nursing studies have documented the consistent concerns that abused women have regarding their children and the influence of these fears in the woman's decision to stay with or leave her abusive partner (Henderson, 1990; Humphreys, 1991, in press; Lubinski, Campbell, & Board, 1995; Ulrich, 1991). Nurses as well as other healthcare professionals must be aware of these issues and serve as advocates when abused women are threatened with prosecution for child endangerment or neglect. Additionally, public health nurses need to be aware of the possibility of such charges as they provide health teaching and advice to families with the potential for violence.

Recommendation #13
The Nursing Profession Should Become an Integral Part of International Initiatives to Address Domestic Violence, including Human Rights Initiatives, Healthcare Enterprises, and Collaborative Research Projects

Domestic violence research on the international level has been very limited. Counts, Brown, and Campbell (1992) used primary ethnographic evidence collected from 14 different societies worldwide representing a range of geographic locations, industrialization, household arrangements, and degree of spousal violence to examine evidence supporting the primary theoretical stances about battering from Western social sciences. Although the feminist (or matriarchal) theoretical premises received considerable support, there were several aspects brought into question. The review suggested that all forms of violence against women could not be considered as aspects of the same phenomenon, and that status of women is an extremely complex, multifaceted phenomenon that may have a curvilinear rather than a direct (inverse) relationship with wife battering. The review also demonstrated the importance of societal influences on individual couples. This study differentiated *wife beating* (occasional, nonescalating, without serious or permanent injury, and seen as ordinary by most members of the culture, and occurring in almost all societies in the world) from *wife battering*, the continuing, usually escalating, potentially and actually injurious pattern of physical violence within a context of coercive control) most often described in Western social sciences and health research. Those factors that were found to discourage the escalation of wife beating to battering across societies included community level sanctions against battering and sanctuary for beaten wives enacted in culturally specific and appropriate forms. It is possible that some of these community-level strategies could be adapted as primary and secondary prevention measures in the United States.

More international nursing research is needed and could be conducted collaboratively through entities such as the International Council of Nursing. In Vienna in 1993, violence against women was first officially recognized as a human rights violation by the international community. International organizations such as the World Health Organization and the Pan American Health Organization are just beginning to conceptualize intimate partner violence as a health problem and strategize how to include domestic violence initiatives in international maternal child and mental health initiatives. Nursing is in a position to take leadership in such initiatives.

Recommendation #14
Nursing Education Programs at All Levels Must Include Content on Domestic Violence and Violence Against Women

Certification examinations must include questions regarding assessment and interventions for victims of domestic violence. Several initiatives are underway for all healthcare professionals to assure that content on domestic violence and violence against women is included in basic as well as advanced and continuing education. An encouraging trend is that most basic nursing textbooks now include a chapter on domestic violence, and specialty journals include current findings on their specific aspects of intimate partner violence. Additional educational recommendations are that, at a minimum, lectures on domestic violence should be incorporated in basic nursing courses. These would include: (a) content on the prevalence of domestic violence, assessment techniques and referral processes in women's health or obstetric courses, (b) content on the outcomes and psychological sequelae as well as appropriate communication and interpersonal approaches in psychiatric nursing courses, and (c) community prevention and intervention programs in community health programs. Shelters and community programs for domestic violence should also be encouraged as sites for clinical placement because they provide experiences in a broad diversity of clinical problems. In a similar manner, graduate education programs must incorporate specialty knowledge and encourage the development of some nurses to become experts in domestic violence so that they can be the designated specialist in their later clinical practice.

Recommendation #15
Research Conducted with Battered Women and Their Children Must Be Sensitive to Ethnic and Cultural Issues

Campbell and colleagues (Campbell, Campbell et al., 1994) reported an important nursing study determining the reliability and factor structure of the ISA with a sample of 504 African-American women. Campbell found three factors with the African-American sample compared with the original two reported by Hudson and McIntosh. The new factor identified with this sample reflected behaviors of an extremely controlling and isolating nature. Campbell interprets this phenomena by using the work of Oliver (1989) which indicates that "when black males engage in violence against black females, it is because they have defined the situation as one in which the female's actions constitute a threat to their manhood" (p. 265). This study further documented the importance of conducting and reporting separate instrument reliability and validity assessments for different ethnic groups and paying attention to ethnic group representation and analysis in both developing and choosing a measurement instrument.

In translating instruments to other languages, researchers need to recognize the inherent complexities, such as reverse translation procedures and standards. Differences in spoken and written dialect within the same language need to be recognized as well (e.g., Spanish language variations among speakers from different countries).

Nursing researchers were among the first to address issues of ethnic influences on battering (e.g., Torres, 1987), a field where the state of the science in relationship to culture is underdeveloped. There have been several clinical nursing articles addressing nursing care of battered women both taking culture into account (e.g., Campbell et al., 1993) and detailing nursing care (not yet tested) specific to various cultural and geographic groups (Bohn, 1993; Campbell, 1993; Fishwick, 1993; Rodriguez, 1993; Torres, 1993). In addition, McFarlane, Parker, & Soeken (1996) specifically examine the prevalence, frequency, and severity of abuse during pregnancy in three different cultural groups and found the former to be significantly lower among Hispanic women while the latter was lowest among African-American couples. Campbell and her colleagues (1994; in press) have investigated the influence of ethnicity (African-American vs. Anglo) on depression and subsequent violence in battered women and found no differences. Overall, these results indicate the importance of continuing to include ethnicity as a variable in nursing research on battering and to report similarities between ethnic groups as well as differences.

Culturally sensitive research also involves careful strategies for recruiting ethnic minority samples and interpreting results within a cultural context (Henderson, Sampselle, Mayes, & Oakley, 1992). Issues of race and ethnicity are sensitive in violence-related research, and it is extremely important to include class and/or income as well as ethnicity in analysis (Hawkins, 1992; Porter & Villarruel, 1993).

Recommendation #16
Nursing Should Take a Leadership Role in Discouraging Legislation on Mandatory Reporting by Healthcare Professionals with Mentally Competent Patients

Several states have adopted legislation that requires healthcare professionals to report suspicions of spouse abuse (mandated reporting). It should be noted that every state requires reports of injuries resulting from "lethal weapons" such as knives or guns, regardless of the relationship between the victim and offender. Proposed legislation regarding "mandated reporting" goes beyond these reports and regards spouse abuse in a similar manner to child or elder abuse.

Proponents of mandatory reporting believe it will increase assessment for abuse and provide more protection for women by placing the onus of responsibility for reporting on healthcare professionals. However, others are concerned that mandatory reporting will decrease the abused woman's disclosures of abuse or seeking of healthcare because of fears of retaliatory violence. In fact, there is anecdotal evidence that many batterers escalate their violence if their partner seeks help or attempts a separation (Hart, 1993).

For healthcare professionals, other issues arise. Some clinicians may believe that simply "reporting" is the only care required. Alternately, providers who believe that reporting will be detrimental to the patient may choose not to inquire about the causes of injury, thereby depriving the patient of education or referral information.

Additionally, programs providing services to victims of abuse are already overwhelmed with the numbers of women and children needing their services. Unless additional resources are funded, there is no guarantee that reports will be followed by a police investigation or the woman taken to safety. Abused women might then have a false sense of security or belief that she is about to be rescued and not seek safety on her own.

Recommendation #17
When Tested Interventions Are Available, Nursing, in Collaboration with Other Disciplines, Should Be Providing These Interventions for Abused Women as Part of Routine Care

The Canadian Nurses Association (1992) has produced an excellent handbook of recommended nursing interventions for intimate partner violence similar to the many U.S. state medical association handbooks recommending medical interventions. There is some debate as to who should be providing interventions as well as which interventions are the most appropriate at different times in the trajectory of violence. There are no completed evaluations of interventions for abuse provided in the healthcare setting (although several are underway) and no evidence as to which kind of provider would be preferred for what intervention. Stage specific interventions such as those suggested by Campbell and colleagues (Campbell, Ulrich, Sheridan, Campbell, & Landenburger, 1993) may be provided by different providers and/or advocates depending on such variables as where the woman is in her process of recovery, how much danger she and her children are experiencing, where and from whom she prefers to receive interventions, what cultural influences are affecting her situation, and what other healthcare problems she is experiencing. These issues can and should be addressed through further research. In the meantime, nursing should be considering which interventions are most appropriate for nursing roles and providing those, versus which may be better in collaboration or as a referral to another discipline.

SUMMARY

In summary, nursing has made significant contributions to the body of research knowledge about battered women and their children. These findings can be used to support healthcare policy initiatives that will improve the health and safety of these women and children through nursing interventions in collaboration with other disciplines. More research is needed, especially in the area of intervention testing and program evaluation, and nursing is in an ideal position to take leadership and/or join in coalitions to undertake this kind of research (Short, Hennessy, & Campbell, 1995). Specific policy-related research is also needed to test the impact of new health-related policies as they are developed. Nursing experts have been and increasingly can be called upon to testify in relationship to various policy initiatives and to become a part of local, state, and national advisory committees and policy formulating bodies related to intimate partner violence. The Nursing Network on Violence Against Women International (NNVAWI) and the American Academy of Nursing Expert Panel on Violence (Campbell, Anderson et al., 1993) both are called upon to support health-related initiatives and consult in various policy arenas. The more nursing research that is available to support those groups and experts, the more informed and influential our policy related efforts will be. Nursing can be proud of the base of research that has been laid in this critical area of women's health, but needs to also be challenged to increase its research and policy contribution.

REFERENCES

American Academy of Nursing. (1993). *Violence: Nursing debates the issues.* Washington, DC: Author.

Attala, J. M., Oetker, D., & McSweeney, M. (1995). Partner abuse against female nursing students. *Journal of Psychosocial Nursing, 33*(1), 17–24.

Bachman, R., & Saltzman, L. E. (1995). *Violence against women: Estimates from the redesigned survey.* Washington, DC: U.S. Department of Justice.

Campbell, D. W., Campbell, J. C., King, C., Parker, B., & Ryan, J. (1994). The reliability and factor structure of the Index of Spouse Abuse with African-American battered women. *Violence and Victims, 9,* 259–274.

Campbell, J. C. (1981). Misogyny and homicide of women. *Advances in Nursing Science, 3*(2), 67–85.

Campbell, J. C. (1986). Nursing assessment of homicide with battered women. *Advances in Nursing Science, 3*(2), 67–85.

Campbell, J. C. (1989a). Women's responses to sexual abuse in intimate relationships. *Women's Health Care International, 8,* 335–347.

Campbell, J. C. (1989b). A test of two explanatory models of women's responses to battering. *Nursing Research, 38,* 18–24.

Campbell, J. C. (Ed.). (1995). *Assessing dangerousness.* Newbury Park, CA: Sage.

Campbell, J. C., Anderson, E., Fulmer, T. L., Girourd, S., McElmurry, B., & Raff, B. (1993). Violence as a nursing priority: Policy implications. *Nursing Outlook, 41*(1), 89–92.

Campbell, J. C., Harris, M. J., & Lee, R. K. (1995). Violence research: An overview. *Scholarly Inquiry for Nursing Practice: An International Journal, 9*(2), 104–125.

Campbell, J. C., & Humphreys, J. C. (1993). *Nursing care of survivors of family violence.* St. Louis: Mosby.

Campbell, J. C., Kub, J., Belknap, R. A. & Templin, T. (in press). Predictors of depression in battered women. *Violence Against Women.*

Campbell, J. C., Oliver, C., & Bullock, L. (1993). Why battering during pregnancy? *AWHONN'S Clinical Issues, 4*(3), 343–349.

Campbell, J. C., & Parker, B. (1992). Review of nursing research on battered women and their children. In J. Fitzpatrick, R. Taunton, & A. Jacox (Eds.), *Annual review of nursing research* (Vol. 10, pp. 77–94). New York: Springer.

Campbell, J. C., & Parker, B. (in press). Clinical nursing research on battered women and their children: A review. In A. S. Hinshaw, J. L. Shaver, & S. L. Feetham (Eds.), *Handbook on clinical nursing research.* Newbury Park, CA: Sage.

Campbell, J. C., Pliska, M. J., Taylor, W., & Sheridan, D. (1994). Battered women's experiences in emergency departments: Need for appropriate policy & procedures. *Journal of Emergency Nursing, 20,* 280–288.

Campbell, J. C., Poland, M. L., Waller, J. B., & Ager, J. (1992). Correlates of battering during pregnancy. *Research in Nursing & Health, 15,* 219–226.

Campbell, J. C., Pugh, L. C., Campbell, D., & Visscher, M. (1995). The influence of abuse on pregnancy intention. *Women's Health Issues, 5*(4), 214–223.

Campbell, R., Sullivan, C. M., & Davidson, W. S. (in press). Depression in women who use domestic violence shelters: A longitudinal analysis. *Women's Studies Quarterly.*

Canadian Nurses Association. (1992). *Family violence: Clinical guidelines for nurses.* Ottawa, Ontario: National Clearinghouse on Family Violence, Health and Welfare, Canada.

Counts, D., Brown, J., & Campbell, J. C. (1992). *Sanctions and sanctuary: Cultural analysis of the beating of wives.* Boulder, CO: Westview Press.

Curry, M. A. (in press). Relationship between domestic violence during pregnancy and infant outcome. In J. Campbell (Ed.), *Violence against women and women's health.* Newbury Park, CA: Sage.

Eby, K., Campbell, J. C., Sullivan, C., & Davidson, W. (1995). Health effects of experiences of sexual violence for women with abusive partners. *Women's Health Care International, 14,* 563–576.

Gielen, A. C., O'Campo, P. J., Faden, R. R., Kass, N. E., & Xue, X. (1994). Interpersonal conflict and physical violence during the childbearing years. *Social Science and Medicine, 39,* 781–787.

Glittenburg, J., Babich, K., & Campbell, J. C. (Eds.). (1995). *Violence: A plague upon the land.* Washington, DC: American Academy of Nursing.

Hadley, S., Short, L., Lesin, N., & Zook, E. (1995). Woman kind: An innovative model of health care response to domestic abuse. *Women's Health Issues, 5*(4), 189–198.

Hamilton, B., & Coates, J. (1993). Perceived helpfulness and use of professional services by abused women. *Journal of Family Violence, 8,* 313–324.

Helton, A. S., McFarlane, J., & Anderson, E. T. (1987). Battered and pregnant: A prevalence study. *American Journal of Public Health, 77,* 1337–1339.

Henderson, A. (1993). Abused women's perceptions of their children's experiences. *Canada's Mental Health 41*(1), 7–10.

Henderson, A. (1990, June/September). Children of abused women: Their influences on their mother's decisions. *Canada's Mental Health,* 10–13.

Henderson, D. J., Sampselle, C., Mayes, F., & Oakley, D. (1992). Toward culturally sensitive research in a multicultural society. *Health Care for Women International, 13,* 339–350.

Herman, J. (1992). *Trauma and recovery.* New York: Basic Books.

Hoff, L. A. (1990). *Battered women as survivors.* London: Routledge.

Humphreys, J. C. (1995). Dependent care by battered women: Protecting their children. *Health Care for Women International, 16*(1), 9–20.

Kerouac, S., Taggart, M. E., Lescop, J., & Fortin, M. F. (1986). Dimensions of health in violent families. *Health Care for Women International, 7,* 413–426.

Landenburger, K. (1989). A process of entrapment in and recovery from an abusive relationship. *Issues in Mental Health Nursing, 10,* 209–227.

Mahon, L. (1981). Common characteristics of abused women. *Issues in Mental Health Nursing, 3,* 137–157.

McFarlane, J., Parker, B., & Soeken, K. (1995). Abuse during pregnancy: Frequency, severity, perpetrator and risk factors of homicide. *Public Health Nursing 12*(5), 284–289.

McFarlane, J., Parker, B., & Soeken, K. (1996). Physical abuse and substance use during pregnancy: Prevalence, interrelationships and effects on birth weight. *Journal of Obstetric Gynecological and Neonatal Nursing, 25*(4), 313–320.

McFarlane, J., Parker, B., Soeken, K., & Bullock, L. (1992). Assessing for abuse during pregnancy: Severity and frequency of injuries and associated entry into prenatal care. *Journal of the American Medical Association, 267,* 2370–2372.

McLeer, S. V., & Anwar, R. A. H. (1989). Education is not enough: A systems failure in protecting battered women. *Annals of Emergency Medicine,18*(6), 651–653.

Newman, K. D. (1993). Giving up: Shelter experiences of battered women. *Public Health Nursing, 10*(2), 108–113.

Page-Adams, D., & Dersch, S. (in press). Physical and nonphysical abuse against women: Assessing prevalence in a hospital setting. In J. Campbell (Ed.), *Violence against women and women's health.* Newbury Park, CA: Sage.

Parker, B., & Campbell, J. C. (1991). Care of victims of abuse and violence. In G. S. Stuart & S. J. Sundeen (Eds.), *Principles and practice of psychiatric nursing* (4th ed., 947–967). St. Louis: Mosby.

Parker, B., McFarlane, J., & Soeken, K. (1994). Abuse during pregnancy: Effects on maternal complications and birth weight in adult and teenage women. *Obstetrics & Gynecology, 84,* 323–328.

Parker, B., McFarlane, J., Soeken, K., Torres, S., & Campbell, D. (1993). Physical and emotional abuse in pregnancy: A comparison of adult and teenage women. *Nursing Research, 42,* 173–178.

Parker, B., & Schumacher, D. (1977). The battered wife syndrome and violence in the nuclear family of origin: A controlled pilot study. *American Journal of Public Health, 67*(8), 760–761.

Parker, B., Ulrich, Y., et al. (1990). A protocol of safety: Research on abuse of women. *Nursing Research, 39*(4), 248–250.

Ratner, P. A. (1993). The incidence of wife abuse and mental health status in abused wives in Edmonton, Alberta. *Canadian Journal of Public Health, 84*(4), 246–249.

Ratner, P. A. (1995). Indicators of exposure to wife abuse. *Canadian Journal of Nursing Research, 27*(1), 31–46.

Rodriguez, R. (1989). Perception of health needs by battered women. *RESPONSE 12*(4), 22–23.

Rodriguez, R. (1993). Violence in transcience: Nursing care of battered migrant women. *AWHONN's Clinical Issues in Perinatal and Women's Health Nursing, 4*(3), 437–440.

Rose, K., & Saunders, D. G. (1986). Nurses' and physicians' attitudes about women abuse: The effects of gender and professional role. *Health Care for Women International, 7,* 427–438.

Sebbio, S., Campbell, J., & Soeken, K. (1996). *Battered women and their relationships with their mates over time.* Unpublished master's thesis.

Short, L., Hennessy, M., & Campbell, J. (1996). Tracking the work. In *Family violence: Building a coordinated response* (pp. 59–72). Chicago: American Medical Association.

Tilden, V. P., Schmidt, T. A., Linardi, B., Chioda, G. T., Garland, M. J., & Loveless, P. A. (1994). Factors that influence clinician's assessment and management of family violence. *American Journal of Public Health, 84*(4), 628–633.

Tilden, V. P., & Shepard, P. (1987). Increasing the rate of identification of battered women in an emergency department: Use of a nursing protocol. *Research in Nursing & Health, 10,* 209–215.

Torres, S. (1987). Hispanic-American battered women: Why consider cultural differences? *Responses, 10*(3), 20–21.

Torres, S. (1991). A comparison of wife abuse between two cultures: Perceptions, attitudes, nature, and extent. *Issues in Mental Health Nursing, 12,* 113–131.

Trimpey, M. L. (1989). Self-esteem and anxiety: Key issues in an abused women's support group. *Issues in Mental Health Nursing, 10,* 297–308.

Ulrich, Y. (1991). Women's reasons for leaving abusive spouses. *Women's Health Care International, 12,* 465–473.

Weingourt, R. (1990). Wife rape in a sample of psychiatric patients. *Image: Journal of Nursing Scholarship, 22,* 144–147.

Westra, B., & Martin, H. (1981). Children of battered women. *Maternal-Child Nursing Journal, 10,* 41–54.

Wilson, M., & Daly, M. (1993). Spousal homicide risk and estrangement. *Violence and Victims, 8,* 3–16.

Yam, M. (1995). Wife abuse: Strategies for a therapeutic response. *Scholarly Inquiry for Nursing Practice, 9,* 147–158.

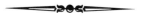

Part XII

Research and Theoretical Issues

Chapter 13

Female Circumcision

Carol D. Christiansen

Female Genital Mutilation

And now hear my appeal! . . . Appeal for my right to live as a whole
. . . Protect, support, and give a hand to innocent little girls who do
no harm . . . Initiate them to the world of love, not to the world of
feminine sorrow.

—Dahabo Elmi Muse (1989)

These words taken from the work of the Somali poet, Dahabo Elmi
Muse (as cited in Hosken, 1993, p. 126), represent the emerging voice
of the millions of women from countries where female genital mutilation (FGM) is routinely practiced. The various procedures comprising the
practice of FGM are mechanisms of social control meant to regulate the reproductive functions of women and to suppress the expression of sexuality
(Jackson, 1991; Levin, 1980). These procedures are often referred to collec-
tively as female circumcision (Armstrong, 1991; Hosken, 1978).

Though known to be an ancient practice, the exact origins of female
circumcision remain obscure (Lightfoot-Klein, 1989a). One theory posits
that female circumcision originated in Africa where clitoral excision was

practiced by the peoples of ancient Egypt (Lowry & Lowry, 1976; Mustafa, 1966; Sami, 1986). From Egypt, the practice may have diffused south, gradually becoming incorporated into the cultures of the tribes surrounding the Red Sea (Lightfoot-Klein, 1989a). Another theory holds that the practice arose independently among different groups at approximately the same time (Slack, 1988).

FGM has frequently and erroneously been compared to male circumcision which, by comparison, is a relatively simple procedure that involves the removal of the foreskin of the penis. In contrast, FGM is much more extreme and involves the cutting away of highly sensitive and healthy organs and tissues (Shaw, 1985). The operations vary according to locale and custom, as does the age at the time of circumcision and the ceremonies surrounding the event (Hosken, 1978).

Toubia (1993) claimed that the most comprehensive estimates available indicated that approximately 114 million women and girls worldwide have been genitally mutilated. Toubia further claimed that an additional 2 million girls a year, or 6,000 a day, are estimated to be at risk for FGM.

These figures may underestimate the actual number of women and girls affected by this traditional practice because statistics monitoring the occurrence of FGM are not maintained. Hosken (1993) and others (Mohamud, 1992; Slack, 1988) have reported that the incidence of FGM may be on the increase in Africa. FGM tends to mirror population growth, and many of the countries practicing FGM are currently experiencing annual growth rates of 2 to 3 percent (Hosken, 1993). Consequently, the number of women and girls affected by FGM is also increasing.

FGM consists of the partial or complete removal of the external genitalia; the severity of the procedure depends on the amount of tissue removed (Brown, Calder, & Rae, 1989). These various procedures have been described and classified in the literature in several different ways (Assad, 1980; Dirie & Lindmark, 1991; El Dareer, 1982; Flannery, Glover, & Airhinenbuwa, 1990; Hosken, 1978; Koso-Thomas, 1987; Lowry & Lowry, 1976; Sami, 1986). The classification system proposed by Sami (1986) is comprehensive and includes the terms most often associated with this phenomenon.

CLASSIFICATION OF PROCEDURES

1. *Sunna:* The mildest form of circumcision which involves excision of the clitoral prepuce. Sunna may also include a pricking of the clitoris which is done to induce bleeding and does not involve the removal of tissue (Clarke et al., 1993).

2. *Excision and clitoridectomy:* The removal of the whole or part of the clitoris, plus or minus part of the labia minora.

3. *Infibulation or pharaonic circumcision:* This involves excision of the clitoris, labia minora, and labia majora, followed by closure of the vaginal orifice. Closure is achieved by approximating the two sides with thorns or sutures.

4. *Intermediate:* A modification of pharaonic circumcision consists of removal of the clitoris with part of the labia minora, preserving the labia majora. Milder variations of intermediate circumcision may include only partial removal of the clitoris and a roughening of the surface of each lip of the labia minora to allow for stitching and subsequent narrowing of the introitus.

5. *Reinfibulation:* This procedure is performed on women who are divorced, widowed, or have given birth. Reinfibulation is often referred to as "tightening" and is done for those who have had previous pharaonic circumcision. The edges of the scar are sewn together in order to simulate the narrow introitus of a virgin.

Infibulation and reinfibulation leave a scar in the midline extending from the fourchette to the region of the clitoris. The introitus is in the posterior part of this scar, approximately one cm from the anal orifice, and is reduced to the smallest possible diameter (Aziz, 1980).

Variation is often found in any of the above classifications that are intended to be broadly descriptive (Clarke et al., 1993). In fact, these procedures are seldom as precise as they have been described. Traditionally performed by an untrained midwife on an unanesthetized and struggling child, the tissue that is removed is usually that which can be grasped by the operator at the moment of excision (Hosken, 1990).

Recently, many countries have begun to medicalize FGM. Specialized training has been made available to nurses as well as midwives and birth attendants and, consequently, circumcisions are being performed in clinics utilizing local anesthesia and antibiotics (Hosken, 1993). While these procedural changes may have decreased the incidence of many short-term life threatening consequences of FGM, the long-term disability and pain associated with FGM continues to drastically and forever alter the lives of the girls and women who have been affected by these procedures.

GEOGRAPHIC SCOPE OF FGM

FGM is most often associated with Africa where it occurs in more than 26 countries in a broad, far-reaching area which parallels the equator—spanning the continent from the Red Sea to the Atlantic Coast. Prevalence rates within these countries range from an estimated low of 5 percent in Uganda and Zaire, to an estimated 98 percent in countries such as Djibouti and Somalia, where the practice is universal (Toubia, 1994). FGM has a much wider geographical distribution, occurring in more than 40 countries worldwide among people of differing races and religions (Hosken, 1993).

Primarily an ethnic practice, FGM is often associated with populations that are not always contained within political boundaries. For example, the occurrence of FGM in a particular country may be limited to specific groups and not considered a custom associated with the population majority (Hosken, 1993). The practice of FGM extends to the southern part of the Arabian Peninsula and the Persian Gulf including Yemen, Oman, and the Arab Emirates. The circumcision of females also occurs in Southeast Asia among the Muslim populations of Indonesia and Malaysia (Abdalla, 1982; Hosken, 1993). FGM is reported to occur with less frequency in diverse populations such as the descendants of West African slaves living in Brazil and among the aboriginal tribes of Australia (Sami, 1986).

The ancient roots of this practice have led historians to believe the FGM has been practiced in some form by the native populations of every continent at some time in their history (Armstrong, 1991). During the nineteenth century, clitoridectomy was known to have occurred in the United States and England (Ragab, 1994). In this era, proponents of the practice claimed that circumcision cured women of a multitude of ills including masturbation and measles. Because of the religious, social, and medical preoccupation with masturbation, clitoral excision was practiced with some frequency in Germany, France, and Britain early in the nineteenth century.

Presently FGM is customarily found in those countries of the world where the economic and social status of women is low and where there is generalized poverty, illiteracy, hunger, inadequate clean water, and inadequate healthcare (Slack, 1988). Regardless of geographic location, the explanations offered for the continuation of the practice of FGM are complex, varied, and deeply embedded within the sociocultural and religious matrices of individual practicing societies (Mays & Stockley, 1983).

HEALTH RISKS

The complications of circumcision are influenced by the conditions under which circumcision takes place as well as the age of the girl at the time of circumcision. For the majority of girls, circumcision occurs before the age of puberty. For example, in Sudan and Somalia, clitoridectomy and infibulation are frequently performed when a girl is 7 or 8 years of age although the procedure may be carried out anytime prior to the onset of menses (Van der Kwaak, 1992). While this age range probably represents the period of time when most cultures circumcise their girls, circumcision may also occur at the time of marriage, pregnancy, or immediately prior to or while a woman is giving birth (Myers, Omorodion, Isenalumhe, & Akenzua, 1985).

Circumcision presents young girls with the risk of immediate death due to shock, hemorrhage, and tetanus, as well as the lifetime potential for the development of chronic and debilitating conditions (Aziz, 1980). The time immediately following circumcision is the most critical because of the possibility of shock and hemorrhage. Shock is not always related directly to blood loss but may also occur because of the intense pain experienced (Aziz, 1980; Mustafa, 1966).

In many situations, circumcisions are performed in villages where aseptic precautions are not observed. Unsterilized items such as knives, scissors, razor blades, and broken glass are instruments frequently utilized by untrained circumcisors (Mays & Stockley, 1983). As a result, injuries to the urethra, bladder, vagina, perineum, and anal canal occur with relative frequency (Rushwan, 1990).

Acute urinary retention is the most frequent complication in the first 48 to 72 hours following circumcision (Abdalla, 1982). Retention is usually the result of edema and scarring but may also occur because of pain associated with urination (Sami, 1986). Additionally, cases of tetanus and sepsis leading to death are common. Severe anemia which may accompany profuse bleeding at the time of the operation coupled with inadequate nutrition has been implicated in the retardation of the physical and mental growth of some children (Mustafa, 1966).

The delayed or long-term complications of circumcision greatly compromise the reproductive health of women. Several authors report that dermoid cysts and abscesses, chronic pelvic infections, dysmenorrhea and hematocolpus, vaginal calculi and vesico-vaginal fistula formation, and infertility are frequent complications (Abdalla, 1982; Aziz, 1980; Cloudsley, 1984; Daw, 1970; Flannery et al., 1990; Hathout, 1963; Tevoedjre, 1981).

The disabling effects of circumcision are most acutely realized during a woman's reproductive and childbearing years. The more extensive forms of circumcision may result in critical distortions of the genitalia as well as in keloid formation and scarring. These are factors that are implicated in the increased maternal and fetal mortality rates of circumcised women (De-Silva, 1989; Slack, 1988). The risk of maternal death is estimated to double in circumcised women, and the risk of stillbirth also increases several fold (World Health Assembly, 1993). Moreover, during childbirth, hemorrhage and infection are common occurrences.

Fetal hypoxia, which may also occur in this same perinatal period, can result in the birth of physically and mentally handicapped infants. Mustafa (1966) reports that in the infibulated populations of Sudan and Somalia, the face and scalp of the newborn may inadvertently be lacerated during delivery when inexperienced midwives cut the circumcision scars in an attempt to facilitate delivery.

SEXUAL AND PSYCHOLOGICAL FACTORS RELATING TO FGM

The complications of FGM most frequently discussed in the literature are those dealing with the physiologic effects of the various procedures. To date, there has been little investigation into the sexual and psychological complications of FGM (Abdalla, 1982; Hosken, 1990; Lightfoot-Klein, 1989a).

Toubia (1993), a Sudanese physician, stated that in the developing countries where FGM occurs, there are few qualified mental health professionals; consequently, there is a lack of research regarding the emotional problems associated with genital mutilation. Also, because there are no culturally acceptable ways for women to express their feelings regarding female circumcision, women frequently develop psychopathologic states. Toubia further stated that in Sudan women were often perceived as malingerers when they presented with complaints related to circumcision.

Lightfoot-Klein (1989b) reported that in Sudan, infibulated women expressed a fear of sex at the time of marriage because vaginal penetration often took anywhere from several days to several months to accomplish. If necessary, women were opened surgically by a midwife to allow for vaginal penetration. In time, the women in Lightfoot-Klein's study became more comfortable with sex. This occurred despite the fact that they could not initiate sexual relations with their husbands or indicate pleasure in the sexual relationship because of cultural restraints.

In a study which was conducted in Somalia, Abdalla (1982) claimed that over 50 percent of the female respondents stated that they were fearful of sex in the first weeks of marriage. This fear was attributed to the anticipated pain of sexual relations which occurred as a result of infibulation. Toubia (1993) stated that the complex issue of sexuality is made even more difficult for circumcised women by the imposition of cultural values which inhibit the expression of emotions. Thus, in Toubia's opinion, because of the significant physical, psychological, and cultural barriers that act to arrest sexual development, circumcised women become sexually objectified in their role as reproductive vehicles for men.

CONTEMPORARY OVERVIEW OF FGM

Until very recently, the Western world was not well acquainted with FGM and the traditions, cultural norms, and complications surrounding these procedures. Even now, for the majority of individuals residing in Western society, including those within the health professions, knowledge of this practice remains obscure and is, for the most part, incorrect.

Today because of political turmoil, educational opportunities, and the general mobility of world population groups, FGM is a phenomenon that is being encountered with increasing frequency in the United States and other Western nations. In recent years, the unrest in Africa and other parts of the world has forced the migration and relocation of tens of thousands of people practicing FGM to the countries of Western Europe, Australia, Canada, and the United States (Hosken, 1990; Lightfoot-Klein & Shaw, 1991). As a result, the ethical, legal, and health issues surrounding the practice of FGM are no longer confined to developing countries. An estimated 200,000 immigrants, emanating from countries where FGM is a known practice, have come to the United States in the past decade (Lightfoot-Klein, 1993).

This recent trend is one of the reasons explaining why FGM is receiving media recognition in the United States. This traditional practice has been brought to the public's attention with increasing frequency. The media is beginning to address the controversial nature of this phenomenon, exposing the ways in which FGM has affected the lives of immigrant women living in the United States and other Western countries (Beck, 1994b; Corbin, 1994). While condemning FGM as a human rights violation, the media has rated that there may be potential difficulties posed by official attempts to eradicate this practice.

Anecdotal evidence exists indicating that circumcisions are currently being performed in many cities of the United States on the daughters of immigrants from Somalia, Sudan, Ethiopia, Nigeria, and Kenya (F. P. Hosken, personal communication, February, 1993). FGM is becoming a concern wherever practicing groups settle. As health providers within the United States and other Western nations encounter the women and children who have been affected by FGM, complex medical, social, ethical, and legal issues will have to be addressed.

Despite the fact that more is now known about the physiological effects and complications of FGM, there is still a lack of comprehensive knowledge and understanding of this phenomenon. This is partially explained by the fact that the populations practicing FGM differ in geographic location, culture, language, and political organization. Nonetheless, following immigration, the women whose lives have been affected by FGM share certain similarities in their physical, emotional, and psychological needs. To date, existing research has not yet fully documented the subjective meanings of FGM and the effects of FGM upon women within the context of their lives. This has impeded health professionals in their attempts to provide culturally sensitive care to circumcised women. Additionally, the majority of studies researching this topic have been conducted in the respondents' countries of origin.

IMPLICATIONS

Circumcised women living in Western cultures are at a higher risk for physical and emotional disorders not only because of circumcision, but because of their status as immigrants. This risk is explained, in part, by differences in language and cultural values. These factors can determine the way in which immigrant women define illness, communicate, and interact with the dominant culture.

Effectively reaching the majority of immigrant and refugee women affected by circumcision requires that healthcare providers plan and implement community-based programs and services directed toward specific populations of women. This recommendation is specifically relevant to the major urban centers where these populations are established.

Understanding the cultural meanings embedded within the phenomenon of circumcision will facilitate the planning and implementation of effective interventions that take into account women's lived experience.

In most instances, cultural barriers prohibit women from discussing issues relating to circumcision and from participating in preventive and health promotion activities. Awareness of this fact is useful for health professionals to be informed, culturally sensitive, and understanding of the physical, emotional, and psychological issues associated with female circumcision. Similarly, health providers must be sensitive to family dynamics and to the husband or father's position with regard to family health decisions.

As a specialized concern of women's health, raising the level of awareness to the issues surrounding circumcision can have a positive impact upon the health and general well being of the women affected by this practice.

REFERENCES

Abdalla, R. (1982). *Sisters in affliction.* London: Zed Press.

Armstrong, S. (1991). Female circumcision: Fighting a cruel tradition. *New Scientist, 2,* 42–47.

Assaad, M. B. (1980). Female circumcision in Egypt: Social implications, current research, and prospects for change. *Studies in Family Planning, 11*(1), 3–16.

Aziz, F. A. (1980). Gynecologic and obstetric complications of female circumcision. *International Journal of Gynaecology and Obstetrics, 17,* 560–563.

Beck, J. (1994a, February 6). We must not ignore the cultural abuse of women and girls. *Chicago Tribune*, Sec. 4, p. 3.

Beck, J. (1994b, September 15). Female mutilation shouldn't be tolerated anywhere. *Chicago Tribune*, Sec. 1, p. 29.

Brown, Y., Calder, B., & Rae, D. (1989). Female circumcision. *Canadian Nurse, 85*(4), 19–22.

Clarke, N., Cornwell, L., Gibson, R., Keyi-Ayema, V., Mohamed, H., & Telfer, S. (1993). *Female genital mutilation.* (Available from Women's Health in Women's Hands, 344 Dupont Street at Spadina, Suite #402, Toronto, Ontario, Canada.)

Cloudsley, A. (1984). *Women of Omdurman: Life, love, and the cult of virginity.* New York: St. Martin's Press.

Corbin, B. (1994, June). The torturous realities of female genital mutilation. *National Now Times, 26*(4), 5, 6, 12.

Daw, E. (1970). Female circumcision and infibulation complicating delivery. *Practitioner, 204,* 559–563.

DeSilva, S. (1989). Obstetric sequelae of female circumcision. *European Journal of Obstetrics, Gynecology and Reproductive Biology, 32,* 233–240.

Dirie, M. A., & Lindmark, G. (1991). Female circumcision in Somalia and women's motives. *Acta Obstetrica et Gynecologica Scandinavica, 70,* 581–585.

El Dareer, A. (1982). *Woman, why do you weep? Circumcision and its consequences.* London: Zed Press.

Flannery, D., Glover, E. D., & Airhinenbuwa, C. (1990). Perspective on female circumcision: Traditional practice or health risk? *Health Values, 14*(5), 34–40.

Jackson, C. (1991). Female circumcision: Should angels fear to tread? *Health Visitor, 64*(8), 252–253.

Hathout, H. M. (1963). Some aspects of female circumcision. *Journal of Obstetrics and Gynaecology of the British Commonwealth, 70,* 505–507.

Hosken, F. P. (1978). The epidemiology of female genital mutilations. *Tropical Doctor, 8,* 150–156.

Hosken, F. P. (1990). Female genital mutilation. *Woman of Power, 18,* 42–45.

Hosken, F. P. (1993). *The Hosken report.* Lexington, MA: Women's International Network News.

Koso-Thomas, O. (1987). *The circumcision of women.* Atlantic Highlands, NJ: Zed Books.

Levin, T. (1980). "Unspeakable atrocities": The psychosexual etiology of female genital mutilation. *The Journal of Mind and Behavior, 1*(3), 197–210.

Lightfoot-Klein, H. (1989a). *Prisoners of ritual: An odyssey into female genital circumcision in Africa.* New York: Haworth Press.

Lightfoot-Klein, H. (1989b). Rites of purification and their effects: Some psychological aspects of female genital circumcision and infibulation (Pharaonic circumcision) in an Afro-Arab Islamic society (Sudan). *Journal of Psychology and Human Sexuality, 2*(2), 79–91.

Lightfoot-Klein, H. (1993). Disability in female immigrants with ritually inflicted genital mutilation. *Women & Therapy, 14,* 187–194.

Lightfoot-Klein, H., & Shaw, E. (1991). Special needs of ritually circumcised women patients. *Journal of Obstetric, Gynecologic and Neonatal Nursing, 20,* 102–107.

Lowry, T. P., & Lowry, T. S. (1976). *The clitoris.* St. Louis, MO: Warren H. Green.

Mays, S., & Stockley, A. (1983). Victims of tradition. *Nursing Mirror, 156*(21), 19–21.

Mohamud, A. (1992, March) Female genital mutilation: A continuing violation of the human rights of young women. *International Council on Adolescent Fertility Passages,* pp. 9–16.

Mustafa, A. Z. (1966). Female circumcision and infibulation in the Sudan. *Journal of Obstetrics and Gynaecology of the British Commonwealth, 73,* 302–306.

Myers, R. A., Omorodion, F. I., Isenalumhe, A. E., & Akenzua, G. I. (1985). Circumcision: Its nature and practice among some ethnic groups in Southern Nigeria. *Social Science and Medicine, 21*(5), 581–588.

Ragab, M. J. (1994, June). Genital mutilation: The case for international duplicity. *National Now Times, 26*(4), 6, 12.

Rushwan, H. (1990, April/May). Female circumcision. *World Health,* 24–25.

Sami, I. R. (1986). Female circumcision with special reference to the Sudan. *Annals of Tropical Pediatrics, 6,* 99–115.

Shaw, E. (1985). Female circumcision: Perceptions of clients and caregivers. *College Health, 33,* 193–197.

Slack, A. T. (1988). Female circumcision: A critical appraisal. *Human Rights Quarterly, 10,* 437–486.

Tevoedjre, I. (1981). Violence and the child in the adult world of Africa. *Child Abuse and Neglect, 5,* 495–498.

Toubia, N. (1993). *Female genital mutilation: A call for global action.* New York: Women, Ink.

Toubia, N. (1994). Female circumcision as a public health issue. *New England Journal of Medicine, 331*(11), 712–715.

Van der Kwaak, A. (1992). Female circumcision and gender identity: A questionable alliance. *Social Science and Medicine, 35*(6), 777–787.

World Health Assembly. (1993). *Female genital mutilation* (Press Release WHA/10) Geneva, Switzerland: Author.

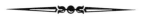

ABSTRACTS

For the following review, articles were selected which will contribute to the reader's understanding of the psychosocial, physical, and emotional needs of circumcised women.

Calder, B. L., Brown, Y. M. R., & Rae, D. I. (1993). Female circumcision/genital mutilation: Culturally sensitive care. *Health Care for Women International, 14,* 227–238.

These researchers conducted a study in Somalia that attempted to identify the complications of circumcision, acceptable interventions for these complications, and caregivers considered acceptable by the respondents. The authors believed that by acquiring this information, they would be able to assist health professionals in providing culturally sensitive and comprehensive care to immigrant women.

The data was collected by a questionnaire that was administered to female students in two schools of nursing and one school of education in Somalia. The physical complications related to circumcision most often reported were those dealing with menstrual difficulties and urinary complaints such as dysuria, incontinence, and urinary infections. Respondents also stated that when faced with circumcision-related problems they would seek advice from

"friend, mother, or grandmother." Nurses, midwives, and female physicians were also considered acceptable, but not male physicians.

Because circumcised women in this study sought the advice of friends and family before seeking professional help, the researchers suggest that it is important to mobilize family resources when planning interventions for women having circumcision-related problems. Also because women claimed to rely upon other women within the community for assistance, the authors believed this presented an opportunity for health professionals to work with community groups to make them aware of local resources and to provide them with correct, general health information.

The researchers reported that many of the interventions routinely recommended for urinary tract complaints were rejected by the respondents. For example, increasing oral fluids in the presence of infection was not acceptable to infibulated women because of the difficulties they experienced in urination. Also, there was a belief that frequent urination would tend to weaken the infibulation scar. In fact, in the presence of infection, respondents frequently decreased the oral intake of fluids.

This study points to the importance of the need for healthcare professionals to have awareness and understanding of specific cultural beliefs, practices, and customs in order to plan and implement relevant interventions.

Christiansen, C. D. (1995). *The lived experience of circumcision in immigrant Somali women: A Heideggerian hermeneutic analysis.* Unpublished doctoral dissertation, University of Illinois at Chicago.

Heideggerian hermeneutic phenomenology provided the philosophical background for this interpretive study that sought understanding of the lived experience of circumcision in the lives of women who had immigrated to the United States from Somalia. Understanding the lived experience required that the subjective meanings of circumcision that were embedded in the everyday practices and experiences of Somali women be made visible.

The interviews of the Somali women who participated in this study were guided by an interest in obtaining descriptions of their life-worlds with respect to their interpretations of the meaning of circumcision within the context of their shared culture. Textual analysis of the data identified the relational themes and constitutive patterns present in the data that uncovered the implicit and explicit meanings common to the lived experience of circumcision.

Data analysis yielded two constitutive patterns and their related themes. The first constitutive pattern, "I Am Forever Changed": Becoming the Same/Becoming Different, brought visibility to the experiences of transformation and discovery in the lives of the women. The second pattern, "Living with My Past While Anticipating My Future," gave meaning and understanding to the structural dimensions of time and the lived experience of circumcision.

Dirie, M. A., & Lindmark, G. (1991). Female circumcision in Somalia and women's motives. *Acta Obstetrica et Gynecologica Scandinavia, 70,* 581–585.

This study, undertaken in Somalia, surveyed 300 women in order to determine the types of circumcision performed, the age at which circumcision took place, and the motives perpetuating the practice. The study reported that 100 percent of the women interviewed had been circumcised and 88 percent had been circumcised with excision and infibulation, the most extensive of all procedures. The majority of the respondents (69 percent) had been circumcised at home by an untrained person.

An interesting finding in this study is that almost 70 percent of the women claimed to justify the continuation of circumcision for religious reasons, believing that the Islamic religion mandated conformity to this practice. Other respondents (20 percent) stated that they had been circumcised to protect their virginal status in order to ensure their future marriageability. The remaining respondents believed that circumcision was performed for reasons of hygiene, as the clitoris was considered to be "unclean."

The attitudes of respondents to circumcising their daughters was also obtained in this study. All of the respondents responded affirmatively by stating that they would continue the practice and have their daughters circumcised. Fifty percent of the women stated that they would have their daughters excised and infibulated, 40 percent stated they favored clitoridectomy, while only 10 percent claimed to prefer the milder Sunna.

The researchers noted that the respondents had a literacy rate of 87 percent, a rate much higher than that of the general population of Somalia. Despite their higher educational status, none of the respondents in this study rejected the practice of circumcision. This finding seemed to support earlier studies that revealed that education and economic status had little influence on the continuation of this practice. The researchers theorized that education may have an effect when people acquire more knowledge about the complications of circumcision.

Hosken, F. P. (1993). *The Hosken report: Genital and sexual mutilation of females.* (4th ed., rev.). Lexington, MA: Women's International Network News.

This report provides a comprehensive review of female genital mutilation from a global perspective. Detailed case histories of many of the countries practicing FGM are included. Information is also given regarding the strategies currently in effect to bring about the changes necessary to save women and girls from practice.

Lightfoot-Klein, H. (1989). The sexual experience and marital adjustment of genitally circumcised and infibulated females in the Sudan. *The Journal of Sex Research, 26*(3), 375–392.

Lightfoot-Klein conducted a study in Sudan over a five-year period in which she interviewed over 300 Sudanese women and 100 Sudanese men on the sexual experiences of circumcised and infibulated women. As with other countries situated on the Horn of Africa, Sudanese circumcision involves excision of the clitoris, labia minora, the lining of the labia majora, and infibulation.

Despite severe genital mutilation and the fact that Sudanese women are culturally prohibited from expressing sexual desire or pleasure, Lightfoot-Klein discovered several factors that made it possible for women to achieve sexual satisfaction. In many instances, Sudanese women were able to rely upon a limited series of covert sexual signals and behaviors that they were able to successfully utilize within the marital relationship to indicate sexual willingness. Also, many women who had undergone pharaonic circumcision reported orgasm on a consistent basis. Based on the detailed reports of the respondents, Lightfoot-Klein theorized that circumcision facilitated the enhancement of other erogenous zones.

Mire, S. (Producer/Director), & Christiansen, C. (Narrator). (1994). *Fire Eyes* [Film]. (Available from Filmakers Library, 124 E. 40th Street, New York, NY 10016.)

Produced by a Somali woman, this documentary deals with female circumcision and provides insight into many of the cultural norms and beliefs surrounding FGM. In the film, the producer recounts her own circumcision and re-enacts the events of a circumcision ceremony for the viewer. Consequently, the viewer is able to gain a new understanding of FGM and the devastating impact of this phenomenon upon the lives of women.

Shaw, E. (1985). Female circumcision: Perceptions of clients and caregiver. *College Health, 33*, 193–197.

This article summarized data from a descriptive study that was undertaken in order to identify the healthcare needs of circumcised women from Sudan, Somalia, and Egypt who had utilized the Western medical system while residing in a university town in the United States. The researcher also surveyed 95 student health services that had a population base of at least 500 foreign students to determine the problems providers encountered while caring for circumcised women.

The study revealed that most of the respondents had sought medical care for pregnancy, dysmenorrhea, dyspareunia, pelvic inflammatory disease, and urinary tract infections. All of the respondents stated that they were fearful of painful pelvic examinations because of their altered anatomy, especially if they had undergone infibulation. For those respondents that were pregnant, most feared the tearing of the infibulation scar during delivery if the required episiotomies were not performed correctly and within the appropriate time period. Several of the respondents stated they had experienced problems in the postpartum period due to improper medical management during delivery and improper suturing following delivery.

All of the respondents stated that healthcare providers should be familiar with the practice of circumcision and the differences in procedures. Women also stated that health professionals must be sensitive to the fact that circumcised women prefer to see female physicians and that permission from male relatives must often be obtained before services can be rendered.

Of the 48 college health services surveys which were returned, 50 percent of the respondents claimed that their professional staffs were familiar with female circumcision. The majority of the health services thus responded reported that physicians and nurses had experienced difficulty in completing pelvic examinations on women who were excised or infibulated. Health providers could not always establish if and when a client was experiencing pain from a pelvic examination because most of the women did not verbally express discomfort. The author believed that this may stem from the fact that many Islamic women are taught not to express pain during pelvic examinations, labor, and delivery. Therefore, pain management should be initiated without relying exclusively on client responses.

Respondents from health services also claimed that clients frequently left clinics without being examined if female physicians were not available. In many cases, staff believed that these clients would have been "lost" in the system if efforts were not made to schedule subsequent visits when female physicians were available.